D0883436

High-risk newborn infants

THE BASIS FOR INTENSIVE NURSING CARE

High-risk newborn infants

THE BASIS FOR INTENSIVE NURSING CARE

SHELDON B. KORONES, M.D.

Professor of Pediatrics, University of Tennessee College of Medicine;
Director, Newborn Center, City of Memphis Hospital,
Memphis, Tennessee

With editorial assistance of, and a chapter by

JEAN LANCASTER, R.N., M.N.

Associate Professor of Nursing of Children, University of Tennessee
College of Nursing; Clinical Supervisor of Nurses, Newborn Center,
City of Memphis Hospital, Memphis, Tennessee

THIRD EDITION

with 148 *illustrations*

The C. V. Mosby Company

ST. LOUIS • TORONTO • LONDON   1981

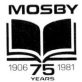

MOSBY

1906 **75** 1981
YEARS

A TRADITION OF PUBLISHING EXCELLENCE

THIRD EDITION

Copyright © 1981 by The C. V. Mosby Company

Previous editions copyrighted 1972, 1976

Printed in the United States of America

The C. V. Mosby Company
11830 Westline Industrial Drive, St. Louis, Missouri 63141

Library of Congress Cataloging in Publication Data

Korones, Sheldon B.
  High-risk newborn infants.

  Includes bibliographies and index.

  1. Infants (Newborn)—Diseases—Nursing.
2. Neonatal intensive care.   3. Intensive care
nursing.   I. Lancaster, Jean.   II. Title.
[DNLM: 1. Infant, Newborn, Diseases—Nursing.
2. Intensive care units.   WY 159 K84h]
RJ254.K67 1981   618.92′01   81-963
ISBN 0-8016-2738-9   AACR2

C/VH/VH 9 8 7 6 5 4 3   03/C/323

To

my **Mother's** inspiring memory and my **Father's** selfless devotion.

To

Judy, who sustains me so steadily, and to **David** and **Susan,**

who grew up so admirably.

Preface

There were numerous moments of reflection during the preparation of this third edition, most of them dwelling on the changes that have occurred in the role of nurses in neonatal intensive care. Almost 10 years have elapsed since the preface for our first edition was written, and at that time a strong case was made for "specially trained nurses" whose activities in a special care unit were "fundamental to its success." Certainly that much has not changed, for it is indeed more valid today than it was a decade ago. Furthermore, the status of "colleague in the intensive care setting" was advocated, and it has materialized significantly. The "expanded role of the nurse" had become cliché, even though it was a new concept. It implied more initiative and independent action, while emphasizing the cooperative nature of both; the nurse should work *with* the physician, not *for* him. It was in that context that this book was first offered. Nurses wanted, and needed, to know the pathophysiologic bases of their indispensable efforts. Now, the "expanded role" continues to expand, because the needs that were urgent a decade ago are even more urgent today. The "nurse clinician/specialist" permeates our ranks because the complexity and sheer volume of work is unmanageable by the physician alone.

The role of these talented individuals requires more precise delineation and nationally recognized certification must also eventuate. The effectiveness of those who already function in these roles is well established. Delivery of acceptable care to sick babies will not be feasible in the future if these developments in nursing are impeded. Since our call for regionalization of perinatal care is being answered throughout the country with vigorous activity and tremendous expenditure, we are now responsible for a large number of very sick patients. Their illnesses are complex, their misadventures occur around the clock, and their intact survival usually demands a rapid therapeutic reaction. Our situation is further complicated by the frequent geographic remoteness of distressed infants—remote from the expertise intended to enhance their chances of intact survival. The transport of infants to regional centers has therefore become a massive endeavor in which qualified nurses are increasingly involved. Their functions vary from supportive to supervisory, depending on locality. That the effectiveness of their supervisory activity has been well documented is noteworthy.

Those recurrent moments of reflection were obviously gratifying. We have come a long way since this book was first published, but we are only at the end of a very significant beginning.

The efforts expended for this revision were motivated by a keen sense of responsibility to those readers who are still creating the changes described in preceding paragraphs. If publication of the first edition was timely, the hope is fervent that this latest version is at least equally appropriate. Extensive changes and additions have been effected in all but a few chapters, which themselves have also undergone some changes. The chapter that was previously confined to acid-base and blood gas material has been expanded to include fluids and electrolytes. A chapter on the pertinent aspects of disorders in the central nervous system has been added. The inevitable need to revise the chapter on lung disorders has been effected enthusiastically. In that chapter, the sections on patent ductus arteriosus, meconium aspiration, and extraneous air syndromes are considerably amplified; a rather detailed treatment of persistent fetal circulation has been included for the first time. Revised and extended remarks have been written concerning glucose metabolism, thermoregulation, and physical examination. The chapter on parent-infant rela-

tionships has been thoroughly rewritten by Jean Lancaster. Furthermore, the number of illustrations has been increased throughout.

A number of individuals have provided valuable support for this revision. Involved more directly than anyone else was Marion Haynes, who patiently and with uncommon expertise was able to prepare this manuscript in spite of the difficulties I unavoidably created. Without Rosalind Griffin's efforts the manuscript and galleys would not have been prepared in time to meet designated deadlines. To Jean Lancaster, R.N., M.N., Penny Slade, R.N., M.N., and Anita Hoskins, R.N., M.S., and Anne Lamb, R.N., my gratitude for editorial and commentary contributions, for supportive friendship, and for wise counsel. Our Pediatric Nurse Associates, Sandy Gates, R.N., M.S., P.N.P., Ellen Keels, R.N., P.N.P., Paula Millen, R.N., M.S.N., P.N.P., and Marilyn Dean, R.N., P.N.P., suggested all the additions in the chapter on physical findings by forcefully presenting me with a "must" list that could not be refused. Kathleen Fletcher, Ph.D., contributed superb editorial advice on several occasions, heedless of the time required.

Thanks, too, to Susan Poo.

Sheldon B. Korones

Contents

High-risk newborn infants

THE BASIS FOR INTENSIVE NURSING CARE

The fetus

Neonatal disorders, especially those that occur soon after birth, are usually the result of prenatal difficulties. Effective management of these illnesses requires familiarity with the intrauterine events that give rise to them. This chapter is concerned with the important aspects of fetal growth and function and the maternofetal relationships on which they depend.

THE PLACENTA: JUXTAPOSITION OF FETAL AND MATERNAL CIRCULATION

Fundamentally, the placenta provides bidirectional passage of substances between the mother and the fetus, whose circulations are contiguous but separate. The placenta is comprised of a maternal contribution called the *decidua basalis* and an embryonic one called the *chorion*. The maternal tissue contains uterine blood vessels, endometrial stroma, and glands; the embryonic tissue is composed of chorionic villi anchored to the chorionic plate.

The placenta (from Latin for "flat cake") is shaped like a round biscuit. At term it is about 15% of the fetal weight, approximately 6 to 8 inches in diameter, and 1 inch thick. Throughout pregnancy it occupies approximately one third of the inner surface of the uterus. One side, the fetal surface, is covered by glistening amniotic membrane, which receives the umbilical cord near its center. The opposite side, the maternal surface, remains embedded in the uterine wall until it begins to separate during labor and is extruded during the third stage (Chapter 2). The placenta is composed of fifteen to twenty-eight grossly visible segments called *cotyledons* (Fig. 1-1), which are of identical structure and are separated from each other by connective tissue septa. Each cotyledon contains fetal vessels, chorionic villi, and an intervillous

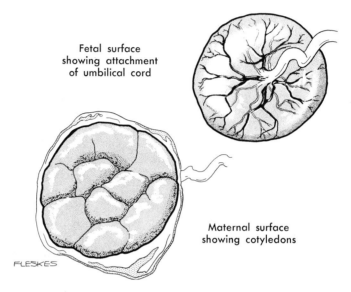

Fetal surface showing attachment of umbilical cord

Maternal surface showing cotyledons

FLESKES

Fig. 1-1. Maternal and fetal surfaces of the placenta. The cotyledons are visible on the maternal surface, which is implanted into the uterine wall. The fetal surface glistens, being covered by amnion. Branches of the umbilical vessels are on the fetal surface. (Modified from Netter: In Oppenheim, E., editor: Ciba collection of medical illustrations, vol. 2, Reproductive system, 1965.)

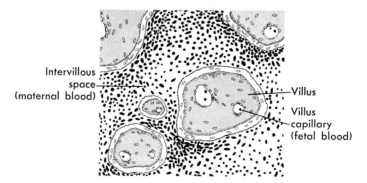

Intervillous space (maternal blood)

Villus

Villus capillary (fetal blood)

Fig. 1-2. Microscopic appearance of the villi in an intervillous space. Fetal capillaries permeate the villi, which are immersed in maternal blood within the intervillous spaces.

space. The dark red color of the placenta is due to fetal hemoglobin rather than maternal blood, which is usually drained by the time the placenta is delivered. Thus, if the placenta appears pale, the fetus was significantly anemic.

Chorionic villi, intervillous space, and placental circulation

Within a week after implantation, the embryo elaborates fingerlike projections of tissue known as the *chorionic villi*, which invade uterine endometrium at the site of implantation. They enlarge and branch considerably, becoming more deeply embedded into uterine tissue as they grow. Each of these projections is ultimately comprised of an outer layer of epithelial cells and a connective tissue core that contains fetal capillaries. During villous invasion of the endometrium, erosion of uterine vessels and supporting tissue occurs, and as a result irregular spaces are formed in the uterine wall. They are filled with maternal blood and surround the chorionic villi. These comprise the intervillous space, and the exchange of substances between maternal and fetal blood takes place at these sites. Transfer of any given substance from the maternal to the fetal circulation thus requires sequential passage from the mother's blood through the outer epithelial layer of the chorionic villus, through the connective tissue, and then through the endothelial wall of the capillary into fetal blood (Fig. 1-2). As pregnancy progresses, the villi decrease in size but in-

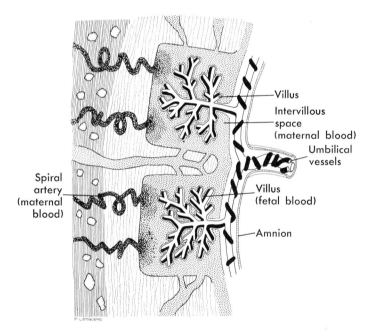

Fig. 1-3. Section through the placenta, showing the spiral arteries that supply maternal blood to the intervillous space, the branching villi immersed in the intervillous space, and the umbilical vessels that branch repeatedly to terminate as villous capillaries. (Modified from Netter: In Oppenheim, E., editor: Ciba collection of medical illustrations, vol. 2, Reproductive system, 1965.)

crease considerably in number. This change in both size and number of villi provides a progressive increase in fetal surface area within the placenta for the greater needs of the growing fetus. The villous surface at term is estimated at 13 to 14 sq M, an area that is ten times greater than the total skin surface of the adult. This enhanced capacity for maternofetal exchange is further implemented by simultaneous thinning of the tissue layer in the villus, thus reducing the distance between fetal capillaries and the intervillous space.

Maternal blood in the uterine arteries enters the base of the intervillous spaces through spiral arterioles. At term there are approximately 100 arteries supplying the placenta. Spurting jets of oxygenated blood diffuse upward and laterally to surround the villi, passing out of the intervillous spaces in a deoxygenated state by way of venous orifices that are situated at the base of the intervillous space adjacent to the spiral arteries. The direction of blood flow is normally maintained by an arteriovenous pressure gradient, that is, from higher arterial pressure to lower venous pressure (Fig. 1-3). Pressure in the spiral arteries is about 70 to 80 mm Hg. In the draining veins it is 8 mm Hg. Lateral flow between cotyledons is negligible.

Fetal blood leaves the body through two umbilical arteries that course through the umbilical cord to the placenta. Once they contact the fetal surface of the placenta, the arteries branch to supply each of the cotyledons. After continued branching and diminution in size, the vessels finally terminate in capillary loops within each chorionic villus. Villous blood receives oxygen from the maternal circulation, returns from capillary loops to venules, and goes thence to larger veins that leave each of the placental cotyledons. Coalescence of veins results in the formation of a single umbilical vein, which passes from the placenta through the length of the umbilical cord to the body of the fetus. A cross section of the umbilical cord reveals two thick-walled muscular arteries and one vein. The vein is noticeably larger than the arteries, although it has a considerably thinner wall (Fig. 1-4). The umbilical vessels are surrounded by a white gelatinous material called Wharton's jelly.

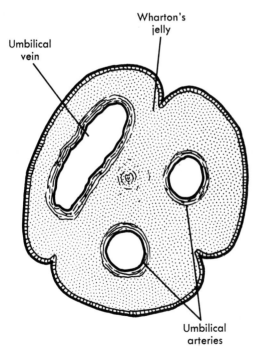

Fig. 1-4. Cross section of umbilical cord. The arteries have thick walls; the lumen of the vein is larger than those of the arteries, and its wall is thin.

FETAL CIRCULATION

Two major circuits, pulmonary and systemic, comprise the circulation in the fetus as well as in the adult. A third component, the placental circuit, is peculiar to the fetus. Pulmonary circulation begins at the pulmonic valve at the origin of the main pulmonary artery, which arises from the right ventricle. It continues through the lungs and terminates at the pulmonary vein orifices in the wall of the left atrium. The systemic circulation includes all other arterial and venous channels elsewhere in the body. The placental circuit is comprised of the umbilical and placental vessels as described earlier.

In any discussion of circulatory patterns a conceptual subdivision into "right" and "left" sides is often invoked. In the mature individual the right-sided circulation contains venous blood and the left side, arterial blood. Anatomically the right side begins at the venous end of capillary beds in all organs except the lungs. It continues through progressively enlarging veins to the inferior vena cava into the right atrium, to the right ventricle, into the pulmonary arteries, and finally to the pulmonary alveolar capillaries, where oxygenation occurs. Blood now continues on to the left side, which begins at the alveolar capillaries and progresses through the pulmonary veins into the left side of the heart, through the aorta to smaller arteries, and to the arterial side of capillary beds in all organs except the lungs. At the arterial side of the capillaries, blood gives up oxygen and continues to the venous side, where it reenters the right side of the circulation.

The normal mature circulation is characterized by flow of unoxygenated (venous) blood into the right side of the heart, which continues into the pulmonary circuit, where oxygenation occurs, and then returns to the left side of the heart for distribution to the rest of the body by way of the aorta. Thus the only

connections between the right and left circulations are at the capillary beds in the lungs and in the capillaries of other organs of the body.

When, as in certain cardiovascular malformations, a connection between the right and left sides exists at sites other than the capillaries, an anatomic shunt is said to be present. Examples of such anomalies are persistent patency of the ductus arteriosus, arteriovenous aneurysm, and numerous malformations of the heart itself. Blood flow through an abnormal vascular channel from the venous to the arterial circulation constitutes a right-to-left shunt. Conversely, flow of blood through an anomalous channel from artery to vein is a left-to-right shunt. In either case blood enters one side of the circulation from the other before reaching the capillary bed for which it is normally destined, and the result is an admixture of oxygenated and unoxygenated blood.

Fetal circulation differs from the neonatal or adult pattern in three major respects: (1) presence of anatomic shunts, one within the heart at the foramen ovale, one immediately outside the heart in the ductus arteriosus, and another at the juncture of the ductus venosus and the inferior vena cava; (2) presence of a placental circulation; and (3) minimal blood flow through the lungs (3% to 7% of cardiac output).

The course of fetal circulation is depicted in Fig. 1-5. (The atria are *inferior* to the ventricles so that the fetal pattern of blood flow can be clearly and simply indicated.) Blood that has been oxygenated in the chorionic villi leaves the placenta through the umbilical vein, which enters the fetal abdomen at the umbilicus and then courses between the right and left lobes of the liver. Some of this blood perfuses the liver through branches of the umbilical vein, whereas the rest continues past it to the ductus venosus and empties into the inferior vena cava at a point just below the diaphragm. Blood now enters the heart through the inferior vena caval orifice, where a direct communication exists between the right and left atria (foramen ovale). Here the caval bloodstream is divided, the major portion flowing directly into the left atrium, whereas the remainder enters the right atrium to join blood from the superior vena cava, which drains the head, neck, and upper extremities. The left atrium also receives blood that has perfused the lungs from pulmonary veins, and this mixture enters successively the left ventricle, the ascending aorta, and the aortic arch, from whence most of it is distributed to the coronary arteries and the vessels of the head and upper extremities.

The smaller quantity of blood directed to the right atrium from the inferior vena cava is added to the superior vena caval

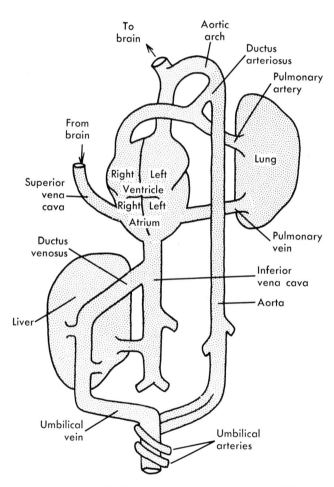

Fig. 1-5. Fetal circulation. (Modified from Lind, J., Stern, L., and Wegelius, C.: Human foetal and neonatal circulation, Springfield, Ill., 1964, Charles C Thomas, Publisher.)

flow and enters the right ventricle and then the main pulmonary artery. Most of it is conveyed to the descending aorta through the ductus arteriosus. Some continues through the pulmonary circuit to perfuse the lungs and return to the left atrium by way of the pulmonary veins. The descending aorta bifurcates at the lower end of the body into the right and left iliac arteries. The two hypogastric arteries are branches off the latter vessels. They each course upward around the bladder and leave the abdomen through the umbilical cord, where they are called the umbilical arteries.

Admixture of blood occurs at three sites in the fetal circulation: (1) the fora-

men ovale, (2) from the pulmonary artery to the descending aorta through the ductus arteriosus, and (3) at the junction of the ductus venosus and inferior vena cava.

THE AMNION AND AMNIOTIC FLUID

The amnion and the amniotic cavity develop in the embryo during the first week, appearing as a small elongated sac adjacent to the dorsal embryonic surface. As the fluid-filled cavity enlarges, it spreads around the embryo in all directions and ultimately comes to surround the fetus. This cavity is traversed only by the umbilical cord, which courses from

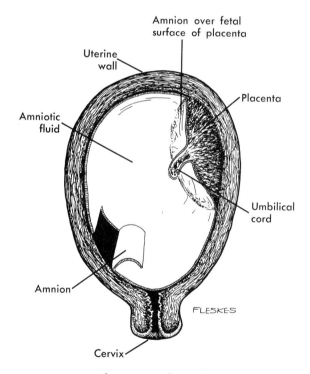

Fig. 1-6. Uterine cavity at term. The amnion lines the uterine wall. It continues over the placenta and reflects from it to envelop the umbilical cord. Amniotic fluid surrounds the fetus to fill the cavity. (Modified from Hillman, L. M., and Pritchard, J. A.: Williams obstetrics, ed. 14, New York, 1971, Appleton-Century-Crofts.)

the umbilicus to its insertion into the placenta. The amniotic membrane is 0.5 mm or less in thickness and is comprised of five microscopic layers. Fully developed, it lines the entire inner surface of the uterine wall, except at the site of placental attachment, where it covers the fetal surface of that organ, reflects onto the umbilical cord, and completely envelops it (Fig. 1-6). The fluid that surrounds the fetus (amniotic fluid) is contained by this membrane, and when the latter ruptures at the onset of labor, the fluid is released.

Amniotic fluid accumulates progressively throughout pregnancy, attaining a volume of approximately 1000 ml at term (normal range: 400 to 1500 ml). It continuously enters and leaves the amniotic cavity in large volumes, creating a constant turnover that involves complex water and solute exchanges not yet precisely delineated. Amniotic fluid is derived primarily from maternal serum early in pregnancy and from fetal urine later. Some fluid orginates in the fetal lung. Egress of fluid occurs largely by absorption into the fetal bloodstream from the gastrointestinal tract, into which it gains entry as a result of repeated fetal swallowing. That the fetus swallows effectively has been shown often by amniography, a procedure that entails injection of radiopaque dye into the aminotic fluid for the primary purpose of demonstrating the site of placental implantation for the possible presence of placenta previa. At term, the fetus is thought to swallow 500 ml per day, but there are reports of tremendous volumes as high as 500 ml per hour. Normal volumes of amniotic fluid are thus largely regulated by contributions of the fetal urinary tract and evacuation through the gastrointestinal tract. Thus, if the elimination of fluid is impaired, the quantity of fluid may be increased abnormally to more than 2000 ml. This increase is called *hydramnios* or *polyhydramnios.* Conversely, if little or no urine is excreted, amniotic fluid may be virtually absent or greatly reduced in quantity. This abnormality is known as *oligohydramnios.*

The elimination of fluid is impaired in any fetus who is unable to swallow, for example, a fetus with gross malformation of the brain (anencephaly, hydrocephalus). Structural obstruction to swallowing of amniotic fluid is also responsible for abnormal accumulations of volume *(polyhydramnios).* These obstructions occur in high gastrointestinal malformations such as esophageal atresia and duodenal atresia. Cardiac failure of the fetus occurs in hydrops fetalis, which is also associated with polyhydramnios.

If impaired swallowing restricts the outflow of amniotic fluid, obstructed micturition severely restricts the inflow. Oligohydramnios thus results from obstructed fetal micturition. Fetal urinary contribution to amniotic fluid is thus diminished or eliminated in renal agenesis or dysplasia and in urethral obstruction. Oligohydramnios (unassociated with urinary tract obstruction) is a frequent occurrence in postmaturity and fetal death.

Amniotic fluid affords a milieu that allows relatively free fetal movement. It protects the fetus from externally inflicted trauma, and it contributes to the stability of fetal body temperature. During early labor, hydrostatic forces created by uterine contractions are mediated by the fluid to aid in normal dilatation of the cervix and descent of the fetus.

MATERNOFETAL EXCHANGE OF GAS ACROSS THE PLACENTA

The placenta has a number of critical functions, but perhaps the most sensitive of all is its role as the fetus' lung. The juxtaposition of maternal and fetal circulations at the placental site, with separation of each circulatory unit by a relatively thin membrane, provides the structural basis for exchange of gases between mother and fetus. The diffusion of gases across placental membranes is similar to gas diffusion across cellular membranes in any other organ of the body. Although the placenta functions as a lung for the fetus, the obvious and fundamental difference is that it accommodates the exchange of gases from one individual's circulation to another. The placenta is not as efficient as the lung, yet it is effective for this purpose; gas diffusion in the placenta is only one fiftieth as efficient as in the postnatal lung.

Fetal respiration occurs by transfer of oxygen from maternal blood in the intervillous space to fetal blood in the villous capillaries and by release of carbon dioxide in the opposite direction from fetus to mother. The normal flow of these gases is governed by their respective partial pressures in maternal and fetal blood and by unimpeded fetal and maternal blood flow in the placenta.

Gases have a tendency to expand, and they exert measurable pressure in the process. This pressure is expressed in millimeters of mercury (mm Hg). Thus pressure exerted by gases in the atmosphere at sea level is 760 mm Hg. In any mixture of two or more gases, the pressure exerted by each of them is called their *partial pressure*. The sum of the partial pressures of each constituent gas in a mixture is the total pressure exerted by that mixture. The expression symbolizing partial pressure of a gas is written P (or p) preceding its chemical formula. The partial pressures of oxygen and of carbon dioxide are written as P_{O_2} and

P_{CO_2}. This terminology is utilized routinely in reports from clinical and research laboratories.

Assuming normal placental blood flow, the differences in the partial pressures of gases (P_{O_2}, P_{CO_2}) that exist between maternal and fetal blood determine the direction in which these gases move. Gases are transferred in response to pressure gradients, that is, from a higher pressure to a lower one. Tissues intervening between the maternal and fetal circulations (normally 3.5 to 5.5 microns in total thickness) seem to offer more resistnace to the movement of oxygen than to carbon dioxide; carbon dioxide is twenty times more diffusable than oxygen. Table 1-1 gives P_{O_2} and P_{CO_2} values of fetal blood in the umbilical artery, maternal blood in the intervillous space, and fetal blood in the umbilical vein as reported by a number of investigators. The acquisition of oxygen and the surrender of carbon dioxide by fetal blood are indicated in the alterations of P_{O_2} and P_{CO_2} that result from the exchange of gases with maternal blood in the intervillous space. The influence of partial pressure gradients can be appreciated by noting, in Table 1-1, that a higher maternal P_{O_2} in the intervillous

Table 1-1. Mean quantitative changes in fetal blood gases resulting from fetomaternal exchange*

	P_{O_2} (mm Hg)	P_{CO_2} (mm Hg)
Umbilical artery (blood from fetus)	16	46
Intervillous space (maternal blood)	40	38
Umbilical vein (blood to fetus)	29	42

*Based on data from Seeds, A. E.: Pediatr. Clin. North Am. **17**:811, 1970.

space moves oxygen into the fetal circulation to raise P_{O_2} from 16 mm Hg in the umbilical artery to 29 mm Hg in blood returning to the fetus by way of the umbilical vein. The flow of oxygen is therefore from mother to fetus. The direction of carbon dioxide transfer is from fetus to mother because P_{CO_2} in the intervillous space (38 mm Hg in maternal blood) is lower than in the umbilical artery (46 mm Hg in fetal blood); thus carbon dioxide moves from fetus to mother with a resultant diminution of P_{CO_2} in the umbilical vein (42 mm Hg) compared with that in the umbilical artery (46 mm Hg).

Maintenance of these pressure gradients depends on normal maternal blood gas levels and normal blood flow in the mother and fetus. A number of disorders may alter maternal blood gas levels sufficiently to hamper gas exchange at the intervillous space. Thus severe pneumonia, asthma, congestive heart failure, and apnea during convulsions (epilepsy, eclampsia) may result in maternal hypoxemia that endangers the fetus. Impairment of blood flow to the intervillous space may occur as a consequence of maternal shock or congestive heart failure. Local impediment to placental perfusion may result from abnormally intense and frequent uterine contractions during labor or from compression of the inferior vena cava by the overlying heavy uterus when the mother is supine (supine hypotension syndrome).

FETAL GROWTH

Growth of the fetus involves an increase in the number of cells (hyperplasia) and an increase in their size (hypertrophy). Growth progresses through three stages: (1) hyperplasia, (2) a declining rate of hyperplasia with increasing hypertrophy, and (3) predominant hypertrophy. Embryonic growth is largely hyperplastic; hypertrophy becomes increasingly prominent later in pregnancy. Growth may be impeded during any or all of these progressive stages, resulting in different types of growth failure. Thus the number of cells may be diminished although their size remains relatively normal, cell size rather than quantity may be reduced, or both size and number may be diminished. The net result is subnormal size and weight of affected organs. These effects depend on the stage of growth during which an insult is inflicted. For example, intrauterine rubella infection, which occurs early in pregnancy, produces a severe reduction in the quantity of cells in many organs. On the other hand, the effects of toxemia, which often appear late in pregnancy, are characterized by a significant reduction in cell size, although cell number is relatively normal. All these changes have been produced in pregnant animals that were starved at various stages of pregnancy. Interference with cellular proliferation (hyperplastic growth) may cause a permanent diminution in the quantity of cells, although impaired hypertrophy is apparently reversible to some extent if proper feeding is instituted after birth. There is evidence that these phenomena may also be operative in humans. The human brain continues to grow by cellular proliferation for at least 8 postnatal months after 40 gestational weeks. Postnatal malnutrition impairs this process. Whether maternal malnutrition permanently limits organ growth in humans has yet to be documented. Data from animal studies and clinical observations of human infants suggest that permanent limitation of growth does indeed occur.

The characteristics of normal cellular growth are of importance in understanding the abnormalities of birth weight and size that are peculiar to prematurity and intrauterine growth retardation. A more detailed discussion of fetal growth is presented in Chapter 5.

ASSESSMENT OF FETAL STATUS (FETAL DIAGNOSIS)

The growing ability to assess fetal conditions in utero continues to be one of the most exciting areas in perinatology. The diagnosis of certain disorders of the fetus is feasible; approximation of fetal maturation is aided significantly by examination of chemical and cellular constituents of amniotic fluid and by accurate estimation of fetal head size. Lung maturation is assessed by lecithin-sphingomyelin (L/S) ratio determination, which indicates the status of surfactant production. Identification of hypoxic stress in utero is possible by monitoring fetal heart rate and by sampling specimens for blood gas and pH determinations. The overall health of the fetus is assessable by estriol determination. The diagnosis of placenta previa can be made by amniography (injection of radiopaque dye into the amniotic cavity) or by ultrasound to demonstrate placental position. Postnatal microscopic examination of the amniotic membrane and the umbilical cord for the presence of neutrophilic infiltration has been used to determine the presence of fetal exposure to intrauterine bacterial infection (Chapter 12). Insofar as intrauterine therapy is concerned, transfusion is the only procedure currently in common use. A description of the most widely used methods for fetal diagnosis and assessment follows.

Examination of amniotic fluid

Amniocentesis. Amniotic fluid may be withdrawn simply and safely by amnio-centesis, that is, insertion of a needle through the abdominal and uterine walls into the amniotic cavity. Amniocentesis has been performed as early as the twelfth gestational week. Amniotic fluid components can be analyzed for the severity of erythroblastosis (Rh incompatibility); for predictions of postnatal appearance of hyaline membrane disease, certain genetic disorders, and inborn errors of metabolism; and for fetal age. Although the complications of amniocentesis are uncommon, a variety of them have been reported. These risks include abortion, maternal hemorrhage, infection, fetal puncture wounds, pneumothorax, laceration of the fetal spleen, damage to placental and umbilical vessels, and sudden death from fetal exsanguination.

Bilirubin. Determination of bilirubin in amniotic fluid is valuable for assessment of the severity of Rh disease. Bilirubin is derived form the breakdown of red blood cells (Chapter 10), and it is thus present at certain levels in normal amniotic fluid. Peak levels are attained between 16 and 30 weeks of gestation, and a steady decline thereafter usually culminates in its disappearance by 36 weeks. In most instances there is no bilirubin in amniotic fluid beyond 36 weeks of gestation. This finding is variable, however, and bilirubin determination is not valuable for estimation of fetal maturity. If, as in fetal erythroblastosis, an excessive rate of hemolysis occurs, bilirubin levels in amniotic fluid rise abnormally. These values are plotted on a graph that delineates three zones of fetal involvement (mild, moderate, and severe), depending on the bilirubin concentration. If the results indicate severe disease, an intrauterine transfusion or an immediate termination of pregnancy is urgently indicated. If moderate involvement is present, repeated frequent determinations are required to monitor the course of fetal disease. Values falling into the zone of mild involvement contraindicate intrauterine transfusion or interruption of pregnancy, since postnatal therapy is effective in these circumstances. The amniotic fluid of hyperbilirubinemic mothers often contains abnormally increased amounts of bilirubin, even in the absence of Rh disease.

Creatinine. Levels of creatinine in the amniotic fluid increase with gestational age and are thus useful in the assessment of fetal maturity. Creatinine in amniotic fluid is derived from fetal urine. It is excreted through the kidneys across the glomeruli, which increase substantially in number during the third trimester. Thus it is reasonable to expect that creatinine levels will rise steadily as pregnancy progresses. In normal pregnancies, 1.6 to 1.8 mg/100 ml of creatinine is indicative of 36 or 37 gestational weeks in approximately 94% of patients. However, the usefulness of this determination for estimation of fetal age is unfortunately limited in complicated pregnancies in which maternal renal function is impaired. Thus, in toxemic mothers, amniotic fluid creatinine concentrations are often misleadingly higher than in normal pregnancies of like duration. The toxemic gravida's impaired kidney function causes some degree of creatinine retention, and therefore her serum level is elevated. This increase (if greater than 1 mg/100 ml) is reflected in amniotic fluid as a high creatinine concentration, which suggests a mature fetus, when in fact the fetus is premature. Higher-than-expected values have been observed in diabetic mothers. On the other hand in Rh disease amniotic fluid creatinine concentration may be lower than expected. For these reasons *the critical question of fetal age cannot be consistently answered solely by determination of amniotic fluid-creatinine concentration.*

Lecithin-sphingomyelin ratio (L/S ratio). In the fetal lung, fluid is secreted into the alveoli, and it is ultimately deposited into amniotic fluid after migration up the respiratory tract and out the glottic opening into the posterior pharynx. This secretion contains surfactant, a complex substance that is comprised of several phospholipids, which lowers surface tension forces of alveolar walls (Chapter 8). This function is indispensable for initial opening of the alveoli during the first breath and for prevention of alveolar collapse (atelectasis) subsequently. Deficiency of surfactant results in the widespread atelectasis that characterizes hyaline membrane disease. The demonstration, in amniotic fluid prenatally, of sufficient surfactant to preclude hyaline membrane disease postnatally is one of the most helpful and reliable of all intrauterine tests for fetal maturity. This procedure actually indicates the maturational status of fetal lungs—that is, the capacity of the lungs to accommodate normal ventilation after birth. There is no consistent relationship between fetal weight, age, and pulmonary maturity. Up to 10% of mature fetuses have been reported to have low L/S ratios, whereas normal ratios have been reported in premature fetuses.

The principal constituent of surfactant is lecithin; it comprises 50% of surfactant phospholipids. Its presence in relation to sphingomyelin is expressed as a ratio that usually changes predictability as pregnancy progresses. Two other phospholipids, while present in considerably smaller quantities than lecithin itself, are essential for effective function of surfactant. These substances are called *phos-*

phatidyl glycerol (PG) and *phosphatidyl inositol (PI)*. They are important in the diminution of surface active forces because they stabilize lecithin in the surfactant layer that lines the alveoli. The presence of PG may well be a more accurate predictor of lung function than the L/S ratio. Surface-active lecithin appears in amniotic fluid at 24 to 26 weeks of gestation, at which time concentrations are very slightly above those of sphingomyelin. Before this time, very little lecithin is measurable; afterward, lecithin increases while sphingomyelin concentration remains relatively unchanged. Surfactant is secreted into the alveolar spaces at approximately 26 to 27 weeks gestation. Between 30 and 32 weeks, lecithin concentrations rise slightly to 1.2 times greater than that of sphingomyelin (L/S ratio = 1.2). At 35 weeks, an abrupt rise in lecithin to at least twice the concentration of sphingomyelin (ratio = 2 or more) signifies pulmonary maturity; this virtually assures that hyaline membrane disease will not occur after birth. Fig. 1-7 depicts the quantitative changes of lecithin and sphingomyelin. It illustrates that the relationship between lecithin and sphingomyelin in amniotic fluid provides a basis for the assessment of fetal pulmonary maturity.

L/S ratios correlate well with gestational age in normal pregnancies. In high-risk pregnancies the correlation is not so straightforward. Lung maturity, as indicated by L/S ratio, may occur early or late in gestation, depending on the exist-

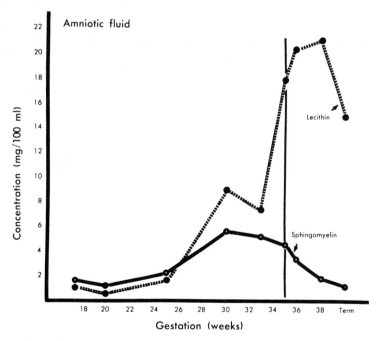

Fig. 1-7. Lecithin (broken line) and sphingomyelin (solid line) concentrations plotted against gestational age. L/S ratio rises to 1.2 at 28 weeks, and to 2 or more at 35 weeks, indicating little chance of hyaline membrane disease postnatally. (From Gluck, L., Kulovich, M. V., Borer, R. C., Jr., et al: Am. J. Obstet. Gynecol.**109**:440, 1971.)

ing maternal disorder. For example, a 3300-gram infant at 38 weeks of gestation has been reported with a ratio of only 0.75, whereas a 920-gram infant at 28 weeks had a normal mature ratio. The older and larger infant had severe hyaline membrane disease, but the smaller infant did not. Following is a list of maternal diseases that have been shown to alter the normal developmental schedule of pulmonary maturity; that is, the attainment of an L/S ratio of 2 or more was either accelerated (pulmonary maturity before 35 weeks) or delayed (pulmonary maturity after 35 weeks). Maternal conditions associated with accelerated development of pulmonary maturity are generally those that cause diminished maternal blood flow to the placenta and therefore an impairment, to some extent, of oxygen transport to the fetus. The resultant fetal distress apparently increases the blood level of corticosteroid, which triggers elaboration of surfactant in Type II alveolar cells.

Disorders associated with alteration from normal time of appearance of mature L/S ratio*

Appearance of mature ratio before 35 gestational weeks (accelerated maturation)

  A. Maternal conditions
    1. Toxemia (early onset)
    2. Hypertensive renal disease
    3. Hypertensive cardiovascular disease
    4. Sickle cell disease
    5. Narcotic addiction
    6. Diabetes, class D, F, R (p. 307)
    7. Chronic retroplacental hemorrhage
    8. Hyperthyroidism
    9. Corticosteroids, aminophylline
    10. Maternal infections
    11. Placental insufficiency
    12. Parabiotic twinning-donor (small) twin

---

*Modified from Gluck, L.: Clin. Obstet. Gynecol. **21:**547, 1978.

  B. Fetal disorders
    1. Prolonged rupture of membranes

Appearance of mature ratio after 35 gestational weeks (delayed maturation)

  A. Maternal condition
    1. Diabetes, class A, B, C (p. 307)
    2. Chronic glomerulonephritis
  B. Fetal condition
    1. Rh disease, particularly with hydrops fetalis
    2. Smaller of identical twins (nonparasitic)

Numerous other variables may affect the outcome of predictions of pulmonary maturity based on the L/S ratio. Some have already been demonstrated, and extensive investigation will no doubt unearth others. The presence of maternal blood in amniotic fluid tends to lower the L/S ratio. Thus a mature ratio in bloody fluid is a valid result; an immature ratio may be artifactual. The presence of meconium in amniotic fluid affects reliable results in an unpredictable fashion; it may either raise or lower the L/S ratio from its true value by a mechanism that is not understood. In some instances a ratio of 2 or more may be associated with postnatal hyaline membrane disease due to events that transpire after collection of the sample. Thus among 425 pregnancies observed in one study, 13 infants whose ratios were normal, nevertheless, had respiratory distress after birth. Twelve of these babies had a low Apgar score of 5 minutes (less than 7), reflecting intrauterine or intrapartum stress that occurred subsequent to the L/S ratio determination. This acute distress may have impaired surfactant activity and therefore induced the occurrence of hyaline membrane disease.

Prolonged rupture of membranes is believed by many to be associated with a significant diminution in the incidence of hyaline membrane disease. The data indicates that this association is prevalent when membranes have ruptured 48 to 72 hours, or longer, prior to delivery. Apparently, prolonged rupture of membranes results in an elevated level of corticosteroids in fetal blood, which stimulates production of surfactant earlier in gestation.

As data accumulate, new insights will evolve regarding accuracies and errors in the predictive value of the ratio. This amniotic fluid analysis is currently indispensable as an aid in deciding whether or not the fetus of a high-risk pregnancy is safer in the uterus or outside it. A ratio of 2 or more reliably predicts the absence of hyaline membrane disease with only occasional inaccuracy. On the other hand, a ratio of less than 2 does not predict the occurrence of hyaline membrane disease as reliably as the ratio greater than 2 predicts its absence. A mature ratio accurately predicts the absence of hyaline membrane disease in approximately 98% of cases. On the other hand, a ratio of less than 2 (immature) has been reported to be associated with hyaline membrane disease in only 40% to 80% of fetuses tested. Apparently the lower the ratio, the more likely the occurrence of hyaline membrane disease.

Shake test on amniotic fluid and neonatal gastric juice. The shake test, or foam test, is a simple procedure that attempts to correlate mature or immature L/S ratios with the presence or absence of foam in prepared samples of amniotic fluid or in the neonate's gastric aspirate collected soon after birth. The sample is mixed with ethanol and shaken for 15 seconds; a reading is made 15 minutes later. The test depends on the ability of lecithin to create a stable foam in ethanol. A positive result is produced by a complete ring of bubbles at the surface that persists for 15 minutes. It appears to be a reliable indication of pulmonary maturity. Hyaline membrane disease has rarely followed a positive foam test. The absence of foam suggests that hyaline membrane disease will occur, but such absence is not as reliably predictive as the low L/S ratio itself. Therefore, the shake test is a good screening procedure for maturity (positive for foam), but in the absence of foam, an L/S ratio should be performed.

Cellular examination to assess fetal maturity. Toward the latter phase of pregnancy, fat-laden cells from fetal skin are exfoliated into amniotic fluid in increasing numbers as term is approached. These cells are thought to originate from the sebaceous glands of fetal skin and perhaps from the respiratory and urinary tracts and amniotic membrane. Lipid in cells is identified by the presence of orange-red droplets on microscopic examination after application of 0.1% Nile blue sulfate solution. Gross groupings according to the percentage of fat-laden cells correlate well with gestational ages. Prematurity is rarely present when 20% of counted cells are fat stained. Clumps of orange cells, or free lipid droplets, are also indicative of a term fetus. In the presence of lower percentages of fat-laden cells, the incidence of false negative results increases. Thus, prematurity is spuriously indicated in a number of infants who are actually mature. The technique of staining may itself alter results considerably. Individual laboratories should carefully analyze their experience before placing reliance on this procedure. This test is valuable in both normal and high-risk fetuses. It is in essence an assessment of the maturity of fetal skin.

Cellular examination for genetic abnormalities. Since the cells in amniotic fluid are of fetal origin, they have been subjected to intensive study in efforts to identify certain genetically transmitted disorders as early in gestation as possible. Fetal involvement, or absence of it, has been correctly predicted in case reports of galactosemia, cystic fibrosis, glycogen storage disease, Marfan's syndrome, and numerous other infrequently encountered disorders. In addition, fetal sex determination is valuable in assessing the risk of sex-linked hereditary abnormalities such as hemophilia, which is manifest only in males. By demonstrating chromatin bodies in the nuclei, and thus identifying a female, the risk of chromatin bodies in a sufficient number of cells indicates a male fetus and thus a 50% risk of having an affected baby.

Meconium-stained fluid. In the term infant, 200 to 600 grams of meconium is contained in the intestine. It is viscous and sticky and varies in color from greenish brown to black. It contains cells from the skin, alimentary tract, lanugo, and vernix caseosa. Meconium may give a positive result for occult blood under normal circumstances, apparently as a result of ingestion of maternal blood or perhaps from clinically inconsequential oozing of alimentary tract vessels. Normal meconium does not contain protein because fetal proteolytic enzymes in the alimentary tract digest it. Rather, the bulk of meconium is comprised of mucopolysaccharides that are the residue of mucous secretions from intramural glands in the alimentary tract (secretions of the salivary, gastric, and intestinal glands). Meconium contains 1 mg of bilirubin per gram of wet weight. If, in the term infant, there are approximately 200 grams of meconium in the intestine, it can be surmised that 200 mg of prenatally excreted bilirubin is available for absorption from the intestinal tract as a contribution to neonatal physiologic hyperbilirubinemia. In 99.8% of normal term infants, the first passage of meconium should occur by 48 hours of age.

The incidence of meconium staining of amniotic fluid is reported to vary from 0.5% to 10.9% of all births. Five percent to 10% is probably a realistic estimate. It occurs most often in term infants; premature infants are rarely involved. Stained fluid usually indicates intrauterine stress.

The release of meconium by the fetus is said to occur in reponse to hypoxia, but this has not been confirmed since it was reported in 1954. The hypothesized mechanism of release involves increased peristalsis of the intestine and relaxation of the anal sphincter in response to hypoxic stress.

The most direct postnatal consequence of meconium release into amniotic fluid is the *meconium aspiration syndrome.* Particles of meconium are drawn into the respiratory tract in utero; the resultant postnatal distress is often sufficiently severe to require mechanical ventilatory support. Prolonged illness is not unusual; occasionally death ensues. The syndrome occurs predominantly in term infants (p. 240).

Presence of meconium in the amniotic fluid of an apparently healthy infant sometimes indicates transient intrauterine hypoxia that is of no ultimate significance to the infant's status at birth. The staining of fetal tissue (nails, skin, umbilical cord) probably indicates that meconium was released into the amniotic fluid at least 4 to 6 hours previously. Meconium is frequently passed by fetuses in the breech presentation even though they have not experienced hypoxia.

Estriol levels in maternal urine

Estriol, a major metabolite of estrogen, is found in relatively large quantities in maternal urine during the latter half of pregnancy. The fetal contribution to maternal urinary estriol concentration is ten times as great as the maternal contribution. Estriol is a valuable indicator of fetal health because its synthesis requires a normal placenta and fetal adrenal cortex. From the placenta it crosses into the maternal blood and eventually is excreted through the kidneys as estriol glucuronide. Intact function of both the fetal adrenal and the placenta are required for excretion of normal quantities of estriol. In pregnancies that are complicated by hypertension, renal disease, or preeclampsia, normal estriol values are a good indication that the fetus is in no danger at the moment. In Rh sensitization, low values are a particularly ominous finding; perinatal mortality up to 65% has been reported in such circumstances. In diabetes low values are a sign of fetal jeopardy, but here the correlation is not always straightforward, since normal findings do not necessarily indicate fetal health. Estriol concentrations are lowest when the fetus is dead or anencephalic. Anencephaly is regularly associated with absence of the fetal adrenal cortex; since there is no fetal adrenocortical function even if the placenta is intact, maternal urinary estriol is absent. Administered to the mother during gestation, steroids cross the placenta to depress fetal adrenal function. Intact activity of the adrenal-placental axis is impaired, and estriol formation is reduced by as much as 50%.

Urinary estriol increases as pregnancy progresses. There is some correlation between length of gestation and estriol determinations, but exceptions are sufficiently frequent to impair utilization of this test for determination of fetal maturity. Its use for monitoring fetal well-being is widespread and valid.

Urinary estriol assay has a significant logistic disadvantage in that a 24-hour urine collection is required. The time consumed in collection and the dependence on recovery of complete daily output impose some limitation on the procedure. Plasma determination may well replace urinary assay because only a single specimen is essential and serial determinations on several blood samples are possible over a short period. Plasma estriol is measurable in several fractions. Total estriol content is measured in a conjugated and an unconjugated fraction. The unconjugated fraction has recently been demonstrated to be more predictive than measurements of the other fractions. Furthermore, unconjugated plasma estriol levels have been found to increase suddenly at approximately 36 weeks of gestation. If this is a consistently demonstrated phenomenon, this determination may constitute another aid in approximating fetal maturity. At present, laboratory methods for plasma determination are cumbersome and time-consuming; which is the principal obstacle to widespread use of plasma for this purpose. Together with other laboratory determinations and careful clinical evaluations, urinary estriol determination is a valuable *adjunct* for identification of fetal illness.

Direct fetal heart rate monitoring

Although 60% to 75% of the fetuses who have difficulty during labor can be identified beforehand on the basis of the high-risk grouping of their mothers, the remainder cannot be similarly anticipated. Thus any healthy fetus of a healthy mother can be sufficiently stressed during labor as to threaten intact survival. The realization that electronic surveillance can rapidly detect the inception of fetal distress has resulted in widespread efforts to monitor the labor of as many women as possible for unanticipated fetal difficulty, regardless of their normal histories. It has been estimated that continuous fetal monitoring can reduce perinatal mortality and brain damage among survivors by 50%. Monitoring of fetal heart rate (FHR) is currently the most valuable available method for this purpose. Continuous beat-to-beat recording of fetal heart action in relation to uterine contractions provides relatively reliable data on the status of the fetus during labor. Ultimately this information furnishes a basis on which the obstetrician can decide whether to allow labor to progress to delivery normally or perform a cesarean section. The traditional intermittent auscultation of fetal heart tones with stethoscope to ears is grossly inadequate by contemporary standards, even when performed every 10 or 15 minutes.

As usually performed, the monitoring procedure involves placement of an electrode on the presenting fetal part (usually the scalp) for reception of a cardiac signal and insertion of a catheter into the amniotic space for recording uterine contractions. This internal technique is limited to women in labor. Both measurements can be made externally, from the maternal abdominal wall, but the internal method is more accurate. As external methods have improved, however, monitoring of the fetus has become more feasible earlier in labor or prior to its onset. Early evaluation of the fetal heart rate before the inception of labor predicts the fetus' capacity to withstand it (see indirect FHR monitoring, p. 21).

Records of fetal heart rate patterns during labor reflect transient acceleration, transient deceleration, tachycardia, bradycardia, and variability of millisecond intervals between each heartbeat.

The most frequent significant heart rate changes involve three types of deceleration that are categorized according to their timing with uterine contractions and the shape of the recorded waveform (Fig. 1-8).

Early deceleration (head compression). *Early deceleration* is probably due to fetal head compression (HC) during contractions. The resultant increased intracranial pressure activates impulses from the medulla through the vagus nerve to the heart, with consequent slowing of cardiac rate. The deceleration begins simultaneously with the onset of uterine contractions; it ceases at the end of the contraction. The waveform on the tracing is similar from one period of deceleration to the next. The heart rate remains in the normal range (120 to 160 beats/min). This pattern does not seem to have clinical significance. It usually occurs when the cervix is dilated 4 to 7 cm. It has not been associated with increased neonatal mortality or morbidity, or with alterations in fetal blood pH that would indicate distress. This fetal response to uterine contraction has been modified experimentally by administration of atropine, which is known to block the transmission of impulses through the vagus nerve.

Late deceleration (uteroplacental insufficiency). *Late deceleration* is thought to indicate uteroplacental insufficiency (UPI). It is an ominous pattern in which the onset of decelerated fetal heart rate occurs *after* the onset of contraction, reaching its slowest rate after the contraction has ended. Thus the temporal relationship of this deceleration to uterine contraction differs from that of *early deceleration*. The shape of the waveform is similar, however. Even though diminished from baseline, the heart rate is usually within normal limits. This type of recording indicates fetal hypoxia due to diminished maternal blood flow through the intervillous space. Animal experiments have demonstrated the association of late deceleration with lowered fetal arterial P_{O_2}. The deceleration can be abolished or diminished by administering high oxygen concentrations to the mother. The *late deceleration* pattern is often noted in pregnancies that are complicated by diabetes, toxemia, hypertension, Rh disease, maternal hypotension in the supine posi-

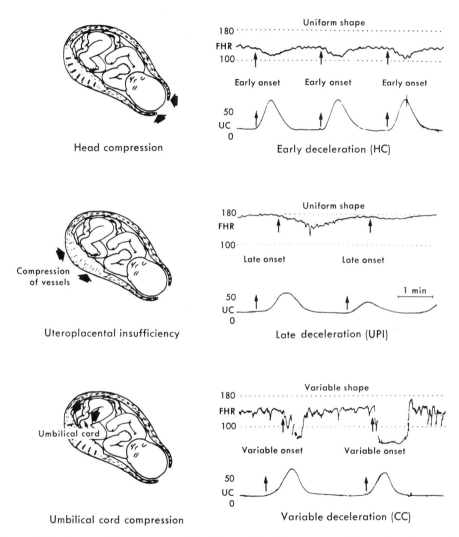

Fig. 1-8. The three major patterns of decelerated fetal heart rates. Note the relationship of onset and end of bradycardia to increased intrauterine pressures (contractions). *FHR*, Fetal heart rate; *UC*, uterine contraction; *HC*, head compression; *UPI*, uteroplacental insufficiency; *CC*, cord compression. See text for full explanation. (From Hon, E. H.: An introduction to fetal heart rate monitoring, Los Angeles, 1973, University of Southern California Press.)

tion, and hypertonicity of the uterus due to excessive oxytocin. Delay in the appearance of fetal cardiac deceleration relative to a uterine contraction ("lag time") is probably a function of the transit time of poorly oxygenated blood from fetal villi to the placenta to the central fetal circulation. In *early deceleration*, there is no such delay. Pressure exerted on the fetal head by the uterine contraction stimulates impulses through the vagus nerve that are instantaneously transmitted to the heart. Deceleration and contraction are thus synchronous, since the circulation is not involved and there is no transit or "lag" time. Also, in contrast to *early deceleration*, this delayed variety is often associated with fetal acidosis, lowered P_{O_2}, elevated P_{CO_2}, and low Apgar scores. *Late deceleration* cannot be eliminated by atropine, but it can be improved by oxygen administration to the mother or by correction of any of the detectable causes of diminished placental blood flow. The lowered cardiac rate that characterizes *late deceleration* is directly related to suboptimal oxygenation of fetal blood, however transient it may be.

Variable deceleration (cord compression). *Variable deceleration* bears no temporal relation to uterine contractions. It is the most common deceleration pattern, occurring in approximately 50% of all records. Its onset may be early or late in relation to uterine contractions. In contrast to the two previously described patterns, this waveform is irregular. The record shows an abrupt fall in heart rate to below 100 beats/min and an equally abrupt rise to preexisting levels (baseline). *Variable deceleration* is thought to result from intermittent compression of the cord between fetal parts. Short periods of compression seem to be benign, but prolonged periods of obstructed blood flow

through the cord may cause severe hypoxia and acidosis. These episodes of deceleration can often be eliminated by change in maternal position to alter the relationships between the cord, the fetal parts involved in compression, and the uterine wall.

Complications of direct FHR monitoring. Several complications of direct, invasive fetal heart rate monitoring have been recorded, including maternal infection, neonatal infection, and maternal and neonatal soft tissue injury.

The status of maternal infection as a complication of invasive fetal heart rate monitoring is controversial. Although it is logical to expect that an invasive catheter that is passed into the uterine cavity through a contaminated field is quite likely to introduce infection in at least some instances, the variables that have influenced outcomes of numerous studies have precluded clear conclusions. Thus, maternal infection during direct monitoring is also influenced by such factors as the length of membrane rupture, cesarean section, predisposal to infection, and high risk for any reason. Numerous published studies have differed so widely in their conclusions that it is impossible to be certain that monitoring causes a significant increase in the incidence of maternal infection.

The risk of neonatal infection is very real, but very small. The most common site of infection is the scalp, as might be expected, from invasive attachment of an electrode. The most common implicated organisms are *E. coli* and group B beta hemolytic streptococcus. The incidence of scalp abscesses varies among a number of reports from 0.1% to 5.4%. These infections are not usually serious. However, a few quite serious infections have been reported, such as osteomyelitis of the skull and septicemia. Usually these have been caused by group B beta hemolytic streptococcus.

Maternal soft tissue injury is largely restricted to uterine perforation and the sequelae thereof. The incidence of this complication is not known; the possibility of occurrence is very real. Uterine perforation may be asymptomatic, but on the other hand intraperitoneal bleeding and abscess have been reported. An infected hematoma of the broad ligament has also been observed.

Fetal and neonatal hemorrhage from the scalp has been noted on several occasions. Significant bleeding from the scalp following the laceration of an artery during the insertion of the needle has been observed. Additionally, bleeding may occur from the scalp of a fetus or neonate in the presence of an inherited or acquired coagulation defect. Thus, bleeding is possible in a fetus or infant whose mother has or has had thrombocytopenic purpura. It is also possible in infants who are at risk for inherited coagulation defects (hemophilia). Invasive fetal heart rate monitoring should be avoided when family history indicates the possibility of a bleeding diathesis. The inadvertent attachment of a scalp electrode at inappropriate sites has also occurred occasionally. Electrodes have been applied to an eyelid and to a posterior fontanelle with drainage of cerebral spinal fluid from the site of attachment for 3 days.

The incidence of all these complications is extremely low. In some instances they are the result of ineptness of the operator. In other instances, such as fetal and maternal infections, they are probably unavoidable. The proponents of universal fetal heart rate monitoring believe that the incidence of these misadventures is so low and the benefits so great that they should not discourage the widespread use of this procedure.

The usefulness of assessment according to the above categories is indicated by the reported predictive value of the data. Normal heart rate patterns recorded 30 minutes or less before delivery are associated with normal 5-minute Apgar scores in approximately 99% of the babies studied. Abnormal patterns are not as specifically predictive. Virtually every baby who is depressed at birth has had an abnormal fetal heart rate but only 20% of the ominous deceleration patterns (late and severe variable decelerations) are associated with low Apgar scores. In many instances, an abnormal record is not indicative of poor fetal outcome. The significance of such records can be verified by pH analysis of fetal blood (see p. 23). Currently there seems to be little disagreement that all high-risk pregnancies should be monitored during labor and that all women who receive oxytocin should also be monitored. Since equipment for noninvasive (external) monitoring seems to be effective, universal monitoring of the apparently normal fetus is feasible. How much benefit will be derived therefrom has not yet been documented.

Indirect fetal heart rate monitoring

Indirect (external) fetal heart rate monitoring derives data from devices that are attached to the maternal abdominal wall. The procedure is noninvasive, which is its principal advantage. It is also advantageous because it can be used before labor, before membranes have ruptured, and during labor. However, the fetal heart rate signal that is transmitted through the maternal abdominal wall is considerably less accurate than the recordings obtained by the direct method. Uterine contractions can also be recorded through the abdominal wall by tocodynamometry, which involves application of a pressure-sensitive device that is strapped in place. Although uterine contractions may be recorded, the precise pressures generated during contractions cannot be measured.

Ultrasound is the most common modality used for the indirect recording of fetal heart rate. This technique utilizes the Doppler principle to continuously record the heart rate. Phonocardiography is also used for fetal heart rate recording. It involves the placement of a small microphone on the maternal abdomen. Phonocardiography has fewer applications than does ultrasound. Finally, the fetal electrocardiogram can be obtained by these same indirect methods. In every instance however, the maternal electrocardiographic signal interferes with the one that emanates from the fetus. Fetal ECG is not frequently used.

In spite of the disadvantages of indirect fetal heart rate monitoring, the technique is the only one available for assessment of fetal cardiovascular status prior to rupture of membranes. It is an addition to the direct method; in its present state, it cannot replace it for the derivation of accurate data.

Contraction stress test (CST); oxytocin challenge test (OCT)

The contraction stress test (CST) is widely used in the prelabor patient to determine the extent of reserve placental function during uterine contractions. By assessing fetal heart rate patterns in response to this stress test, a prediction can be made in regard to the safety with which the fetus will withstand labor.

Each uterine contraction during normal spontaneous or stimulated labor decreases blood flow in the intervillous space to some degree. If placental reserve is adequate, the normal fetus will not be stressed significantly, since in this instance diminished blood flow in the intervillous space does not impair fetal oxygen supply. The fetal heart rate patterns will thus be normal. If, however, placental circulation is marginal or impaired in the resting state, decreased blood flow in the intervillous space during uterine contractions will diminish fetal oxygen supply. The resultant stress is reflected in a fetal heart rate pattern of *late deceleration*.

Cardiologists have for years tested reserve function of the adult heart by subjecting the patient to exercise while recording the electrocardiogram. Potential catastrophe is demonstable during such stress even though a perfectly normal electrocardiogram is produced in the resting state. The oxytocin challenge test imposes the same conditions on the fetus before the onset of labor, in an attempt to predict whether there will be jeopardy after labor begins. During the procedure, fetal heart rate is recorded externally for 15 to 30 minutes in the maternal resting state. Oxytocin is then administered intravenously to the mother at a constant rate of 0.5 mU/min, after which it is gradually increased until three firm uterine contractions occur within 10 minutes. The test is positive (indicating impending fetal danger during labor) if at least two episodes of *late deceleration* are produced. The test is negative if the fetal heart rate is stable and there is no evidence of deceleration. Negative (normal) results occur in 85.9% of tests administered. Positive (abnormal) patterns are seen in 3% to 10%; equivocal results in

5% to 10% and unsatisfactory tracings in another 5% to 10% of tests. If labor begins within 6 or 7 days after the test, a negative result predicts fetal survival in more than 99% of all instances and absence of asphyxia during labor in the vast majority. Of the tests that are positive, 57% to 75% of the outcomes are abnormal (stillbirth, asphyxia at birth, and signs of chronic placental insufficiency). Thus, in the presence of a negative (normal) test result, there is reasonable assurance that the fetus is not in jeopardy. The interpretation of a positive (abnormal) result is not as clear. Although a large number of fetuses are accurately identified as being at risk, there is nevertheless a substantial incidence of false positive results. With cautious assessment, successful vaginal delivery of such fetuses is frequently possible. A positive contraction stress test is not necessarily an indication for cesarean section.

The contraction stress test cannot be administered in cases of placenta previa, vaginal bleeding of any type, previous cesarean section, or high risk for premature labor such as in multiple pregnancy, ruptured membranes, or incompetent cervix. Administration of the test is not simple. It requires $1\frac{1}{2}$ to 2 hours for completion. An intravenous drip for administration of oxytocin with an infusion pump is essential. The test should be performed only in a hospital.

Nonstress test (NST)

The association of accelerated heart rate with fetal movement is the basis of the NST. This procedure involves the recording of fetal heart rate by the same external methods that are used for the CST. Drugs are not administered, and usually the mother and fetus are not disturbed during the procedure. A "reactive pattern" (normal) is said to exist when several accelerations of 15 or more beats per minute occur at the time of fetal movement during a 20-minute period of observation. Absence of this pattern is called *nonreactive* (abnormal). This procedure is an extremely valuable screen that eliminates a large number of contraction stress tests. The interpretation of results is relatively simple; there are no known contraindications to its administration, and the test can be given in an outpatient setting. A reactive pattern during the NST is thought to rule out a need for the CST. The NST, in these circumstances, is repeated 1 week later. If a nonreactive pattern appears, a CST is necessary. In the vast majority of instances, the CST will be normal. Thus, the normal (reactive) nonstress test is as effective in the identification of normal intrauterine status as is the normal contraction stress test.

Fetal blood sampling

Fetal acid-base balance and blood gas content depend on the status of gas exchange across the placenta. When fetoplacental exchange is disrupted for any reason, blood oxygen tension (P_{O_2}) falls, carbon dioxide tension (P_{CO_2}) rises, and pH falls. Usually disruption of gas exchange is the result of inadequate placental blood flow (hypoperfusion). The disorders that are most frequently associated with diminished placental perfusion are toxemia, maternal hypotension due to supine hypotension syndrome, hemorrhage, anesthesia, umbilical cord compression, and hyperactive uterine contractions. The decline in pH is a consequence of fetal attempts to maintain energy needs by metabolizing glycogen to glucose in hypoxic circumstances (anaerobic glycolysis). This emergency metabolic pathway causes lactic acid accumulation, which results in metabolic acidosis. The decline in fetal blood pH is also due to accumulation of carbon dioxide because of impaired placental gas exchange, and the result is respiratory acidosis. These acid-base imbalances are discussed in Chapter 7. These changes can be demonstrated and usefully applied to fetal management during labor by sampling capillary blood from the presenting fetal part, usually the scalp. The pH, rather than blood gas content, has been found to correlate best with intrauterine status and with the infant's condition at birth because blood gas changes have a greater tendency to be transient. Several studies have established the comparability of fetal capillary blood pH with that of the umbilical vessels; the collection of capillary blood from the presenting fetal part (usually the scalp) is thus a valid sampling procedure. The technique is simple, and undesirable side effects are rare. Excessive bleeding from the scalp may occur in utero and postnatally, occasionally requiring sutures to the scalp incision after birth. Compression of the collection site usually controls bleeding. Scalp abscess has also been reported as a complication.

Normally, fetal capillary blood pH is approximately 7.35 during the first stage of labor and approximately 7.25 during the second stage. Values below 7.20 correlate with fetal and neonatal distress. Normal P_{O_2} is 18 to 22 mm Hg, P_{CO_2} is 40 to 50 mm Hg, and base deficit may vary from 0 to 10 mEq/L. Serial determinations are required during all stages of labor if the dynamic changes of fetal distress are to be appreciated; single values are misleading. If a pH between 7.20 and 7.25 is present, repeated sampling is necessary. If pH is below 7.20 in two or more specimens, interference with labor is usually required. Blood pH does not regularly and accurately predict condition at birth; that is, a low pH in utero may be followed by normal postnatal status, or a normal pH may be followed by the birth of a distressed infant. Maternal acidosis (transmitted to the fetus) is the most frequent misleading circumstance in which a low fetal pH is followed by delivery of a normal infant. Maternal acidosis may result from inadequate fluid therapy during labor or from prolonged labor and excessive muscular effort. Thus, if fetal pH is low, maternal acid-base status must be determined before interference with labor is seriously contemplated.

Obviously all labors cannot be monitored by fetal blood sampling. Preselection of patients for this procedure is based on a history that suggests high-risk pregnancy or on the sudden unanticipated appearance of fetal stress during labor, as indicated by abnormal fetal heart rate patterns. Ominous fetal heart rate patterns plus abnormalities of fetal scalp blood pH are often associated with poor fetal outcome (low Apgar scores), diminished neonatal survival, and increased incidence of subsequent neurologic deficit among survivors.

Fetal scalp sampling and continuous fetal heart monitoring together comprise the most effective available procedures for intrapartum surveillance. Fetal heart responses may be an indication for scalp blood analysis, which in turn provides critical information for interpretation of the significance of abnormal heart rate patterns.

Continuous monitoring of fetal blood pH is now possible with implantation of an electrode into the scalp. This method is not yet generally available, however.

Ultrasound

Ultrasonic diagnosis is a useful method for assessment of fetal maturity and growth. It is also helpful in the demonstration of fetal presentation (Fig. 1-9), multiple pregnancy (Fig. 1-10), certain fetal anomalies (Fig. 1-11), fetal death, and localization of the placenta. Whereas radiologic diagnosis is almost totally dependent on the radiopaque appearance of fetal bone (which becomes apparent late in pregnancy), ultrasound demonstrates soft tissue structures at a very early gestational age. It is thus an attractive diagnostic tool because the need for radiologic diagnosis (and its radiation hazards) is eliminated; it produces no maternal discomfort, and it is not harmful to the fetus.

The procedure involves rebound (echo) of very high frequency sound waves from the interfaces of various tissue layers. The reflected sound waves are converted to visible signals on a screen and are then photographed for a permanent record. The sound waves are transmitted at extremely short intervals (pulses) from an ultrasound scanner that is in direct contact with the maternal abdominal wall. Parts of these waves are reflected back to the apparatus as they cross boundaries of different tissues; the remainder continue to penetrate more deeply, and they in turn are reflected as they cross deeper tissue interfaces. Echoes of sound waves are displayed as hundreds of spots of light that coalesce to make up the image of the tissue that is being scanned. The resultant scans show, in transverse (Fig. 1-12) or longitudinal

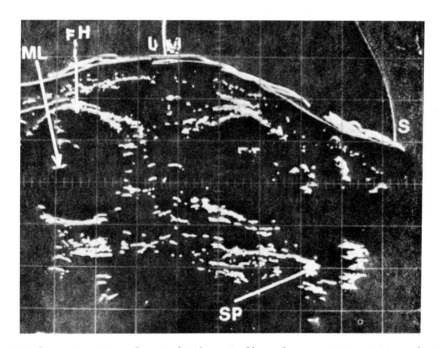

Fig. 1-9. Ultrasonic picture (longitudinal scan) of breech presentation at 30 weeks. *FH,* Fetal head; *ML,* midline of head; *SP,* sacral promontory; *S,* sacrum. (From Thompson, H. E.: Clin. Obstet. Gynecol. **17:**1, 1974.)

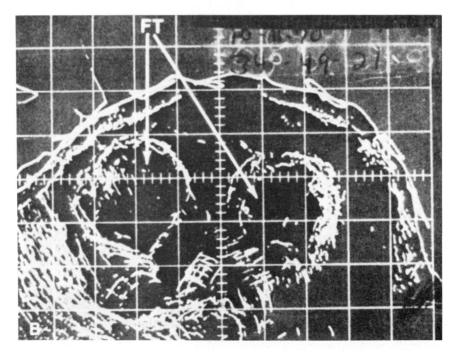

Fig. 1-10. Transverse scan of twin pregnancy taken at level of fetal thoraces *(FT)*. The heads are not shown, since they are 12 cm above the level of the thoraces on this transverse view. (From Thompson, H. E.: Clin. Obstet. Gynecol. 17:1, 1974.)

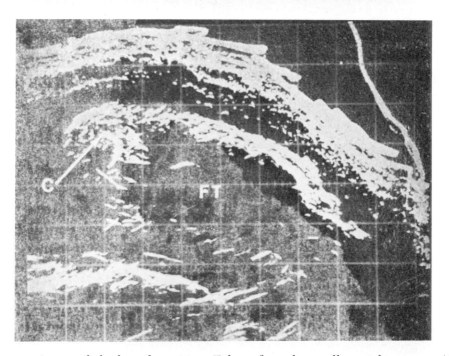

Fig. 1-11. Anencephaly, breech position. Echoes from the small cranial structure *(C)* are seen with the fetal trunk and thorax *(FT)* because this scan is longitudinal. (From Thompson, H. E.: Clin. Obstet. Gynecol. **17**:1, 1974.)

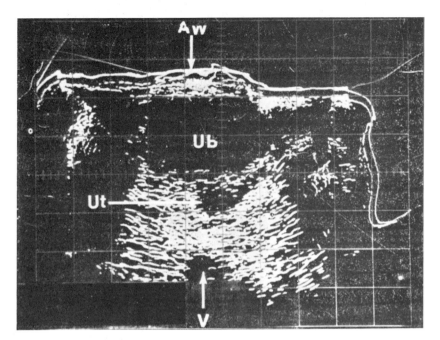

Fig. 1-12. Normal nonpregnant structures, transverse scan. *Aw*, Abdominal wall; *Ub*, urinary bladder; *Ut*, uterus; *V*, vertebral body. The urinary bladder and uterus are non–echo-producing structures. The vertebra is an inverted U. (From Thompson, H. E.: Clin. Obstet. Gynecol. **17**:1, 1974.)

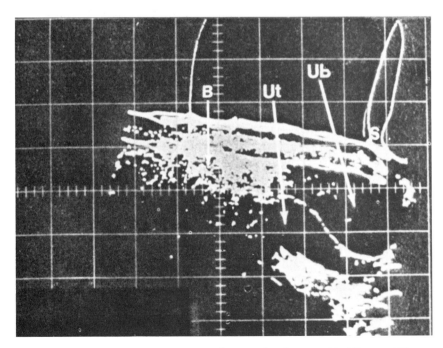

Fig. 1-13. Normal nonpregnant structures, longitudinal scan. *Ut*, Uterus; *Ub*, urinary bladder; *S*, symphysis pubis; *B*, bowel. Bladder and uterus are cystic and non–echo-producing; they are situated below the symphysis pubis. Bowel is nondescript pattern. (From Thompson, H. E.: Clin. Obstet. Gynecol. **17**:1, 1974.)

(Fig. 1-13) views, the anterior abdominal wall, symphysis pubis, urinary bladder, uterus and its contents, and sacrum and vertebrae. The bladder appears as a non–echo-producing image (black), as does the nongravid uterus beneath it. Pregnancy is identifiable as early as 5 weeks, when a group of dense circular echoes (white) form the "pregnancy ring," also called the gestational sac, which completely fills the uterus by the twelfth or thirteenth week. Embryonic structures within the sac are visible some time before. Gestational (menstrual) age may be estimated at about this time by measuring the sac and referring to an appropriate chart that relates sac size to age. Later, the fetal head becomes visible, and at 20 to 24 weeks the thorax can be identified.

Ultrasound technology has advanced considerably during the past few years. Images, formerly produced only in extremes of black and white, are now available in graduated scales between these extremes. These are known as *gray-scale*

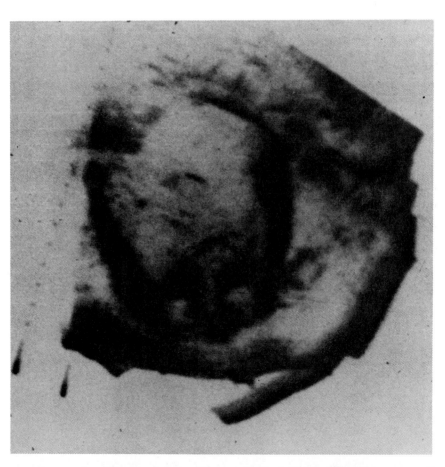

Fig. 1-14. Gray-scale echogram is virtually a portrait of the fetal face from upper lip to coronal suture. (From Carlson, E. N.: Clin. Obstet. Gynecol. 20(2):243, 1977.)

images. They convey rather realistic pictures of soft tissues. Fig. 1-14 is a grayscale echogram that strikingly depicts a fetal face from the upper lip to the coronal suture—a veritable fetal portrait.

Real-time imaging is now widely used for the examination, and preservation on film, of fetal motion in utero. It is thus possible to visualize fetal cardiac activity, or its absence in the event of fetal death. Direct visualization of needle insertion during amniocentesis or for intrauterine transfusions is also feasible. Fetal breathing and movements, activity of heart valves and chambers, fetal swallowing, and bladder filling are all now being studied by real-time techniques.

A normal pregnancy is discernible 4 weeks after the last menstrual period. At 6 to 7 weeks, fetal parts are recognizable and crown-rump measurement for estimation of fetal age is feasible (Fig. 1-15). If this is done before the fourteenth week, the date of a term delivery is predictable within 4 to 5 days in 95% of patients. Utilizing real-time imaging, fetal movement may be discerned as early as 7 weeks; cardiac activity is recognizable at 7 to 8 weeks. At 14 weeks, maturity is assessed by measuring the biparietal diameter of the fetal head (ultrasound cephalometry). A true cross section of the head must be visualized before the biparietal measurement can be made. This point of optimal visualization is identified by the presence of a straight midline echo that runs in an anteroposterior direction, representing the space between cerebral hemispheres (Fig. 1-16). After 28 weeks, interpretation of head measurements be-

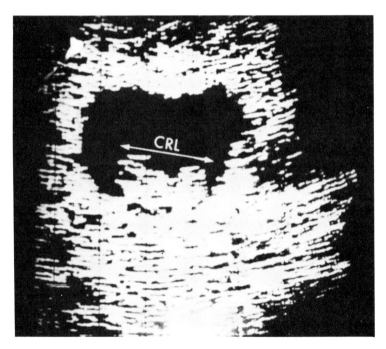

Fig. 1-15. Echogram (longitudinal section) of embryo at 9 weeks' menstrual age. *CRL* indicates correct crown-rump length for accurate measurement. (From Campbell, S.: Clin. Perinatol. 1:507, 1974.)

comes less reliable because of an increased variation in the rate of growth. The biparietal diameter is used alone or in combination with the thoracic diameter for estimation of fetal age by reference to one of several charts available for the purpose. In the absence of serial scans, a single measurement relating fetal head and chest is more accurate than measurement of the head alone for identification of growth abnormalities—retardation or acceleration. For example, the fetal growth failure that is associated with maternal toxemia typically involves preferential sparing of the brain with curtailed growth of the rest of the body. Thus the biparietal diameter may be normal, and the thoracic diameter may be small. One could estimate fetal age because the head is unaffected, but estimation of weight and identification of fetal growth retardation would be inaccurate unless a thoracic measurement was also made. Growth failure cannot be diagnosed un-

less both age and weight are known. If there has been normal growth, weight can be estimated by head measurement alone. In these circumstances it has been found that a biparietal diameter of 8.3 cm or more, taken a week before delivery, indicates a birth weight of at least 2000 grams; at 8.7 cm or more, birth weight is at least 2500 grams. However, if there has been fetal growth failure, these predictions miss the mark grossly because the disproportionately smaller body cannot be perceived without measurement of the thorax. In contrast, fetal growth acceleration requires consideration in pregnant diabetic women. The biparietal diameter does not become larger than normal in this situation until after the thirty-seventh week. Before this time, head measurements alone would miss the fetal overgrowth that is so characteristic of most pregnancies of diabetic women.

The use of ultrasound has considerably

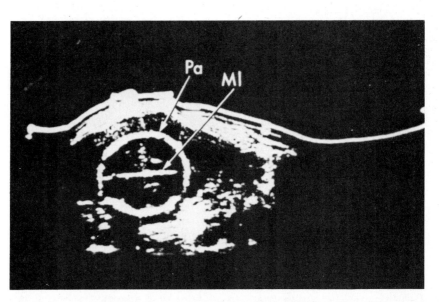

Fig. 1-16. Echogram at 24 weeks menstrual age. The midline echo indicates correct transverse section of fetal head for accurate measurement of biparietal diameter. *Pa,* Parietal bone; *MI,* midline echo. (From Campbell, S.: Clin. Perinatol. 1:507, 1974.)

enhanced the effectiveness of fetal diagnosis. Interpretation of results is often subject to the same pitfalls that are encountered when measurements are obtained postnatally. Early ultrasound examination does, however, provide the best available estimate of fetal age.

Considerations of fetal growth and its implications in management of the neonate are presented in Chapter 5.

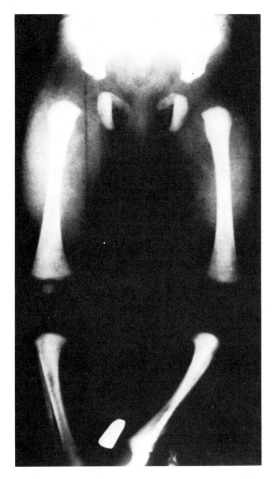

Fig. 1-17. Postnatal x-ray film of lower extremities. Small, round ossification centers at distal femurs are visible bilaterally. This neonate was at least 36 weeks at birth. Proximal tibial centers are not present.

Radiologic diagnosis

Fetal maturity may be ascertained when an ossification center is present at the distal end of the femur or proximal tibia (Fig. 1-17). However, if these small opacities are absent, the fetus is not necessarily immature because growth retardation in a mature fetus may result in absence of these ossification centers. Calcification of fetal teeth has also been used to estimate fetal maturity. Multiple births, hydrocephalus, anencephalus, conjoined twinning, and fetal death are identifiable on plain films. Severe erythroblastosis with hydrops fetalis is demonstrable by extensive edema, which elevates fat layers beneath the skin to produce a "halo sign." The so-called "Buddha position" is also indicative of hydrops fetalis. Because most of these procedures are often not reliable and because of concern for the risk of radiation, ultrasound will largely replace x-ray films as a procedure for fetal diagnosis.

Microscopy of the amniotic membrane and the umbilical cord

Several diagnostic tests are used to determine at birth the presence of bacterial infections that were acquired in utero. The pathogenesis of these infections and the rationale for these diagnostic procedures are discussed in Chapter 12. Within the context of the present discussion on fetal diagnosis, it is appropriate to mention examination of the amnion and umbilical cord. The cellular response of these structures to invasion by bacterial agents is characterized by infiltrations of polymorphonuclear leukocytes. If these cells are noted, the fetus may have an infectious disease, but more often there has merely been exposure to infected amniotic fluid (amnionitis), although the fetus is unaffected. Thus a positive result is most often associated with a normal infant who was exposed to infection before delivery. Infection occurs most frequently after early rupture of membranes. High-risk infants with such findings are often given antibiotics, whether or not they are symptomatic. Although inflammatory cells do not necessarily indicate an affected infant, it is almost always true that among diseased babies amnionitis and inflammation of the umbilical cord are the rule.

HIGH-RISK PREGNANCY

Neonatal intensive care programs have diminished mortality and the incidence of brain damage among survivors, but much if not most of their activity could be eliminated by optimal delivery of prenatal care. Usually the sick neonate was a distressed fetus whose mother's vulverability to perinatal misadventure could have been identified in 60% to 75% of cases. The ideal medical facility for the management of reproductive events is not a neonatal center nor an obstetric center, but it is rather a *perinatal center* capable of providing continuous care for the well-known biologic continuum that is comprised of conception, gestation, labor, birth, and neonatal life.

Identification and special care of patients at high risk early in pregnancy have constituted a fruitful approach to the diminution of perinatal misadventure. The high-risk pregnancy is characterized by one or more maternal conditions that impose considerable hazard to intact survival of the fetus or newborn infant. A list of the most common antepartum factors that identify such pregnancies is presented below. A similar but more extensive tabulation of maternal disorders and their associated fetal or neonatal effects is presented in Chapter 2.

Preselection is most effectively accomplished early by considering the historic factors with which a woman enters gestation. The following is a listing of most of these factors.

Antepartum maternal factors that indicate high risk for adverse fetal outcome
Previous pregnancy misadventure
    Grand multiparity (more than 5 pregnancies)
    Cesarean section
    Midforceps delivery
    Prolonged labor
    Fetal loss before 28 weeks (two such)
    Fetal loss after 28 weeks
    Premature infant
    Postterm infant (42 weeks or over)
    Abnormal fetal position
    Polyhydramnios
    Multiple pregnancy
    Neonatal death
    Infant over 10 pounds at birth
    Fetal or neonatal exchange transfusion
    Congenital anomalies
    Bleeding in second or third trimester
    Toxemia, eclampsia
Abnormalities of reproductive anatomy
    Uterine malformation
    Incompetent cervix
    Small bony pelvis
Metabolic and endocrine disorders
    Family history of diabetes
    Gestational diabetes
    Diabetes
    Thyroid disorder
    Hyperparathyroidism
Cardiovascular disorders
    Toxemia
    Chronic hypertension
    Rheumatic heart disease
    Congenital heart disease
    Congestive heart failure
Renal disorders
    Chronic glomerulonephritis
    Acute pyelonephritis
    Acute cystitis
    Renal insufficiency

Hematologic disorders
  Sickle cell disease
  Rh sensitization
  Anemia (hemoglobin less than 10 grams)
  Idiopathic thrombocytopenic purpura
Other factors
  Age: Under 16 or over 35 years
        Over 30 years (primipara)
  Weight: Less than 100 or more than 200
    pounds
  Syphilis
  Tuberculosis
  Hereditary CNS disorder
  Epilepsy
  Drug addiction
  Smoking (more than one pack daily)
  Alcoholism
  Maternal malnutrition

Neonatal mortality is lowest if the mother is between 20 and 30 years of age. The risk of poor outcome is considerably increased below 16 and over 40 years of age. Neonatal mortality and morbidity are significantly greater among diabetic gravidas. Prematurity, stillbirth, and low birth weight for gestational age (Chapter 4) are considerably more common among mothers with toxemia and hypertensive cardiovascular disease. Neonatal thyroid difficulty is more often associated with maternal thyroid disorder as a consequence of treatment than as a result of the maternal dysfunction itself. Previous Rh sensitization increases the possibility that an erythroblastotic infant will result from the current pregnancy. Hydramnios may be associated with congenital malformations of the gastrointestinal tract or the brain. It is also common in diabetic pregnant women. Bleeding during the second and third trimesters usually follows disruption of placental attachment, which then poses a serious threat to fetomaternal gas exchange. Multiple pregnancy (twins, triplets) may be fraught with difficulty because at least one of the twins is often delivered from the breech position or is retarded in the rate of intrauterine growth. Excessive cigarette smoking (consumption of more than twenty cigarettes daily) is associated with an increased incidence of low birth weight. Rubella is responsible for severe congenital anomalies and for other tissue changes that are usually incompatible with survival or with a normal postnatal course (p. 331). Maternal hyperparathyroidism may cause severe hypocalcemia in the neonate. Idiopathic thrombocytopenic purpura often results in severe thrombocytopenia in the fetus and newborn.

Although these are only some of the conditions that impose a high risk on pregnancy, they involve the majority of high-risk gravidas. In separating these special pregnancies from the uncomplicated ones, it becomes possible to refer a relatively small number of patients (among whom the bulk of perinatal deaths occur) to medical centers that are equipped and staffed to manage them. There remain the unanticipated events for which preparation is difficult, such as the sudden appearance of complications during labor or delivery in a previously uneventful pregnancy or the first occurrence of premature labor, fetal loss, and neonatal death. Nevertheless, with optimal prenatal management, perinatal mortality can be reduced considerably. This has been demonstrated repeatedly in organized programs of prenatal and postnatal care.

REFERENCES

Abramovici, H., Brandes, J. M., Fuchs, K., and Timor-Tritsch, I.: Meconium during delivery: a sign of compensated fetal distress, Am. J. Obstet. Gynecol. **118**:251, 1974.

Amarose, A. P., Wallingford, A. J., and Plotz, E. J.: Prediction of fetal sex from cytologic examination of amniotic fluid, N. Engl. J. Med. **275**:715, 1966.

Aubry, R. H., and Pennington, J. C.: Identification and evaluation of high-risk pregnancy: the perinatal concept, Clin. Obstet. Gynecol. **16**:3, 1973.

Barden, T. P.: Intrapartum fetal monitoring. In Behrman, R. E., editor: Neonatal-perinatal medicine: diseases of the fetus and infant, ed. 2, St. Louis, 1977, The C. V. Mosby Co.

Beard, R. W.: The detection of fetal asphyxia in labor, Pediatrics **53**:157, 1974.

Behrman, R. E., Parer, J. T., and de Lannoy, C. W.: Placental growth and the formation of amniotic fluid, Nature **214**:678, 1967.

Benirschke, K.: What pediatricians should know about the placenta. In Gluck, L., editor: Current problems in pediatrics, Chicago, 1971, Year Book Medical Publishers, Inc.

Brown, J. B.: The value of plasma estrogen estimations in the management of pregnancy, Clin. Perinatol. **1**:273, 1974.

Campbell, S.: The assessment of fetal development by diagnostic ultrasound, Clin. Perinatol. **1**:507, 1974.

Campbell, S.: Fetal growth, Clin. Obstet. Gynecol. **1**:41, 1974.

Carlsen, E. N.: Capabilities of gray-scale imaging in obstetrics and gynecology, Clin. Obstet. Gynecol. **20**:243, 1977.

Clements, J. A., Platzker, A. C. G., Tierney, D. F., et al.: Assessment of the risk of the respiratory distress syndrome by a rapid test for surfactant in amniotic fluid, N. Engl. J. Med. **286**:1077, 1972

Committee on Maternal and Fetal Medicine and Committee on Technical Bulletins of the American College of Obstetricians and Gynecologists: Fetal heart rate monitoring: guidelines for monitoring, terminology, and instrumentation, ACOG Technical Bulletin No. 32, June 1975.

Cook, L. N., Shott, R. J., and Andrews, B. F.: Fetal complications of diagnostic amniocentesis: a review and report of a case with pneumothorax, Pediatrics **53**:421, 1974.

Dancis, J., and Schneider, H.: Physiology: transfer and barrier function. In Gruenwald, P., editor: The placenta, Baltimore, 1975, University Park Press.

Desmond, M. M., Lindley, J. E., Moore, J., and

Brown, C. A.: Meconium staining of newborn infants, J. Pediatr. **49**:540, 1956.

DeVoe, S. J., and Schwarz, R. H.: Determination of maturity and well-being using maternal and amniotic fluids. In Gruenwald, P., editor: The placenta, Baltimore, 1975, University Park Press.

Fox, H. E., and Hohler, C. W.: Fetal evaluation by real-time imaging, Clin. Obstet. Gynecol. **20**:339, 1977.

Freeman, R. K.: Estimation of placental function. In Behrman, R. E., editor: Neonatal-perinatal medicine: diseases of the fetus and infant, ed. 2, St. Louis, 1977, The C. V. Mosby Co.

Fuchs, F.: Volume of amniotic fluid at various stages of pregnancy, Clin. Obstet. Gynecol. **9**:449, 1966.

Gabbe, S. G., and Hagerman, D. D.: Clinical application of estriol analysis, Clin. Obstet. Gynecol. **21**:353, 1978.

Gardner, L. I.: Genetically expressed abnormalities in the fetus, Clin. Obstet. Gynecol. **17**:171, 1974.

Gibbons, J. M., Jr., Huntley, T. E., and Corral, A. G.: Effect of maternal blood contamination on amniotic fluid analysis, Obstet. Gynecol. **44**:657, 1974.

Gluck, L.: Evaluating functional fetal maturation, Clin. Obstet. Gynecol. **21**:547, 1978.

Gluck, L., Kulovich, M. V., Borer, R. C., Jr., et al.: Diagnosis of the respiratory distress syndrome by amniocentesis, Am. J. Obstet. Gynecol. **109**:440, 1971.

Gluck, L., Kulovich, M. V., Eidelman, A. I., et al.: Biochemical development of surface activity in mammalian lung. IV. Pulmonary lecithin synthesis in the human fetus and newborn and etiology of the respiratory distress syndrome, Pediatr. Res. **6**:81, 1972.

Goldstein, A. S., Fukunaga, K., Malachowski, N., and Johnson, J. D.: A comparison of lecithin/sphingomyelin ratio and shake test for estimating fetal pulmonary maturity, Am. J. Obstet. Gynecol. **118**:1132, 1974.

Goodlin, R. C.: Amniotic fluid. In Care of the fetus, New York, 1979, Masson Publishing Co.

Goodlin, R. C., and Clewell, W. H.: Sudden fetal death following diagnostic amniocentesis, Am. J. Obstet. Gynecol. **118**:285, 1974.

Gottesfeld, K. R..: Ultrasound in obstetrics, Clin. Obstet. Gynecol. **21**:311, 1978.

Greene, J. W., Jr., and Beargie, R. A.: The use of urinary estriol excretion studies in the assessment of the high-risk pregnancy, Pediatr. Clin. North Am. **17**:43, 1970.

Hobel, C. J., Hyvarinen, M. A., Okada, D. M., and

Oh, W.: Prenatal and intrapartum high-risk screening, Am. J. Obstet. Gynecol. **117**:1, 1973.

Hon, E. H.: An introduction to fetal heart rate monitoring, New Haven, Conn., 1969, Hearty Press, Inc.

James, L. S., Morishima, H. O., Daniel, S. S., et al.: Mechanism of late deceleration of the fetal heart rate, Am. J. Obstet. Gynecol. **113**:578, 1972.

Jepson, J. H.: Factors influencing oxygenation in mother and fetus, Obstet. Gynecol. **44**:906, 1974.

Ledger, W. J.: Complications associated with invasive monitoring, Seminars Perinat. **2**:187, 1978.

Lemons, J. A., Kuhns, L. R., and Poznanski, A.: Calcification of fetal teeth as an index of fetal maturation, Am. J. Obstet. Gynecol. **114**:628, 1972.

Levi, S.: Uses of ultrasonography in fetal and perinatal medicine, Reviews Perinat. Med. **3**:155, 1979.

Liley, A. W.: Intrauterine transfusion of foetus in haemolytic disease, Br. Med. J. **2**:1107, 1963.

Lind, J., Stern, L., and Wegelius, C.: Human foetal and neonatal circulation, Springfield, Ill., 1964, Charles C Thomas, Publisher.

Mendez-Bauer, C., Poseiro, J. J., Arellano-Hernandez, G., et al.: Effects of atropine on the heart rate of the human fetus during labor, Am. J. Obstet. Gynecol. **85**:1033, 1963.

Miller, F. C., and Paul, R. H.: Intrapartum fetal heart rate monitoring, Clin. Obstet. Gynecol. **21**:561, 1978.

Naeye, R. L.: Structural correlates of fetal undernutrition. In Waisman, H. A., and Kerr, G., editors: Fetal growth and development, New York, 1970, McGraw-Hill Book Co.

Nelson, N. M.: Respiration and circulation before birth. In Smith, C. A., and Nelson, N. M., editors: The physiology of the newborn infant, Springfield, Ill., 1976, Charles C Thomas, Publisher.

Nesbitt, R. E. L., Jr.: Prenatal identification of the fetus at risk, Clin. Perinatol. **1**:213, 1974.

Parer, J. T.: Introduction—benefits and detriments of fetal heart rate monitoring, Seminars Perinat. **2**:113, 1978.

Paul, R. H., and Hon, E. H.: Clinical fetal monitoring, Am. J. Obstet. Gynecol. **118**:529, 1974.

Paul, R. H., and Miller, F. C.: Antepartum fetal heart rate monitoring, Clin. Obstet. Gynecol. **21**:375, 1978.

Pitkin, R. M.: Estimation of fetal maturity. In Behrman, R. E. editor: Neonatal-perinatal medicine: diseases of the fetus and infant, ed. 2, St. Louis, 1977, The C. V. Mosby Co.

Potter, E. L.: Bilateral absence of ureters and kidneys, Obstet. Gynecol. **25**:3, 1965.

Quilligan, E. J., and Paul, R. H.: Fetal monitoring: is it worth it? Obstet. Gynecol. **45**:96, 1975.

Roopnarinesingh, S.: Amniotic fluid creatinine in normal and abnormal pregnancies, Obstet. Gynaecol. Br. **77**:785, 1970.

Saling, E.: Blood chemistry as a method of detection of fetal distress. In Wood, C., and Walter, W. A. A., editors: Fifth World Congress of Gynecology and Obstetrics, Sydney, 1967, Butterworth & Co. (Australia), Ltd.

Seeds, A. E.: Fetal scalp acid-base monitoring. In Behrman, R. E., editor: Neonatal-perinatal medicine: diseases of the fetus and infant, ed. 2, St. Louis, 1977, The C. V. Mosby Co.

Seeds, A. E.: Maternal-fetal acid-base relationships and fetal scalp-blood analysis, Clin. Obstet. Gynecol. **21**:579, 1978.

Shenker, L.: Clinical experiences with fetal heart rate monitoring of one thousand patients in labor, Am. J. Obstet. Gynecol. **115**:1111, 1973.

Stocker, J. Mawad, R., Deleon, A., and Desjardins, P.: Ultrasonic cephalometry, Obstet. Gynecol. **45**:275, 1975.

Thompson, H. E.: Evaluation of the obstetric and gynecologic patient by the use of diagnostic ultrasound, Clin. Obstet. Gynecol. **17**:1, 1974.

Winick, M.: Malnutrition and brain development, New York, 1976, Oxford University Press.

Wood, C.: Fetal scalp sampling: its place in management, Seminars Perinat. **2**:169, 1978.

CHAPTER 2

Fetal and neonatal consequences of abnormal labor and delivery

The condition of an infant at birth is determined by numerous antecedent factors such as genetic endowment, maternal health before and during gestation, maternal complications of pregnancy, development of the embryo, growth of the fetus, and the course of labor and delivery. This chapter addresses itself to the fetal effects of labor and delivery, normal and abnormal. Although some of the abnormal conditions have their inception well before the onset of labor (placenta previa, for instance), they are discussed here because their presence usually becomes manifest during the birth process. No attempt is made to discuss maternal medical disorders such as diabetes, toxemia, or infectious diseases. These are considered elsewhere in relation to their associated neonatal abnormalities. However, Table 2-1 lists a majority of maternal disorders and the fetal or neonatal effects they are known or presumed to produce.

MECHANICS OF NORMAL LABOR

A review of normal labor is essential for an understanding of the abnormalities that play a role in fetal or neonatal difficulties. The classic division of labor into three stages is as follows:

First stage: Cervical dilatation is initiated with the first contraction and ends when the cervix is completely dilated.
Second stage: Fetal expulsion begins when the cervix is completely dilated and ends with birth of the infant.
Third stage: Placental expulsion starts after birth of the baby and terminates with delivery of the placenta.

Text continued on p. 44.

Table 2-1. Maternal abnormalities and associated fetal and neonatal disorders

Maternal factors	Fetal, neonatal disorders
Antepartum	
Metabolic	
Diabetes mellitus	Prematurity*
	Hyaline membrane disease
	Hyperbilirubinemia
	Hypoglycemia
	Macrosomatia
	Hypocalcemia
	Renal vein thrombosis
	Polyhydramnios
	Congenital anomalies
	Intrauterine growth retardation
Gout	Hyperuricemia (transient, asymptomatic)
Malnutrition	Intrauterine growth retardation
Porphyria	Porphyrinuria (transient, asymptomatic)
Endocrine	
Addison's disease	Prematurity
	Intrauterine growth retardation
Chronic hypoparathyroidism	Hyperparathyroidism (intrauterine and postnatal)
Primary hyperparathyroidism	Neonatal tetany (hypocalcemia)
	Hypomagnesemia
Thyroid	
Goiter (nontoxic)	Goiter
Hyperthyroidism (untreated)	Hyperthyroidism (goitrous or nongoitrous)
Hyperthyroidism (treated)	Goiter (nontoxic)
	Hyperthyroidism (goitrous or nongoitrous)
	Hypothyroidism (goitrous or nongoitrous)
Hypothyroidism	CNS defects
	Hypothyroidism
Cardiac	
Congestive failure	Prematurity
	Asphyxia†
Hypertensive cardiovascular disease	Asphyxia
	Intrauterine growth retardation
Pulmonary	
Asthma (intractable) or any disorder associated with hypoxemia and hypercapnia	Asphyxia
	Prematurity
	Intrauterine growth retardation
Gastrointestinal	
Regional ileitis	Prematurity

Continued.

*Prematurity = gestational age less than 37 completed weeks.
†Asphyxia = hypoxemia, hypercapnia, low pH.

Table 2-1. Maternal abnormalities and associated fetal and neonatal disorders—cont'd

Maternal factors	Fetal, neonatal disorders
Antepartum	
Renal	
Polycystic kidney disease	Polycystic kidney disease
Chronic glomerulonephritis	Prematurity
	Intrauterine growth retardation
	Asphyxia
Neurologic	
Myasthenia gravis	Myasthenia gravis
Status epilepticus	Asphyxia
Hematologic	
Blood incompatibility (Rh, ABO, other)	Erythroblastosis fetalis
Idiopathic thrombocytopenic purpura	Idiopathic thrombocytopenia purpura (transient)
Leukemia (acute)	Prematurity
Megaloblastic anemia	Hazards of abruptio placentae
Sickle cell anemia	Low birth weight
	Intrauterine growth retardation
	Abruptio placentae
	Fetal loss
Anemia (iron deficiency)	Low birth weight, prematurity
Skin	
Pemphigus	Bullae (transient)
Neoplastic	
Hodgkin's disease	Hodgkin's disease
Ovarian tumors (complicated)	Prematurity
Collagen disease	
Lupus erythematosus (acute)	Systemic lupus erythematosus
Lupus erythematosus (subacute)	Syndrome of congenital heart block, fibroelastosis, fibrosis of liver, spleen, kidney, adrenals
Infection (antepartum or intrapartum)	
Viral	
Coxsackie	Coxsackie infection (encephalomyocarditis)
Cytomegalic inclusion disease	Cytomegalic inclusion disease
Hepatitis (SH)	Neonatal hepatitis
Herpesvirus infection	Herpesvirus infection
Measles	Measles
Mumps	?Congenital anomalies
Poliomyelitis	Poliomyelitis
Rubella	Congenital rubella syndrome
Smallpox	Smallpox
TRIC agent (cervicitis)	Inclusion blennorrhea
Vaccinia (primary vaccination)	Generalized vaccinia

Prematurity = gestational age less than 37 completed weeks.
Asphyxia = hypoxemia, hypercapnia, low pH.

Table 2-1. Maternal abnormalities and associated fetal and neonatal disorders—cont'd

Maternal factors	Fetal, neonatal disorders
Antepartum	

Infection—cont'd
    Varicella — Varicella
    Western equine encephalomyelitis — Western equine encephalomyelitis
  Protozoan
    Candidiasis (vaginal) — Thrush
    Malaria — Malaria
    Toxoplasmosis — Toxoplasmosis
    Trypanosomiasis — Trypanosomiasis
  Bacterial
    Acute pyelonephritis — Prematurity; Bacterial infections
    Enteropathogenic *E. coli* (carrier) — Diarrhea (enteropathogenic *E. coli*)
    Gonorrhea — Gonorrheal infection (usually ophthalmia)
    Listeriosis — Listeriosis
    Pneumococcal meningitis — Pneumococcal meningitis
    Salmonellosis — Salmonellosis
    Septicemia (any organism) — Septicemia (any organism)
    Shigellosis — Shigellosis
    Syphilis — Congenital syphilis
    Tuberculosis — Tuberculosis
    Typhoid fever — Typhoid fever

Obstetric and gynecologic
  Amputated cervix — Prematurity
  Incompetent cervix — Prematurity
  Toxemia — Prematurity; Intrauterine growth retardation; Hypoglycemia; Hypocalcemia; Aspiration syndrome; Polycythemia; Asphyxia

Pharmacologic
  Alcohol (I. V. or oral) — Hypoglycemia
  Alcohol (chronic alcoholism) — Fetal alcohol syndrome
    Low birth weight
    Developmental delay
    Microcephaly
    Small palpebral fissures
    Maxillary hypoplasia
    Cardiac anomaly (ventricular septal defect, patent ductus arteriosus)
    Abnormal palm creases

Continued.

Table 2-1. Maternal abnormalities and associated fetal and neonatal disorders—cont'd

Maternal factors	Fetal, neonatal disorders
Antepartum	

Pharmacologic—cont'd

Maternal factors	Fetal, neonatal disorders
Aminopterin and amethopterin	Multiple anomalies
	Abortion
	Intrauterine growth retardation
Ammonium chloride	Acidosis
Amphetamines	Transposition of great vessels
Androgen (methyl testosterone)	Masculinization of females
	Advanced bone age
Barbiturates	Withdrawal syndrome
	Diminished sucking
	Diminished serum bilirubin
Cephalothin	Direct Coombs' positive test
Chlorambucil	?Renal agenesis
Chlorothiazides	Thrombocytopenia
	Salt and water depletion
Chloroquine	?Retinal damage
	Death
	Mental retardation
Chlorpromazine	Depression
	Lethargy
	Extrapyramidal dysfunction
Chlorpropamide	Hypoglycemia
	Increased fetal wastage
Cigarette smoking	Intrauterine growth retardation
	Increased neonatal hematocrit
Diazepam (Valium)	Hypothermia
Dicumarol	Fetal hemorrhage and death
Diphenylhydantoin (Dilantin)	Hypoplastic phalanges
	Diaphragmatic hernia
	Cleft lip
	Coloboma
	Pulmonary atresia
	Patent ductus arteriosus
Estrogen	Masculinization of females
	Carcinoma of vagina and cervix (years later)
	Advanced bone age
Ethchlorvynol (Placidyl)	Irritability, jitteriness (withdrawal symptoms)
Hexamethonium bromide	Paralytic ileus
Insulin shock	Death

Table 2-1. Maternal abnormalities and associated fetal and neonatal disorders—cont'd

Maternal factors	Fetal, neonatal disorders
Antepartum	
Pharmacologic—cont'd	
Intravenous fluid (copious, hypotonic)	Hyponatremia
	Convulsions
	Edema
Isoxsuprine (and some other betamimetic tocolytics)	Hypoglycemia
	Hypocalcemia
	Ileus
	Hypotension
	Death
Lithium	Lithium toxicity (cyanosis, hypotonia)
	Cardiac anomalies (especially Ebstein's)
Lysergic acid diethylamide	Chromosome damage
Magnesium sulfate	Hypermagnesemia
	CNS depression
	Peripheral neuromuscular blockage
Meperidine (Demerol)	Placental vasoconstriction
	CNS and respiratory depression
Mepivacaine, lidocaine, other "amides"	Bradycardia
	Convulsions
	Apnea
	Death
	Depression
	Tachycardia
	Flaccidity
	Metabolic acidosis
	Hypoxemia
Methimazole	Goiter
Morphine, heroin, methadone	Withdrawal symptoms (tremors, dyspnea, cyanosis, convulsions, death)
	Intrauterine growth retardation
	Lower serum bilrubin
Naphthalene (mothballs)	Hemolytic anemia (in G-6-PD deficiency)
Nitrofurantoin	Hemolytic anemia (in G-6-PD deficiency)
Nortriptyline	Urinary retention (bladder)
Pentazocine (Talwin)	Neonatal depression
Potassium iodide	Goiter
Prilocaine	Methemoglobinemia; others as in mepivacaine
Primaquine	Hemolytic anemia (in G-6-PD deficiency)
Progestins	Masculinization of female infants
	Advanced bone age

Continued.

Table 2-1. Maternal abnormalities and associated fetal and neonatal disorders—cont'd

Maternal factors	Fetal, neonatal disorders
Antepartum	
Pharmacologic—cont'd	
Propranolol	Low Apgar scores
	Bradycardia,
	Hypoglycemia
Propoxyphene (Darvon)	Hyperactivity
	Sweating
	Convulsions
	Withdrawal symptoms
Propylthiouracil	Goiter
Quinine	Thrombocytopenia
	Abortion
Radioactive iodine	Hypothyroidism
	Thyroid destruction
Reserpine	Obstructed respiration due to nasal congestion
	Lethargy
	Bradycardia
	Hypothermia
Salicylates	Neonatal hemorrhage due to platelet dysfunction
Sedatives (excessive during labor)	CNS depression and respiratory distress
Steroids (adrenocortical)	Increased incidence of fetal death
	Adrenal suppression
	Accelerated fetal lung maturation
	?Cleft palate
Streptomycin	Deafness, eighth nerve damage
Stilbestrol	Adenocarcinoma of vagina in adolescents
Sulfonamides (long-acting)	Kernicterus at low bilirubin levels
Tetracyclines (after first trimester)	Tooth stain, enamel hypoplasia (primary teeth)
	Temporary inhibited linear growth (premature infants)
Thalidomide	Phocomelia and other anomalies
	Death
Tolbutamide (Orinase)	Thrombocytopenia, bilirubin displacement from albumin, hypoglycemia
Vitamin D (excessive)	?Hypercalcemia (supravalvular aortic stenosis, mental retardation, osteosclerosis)
Vitamin K (excessive)	Hyperbilirubinemia
Warfarin	Mental retardation
	Optic atrophy
	Hemorrhage
	Fetal death

Prematurity = gestational age less than 37 completed weeks.
Asphyxia = hypoxemia, hypercapnia, low pH.

Table 2-1. Maternal abnormalities and associated fetal and neonatal disorders—cont'd

Maternal factors	Fetal, neonatal disorders
	Intrapartum

Cord pathology

Maternal factors	Fetal, neonatal disorders
Inflammation	Bacterial infection
	Umbilical vein thrombosis (asphyxia)
Meconium staining	Asphyxia
Prolapsed cord	Asphyxia
Single umbilical artery	Congenital anomalies
	Intrauterine growth retardation
True knot	Asphyxia
Velamentous insertion, vasa previa	Intrauterine blood loss
Rupture of normal cord (precipitous delivery), varices, aneurysm	Intrauterine blood loss

Fetal membrane, amniotic fluid

Maternal factors	Fetal, neonatal disorders
Amnion nodosum	Renal agenesis
	Severe obstructive uropathy (bilateral)
	Intrauterine parabiotic syndrome (small twin)
Amnionitis	Infection, usually bacterial
Early membrane rupture	Bacterial infection
	Prematurity
	Prolapsed cord
Meconium stain (fluid or membranes)	Asphyxia
	Aspiration syndrome
	Pneumonia
Oligohydramnios	Postmaturity
	Renal agenesis and dysplasia
	Polycystic kidney
	Urethral obstruction
	Intrauterine parabiotic syndrome (small twin)
	Fetal death
Polyhydramnios	High gastrointestinal obstruction
	Spina bifida
	Hydrocephalus
	Anencephaly
	Achondroplasia
	Hydrops fetalis
	Intrauterine parabiotic syndrome (large twin)

Placenta

Maternal factors	Fetal, neonatal disorders
Placenta previa	Prematurity
	Asphyxia
	Prolapsed cord
	Intrauterine blood loss

Continued.

Table 2-1. Maternal abnormalities and associated fetal and neonatal disorders—cont'd

Maternal factors	Fetal, neonatal disorders
Intrapartum	
Placenta—cont'd	
Abruptio placentae	Prematurity
	Asphyxia
	Intrauterine blood loss
Fetomaternal transfusion	Intrauterine blood loss (chronic or acute)
	Asphyxia
Incision during cesarean section	Intrauterine blood loss (acute)
Placental insufficiency	Asphyxia
	Intrauterine malnutrition
Multilobed placenta (rupture of communicating vessels)	Intrauterine blood loss (acute)
Complications of labor	
Breech delivery	Asphyxia
	Intracranial hemorrhage
	Visceral hemorrhage (adrenal, kidney, spleen)
	Spinal cord trauma
	Brachial plexus injury
	Bone fracture (clavicle, humerus, femur)
	Epiphyseal injury (proximal femur or humerus)
	Characteristic posture
	Edema, ecchymosis of buttocks, genitalia, and lower extremities
Face and brow presentation	Edema, ecchymosis of face
	Asphyxia
	Characteristic posture (head retraction)
Transverse presentation	Asphyxia, trauma

Prematurity = gestational age less than 37 completed weeks.
Asphyxia = hypoxemia, hypercapnia, low pH.

Before considering each stage of labor, a discussion of uterine contractions is appropriate.

Characteristics of uterine contractions

Contractions provide the force necessary for descent of the fetus; they accentuate differentiation of the uterine wall into upper and lower segments, and they bring about dilatation and effacement of the cervix (see later). During the first stage, intrauterine pressure ranges from 20 to 50 mm Hg. At these pressures the cervix seems to dilate easily. During the second stage, with the addition of conscious maternal expulsive efforts (bearing down), pressures may rise to 70 mm Hg. At the onset of the first stage of labor, contractions appear every 10 minutes, increasing in frequency to every 1 or 2 minutes during the second stage. They normally last for 30 to 90 seconds. Alternation of contraction and relaxation is indispensable to fetal well-being because the flow of blood through the intervillous space is greatly impeded during a contraction, returning to normal during relaxation. The significance to the fetus

Table 2-1. Maternal abnormalities and associated fetal and neonatal disorders—cont'd

Maternal factors	Fetal, neonatal disorders
Intrapartum	
Complications of labor—cont'd	
Precipitate delivery	Asphyxia, trauma
	Intracranial hemorrhage
Prolonged labor	Asphyxia, trauma
	Bacterial infection
Uterine inertia	Hazard of prolonged labor
Uterine rupture	Asphyxia
Uterine tetany	Asphyxia
Shoulder dystocia	Asphyxia
	Brachial plexus injury
	Fractured clavicle
	Fractured humerus
Manual version, extraction	Asphyxia
	Bone fractures
	Brachial plexus injury, spinal cord trauma
Forceps (high or mild)	Asphyxia
	Cephalhematoma
	Intracranial hemorrhage
Multiple gestation	Asphyxia (usually second twin)
	Prematurity
	Intrauterine growth retardation
	Intrauterine parabiotic syndrome (fetofetal transfusion)
	Hypoglycemia (smaller twin)
	Congenital anomalies
	Bacterial infection (first or both twins)

of abnormally long and vigorous contractions is thus apparent; that is, sustained reduction of placental blood flow impairs maternofetal gas exchange, and fetal hypoxia may ensue.

As labor proceeds, increasing differentiation of the uterine wall into a thick muscular superior segment and a thin inferior one (Fig. 2-1) assures that most of the force produced by contractions emanates from the upper segment. The lower one remains relatively passive and distensible. This arrangement is essential if fetal descent is to be accomplished. If the entire uterine wall were as thick and muscular as the upper segment, the force of each contraction would be applied to the fetus equally from all sides rather than from above. The fetus would get nowhere. Furthermore, as will be seen in the description of the first stage, the cervix would neither efface nor dilate.

First stage of labor. As the upper and lower segments become more sharply differentiated with each contraction, cervical effacement (thinning) and dilatation progresses gradually. At the onset of labor, the cervical wall is approximately 2

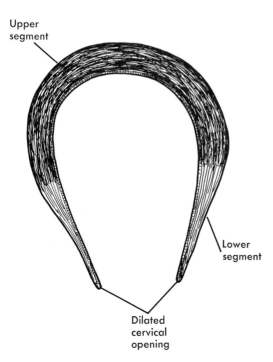

Upper
segment

Lower
segment

Dilated
cervical
opening

Fig. 2-1. Upper (dark shading) and lower uterine segments are shown delineated from each other. Most of the force that propels the fetus originates from the thick muscular upper segment. (Modified from Hellman, L. M., and Pritchard, J. A.: Williams obstetrics, ed. 14, New York, 1971, Appleton-Century-Crofts.)

cm in thickness, surrounding a thin canal of equal depth. Fully effaced at the end of the first stage, the wall of the cervix is only a few millimeters thick. It becomes incorporated into and indistinguishable from the uterine wall of the lower segment. Fully dilated, the cervical canal becomes a shallow, wide orifice that is 10 cm in diameter (Fig. 2-2). The canal becomes wider and thinner as the wall of the cervix retracts to become part of the uterine wall. Thinning and widening of the cervix occurs in response to downward pressure on the fetus that is provided by repeated contractions. Most of the effacement is accomplished during the early part of the first stage, when dilatation is minimal. Later, with effacement almost complete, dilatation progresses more rapidly to completion, marking the onset of the second stage (Fig. 2-3).

Second stage of labor. Although variations are numerous, significant descent of the fetus usually does not occur until the cervix is completely dilated. During the second stage, fetal descent is brought about not only by uterine contractions

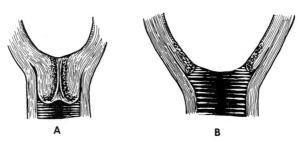

A   **B**

Fig. 2-2. Effacement and dilatation of the cervix. **A,** Appearance of the cervix before onset of labor. The cervical canal is only a few millimeters wide. **B,** Appearance of the cervix late in labor. The cervix is effaced and dilated, having been drawn upward and incorporated into the wall of the lower uterine segment. The cervical canal has widened to approximately 10 cm. (Modified from Hellman, L. M., and Pritchard, J. A.: Williams obstetrics, ed. 14, New York, 1971, Appleton-Century-Crofts.)

but also by periodic increases of intraabdominal pressure. The latter is accomplished by the mother during voluntary contraction of abdominal muscles and fixation of the diaphragm. Maternal oversedation may reduce or eliminate voluntary cooperation.

As fetal descent proceeds, the head rotates to accommodate to the contour of the bony pelvis and thus is normally delivered face downward. Delivery of the shoulders is accomplished when the unextruded body rotates 90 degrees to change their internal position from a horizontal to an anteroposterior one. The face is now turned to one side (Fig. 2-4).

The anterior (upper) shoulder is delivered first, then the posterior (lower) shoulder, and rapidly thereafter, the rest of the body. The cord is cut by the operator after extrusion of the body, the proximal end remaining attached to the undelivered placenta while the distal segment is attached to the infant.

Third stage of labor. After birth of the baby, the placenta separates and is extruded by continued contractions that pry it loose from its attachment to the uterine wall. There is thus a smooth transition from intrauterine placental respiration in a liquid environment to extrauterine pulmonary respiration in a gaseous one. If

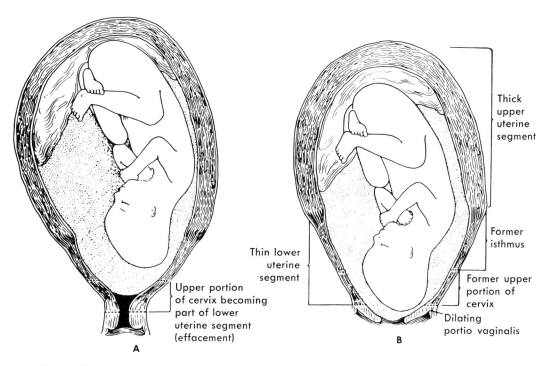

Fig. 2-3. Pregnant uterus. **A,** Late pregnancy. Bracket marks part of cervix that is incorporated into lower uterine segment during effacement. **B,** During labor. Effacement is complete, and dilatation is in progress. Upper segment is thicker, whereas lower segment is longer and thinner. (From Reid, D. E., Ryan, K. J., and Benirschke, K.: Principles and management of human reproduction, Philadelphia, 1972, W. B. Saunders Co.)

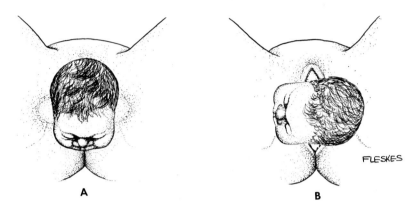

FLESKES

A   B

Fig. 2-4. Rotation of the shoulders prior to delivery. **A,** The head has just been delivered. The shoulders are in a horizontal direction. **B,** Ninety-degree rotation of the entire body has now placed the shoulders in a vertical (anteroposterior) direction while the face has turned to one side. (Modified from Hellman, L. M., and Pritchard, J. A.: Williams obstetrics, ed. 14, New York, 1971, Appleton-Century-Crofts.)

extensive separation of the placenta occurs during the first or second stage, the reduction of surface area available for gas exchange produces hypoxia, which cannot be relieved until the head is delivered.

DYSTOCIA (DIFFICULT LABOR)

Prolongation of labor due to mechanical factors is called dystocia. Precise time limits for the normal duration of labor are difficult to fix. However, it is generally agreed that the combined length of the first and second stages should not exceed approximately 20 hours and that the second stage itself is abnormal if it surpasses 2 hours in primiparas and 1 hour in multiparas. If labor is prolonged, perinatal mortality and morbidity increase because (1) separation of the placenta during the second stage is more likely, and severe fetal hypoxia may ensue; (2) compression of the cord is more likely, and it causes profound fetal hypoxia because blood flow in the umbilical vessels is ob-

structed; and (3) the incidence of intra-uterine bacterial infection rises sharply as labor becomes more protracted, especially if the amniotic membranes have ruptured early (Chapter 12).

Dystocia may be caused by one or more of the following factors: (1) uterine dysfunction (inertia), which involves abnormal contractions of uterine muscle; (2) abnormal presentation, excessive fetal size, or congenital anomalies (such as hydrocephalus), which obstruct fetal descent during the birth process; or (3) abnormal size or shape of the birth canal, which impedes fetal passage. A contracted pelvis is the most common manifestation of this abnormality.

Uterine dysfunction

Uterine dysfunction may be hypotonic (weak contractions) or hypertonic (excessive contractions and muscle tone). The former, which is by far the most common variety, is usually due to impairment of normal fetal descent (contracted pelvis or abnormal fetal presentation). In some labors hypotonic dysfunction is due to overdosage of anesthetic and analgesic agents. This type of dysfunction generally appears during the latter part of the first stage. Progressive dilatation of the cervix is retarded or halted, and contractions weaken or cease altogether. Dangers of prolonged labor to the fetus were described earlier.

The hypertonic variety of dysfunction is infrequent. It appears early in the first stage of labor. Contractions are inordinately painful and sustained. Progress of labor is either slowed or nonexistent. In these circumstances, fetal hypoxia is due to impaired placental blood flow from continuously increased intrauterine pressure. The effects of diminished placental blood flow on maternofetal gas exchange are discussed on p. 53.

Contracted pelvis

An abnormal contour of the bony pelvis often involves a constricted birth passage that impedes normal descent of the fetus; complete obstruction is a rare phenomenon. Pelvic contraction occurs in approximately 5% of white women and in about 15% of black women. Pelvic size may be diminished in the anteroposterior diameter, the transverse diameter, or both. The slowed fetal descent caused by a narrow birth canal causes hypotonic uterine dysfunction and prolonged labor. The fetal dangers of protracted labor have already been enumerated, but in addition, trauma often occurs as a consequence of pressure exerted by the bony pelvis on a tightly fitting fetal part. For instance, cephalopelvic disproportion may cause molding of the fetal head, which is characterized by a misshapen skull, usually in the anteroposterior dimension. Occasionally pressure marks on the scalp are also

seen at the point of contact with the maternal sacrum. In the extreme, a depressed fracture that is grossly visible as an indentation in the surface of the skull may result from excessive pressure against the bony pelvis.

Abnormal fetal presentation

The normal vertex presentation (head first) occurs in 95% of all deliveries. Abnormal presentations include breech, face, brow, and shoulder. Breech deliveries comprise approximately 4% whereas the others comprise 1% of all births.

Face and shoulder presentations can in themselves prolong labor by impeding fetal passage, even if the pelvis is normally constituted. Breech presentations do not in themselves prolong labor unless pelvic narrowing is also present.

Face presentations are not common. They are more likely to occur when the maternal pelvis is contracted, when maternal abdominal musculature is lax (in multipara), and when the fetus is large. Characteristically the head is drawn back so that the occiput almost touches the upper spine. The resultant misfit of the head in the birth canal usually precludes normal passage, and delivery may be considerably delayed. At birth, facial edema and ecchymosis impart a characteristically grotesque appearance, which disappears in about a week (Fig. 2-5). Just as it was in utero, the head is held backward as the infant lies in the crib. Fetal and neonatal mortality are increased severalfold, primarily because of the hypoxic effects of prolonged labor and trauma.

A shoulder presentation occurs when the fetus lies transversely across the pelvis (transverse lie). In this position the long axis of the body is perpendicular to

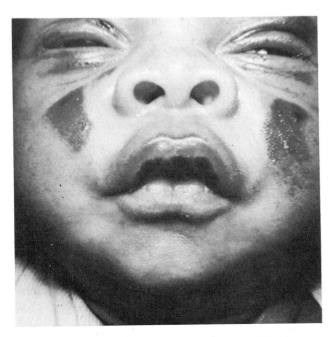

Fig. 2-5. Typical facial appearance after a face presentation. There is generalized swelling, most pronounced in the upper lip. Ecchymoses and abrasions are the result of birth trauma.

the axis of the birth canal; the head is on one side of the pelvis and the buttocks on the other, with one shoulder up and the lower one protruding through the cervical orifice (shoulder presentation). Prolongation of labor is inevitable because fetal passage is obstructed. A considerable degree of obstetric skill is required for correction of a transverse lie; if correction fails, the only alternative is delivery by cesarean section. Shoulder presentations increase in frequency with multiparity. It is thus ten times more frequent in women with parity of four than during first pregnancies. Placenta previa and contracted pelvis may shift fetal position to a transverse one.

BREECH PRESENTATION

The breech position does not in itself impede progress of labor unless pelvic size is diminished. Depending on the part of the body that presents at delivery, breech presentations may occur in one of three varieties. In *frank breech* the buttocks are the presenting part, the lower extremities being flexed upward against the body. In a *complete breech* the buttocks and lower extremities present simultaneously, since the latter are not flexed upward but are approximately on the same plane as the buttocks. *Footling (incomplete) breech* refers to presentation of the feet and legs first, the buttocks later (Fig. 2-6).

The fetal and neonatal hazards of breech delivery are trauma, asphyxia, and prematurity. As a consequence, perinatal mortality may be increased four to ten times over vertex deliveries. The most serious traumatic event, and one that is twice as frequent as in vertex de-

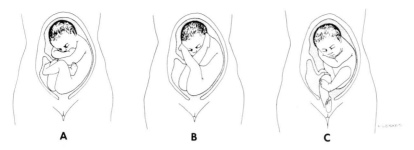

Fig. 2-6. Breech presentations. **A,** Complete breech: the legs, feet, and buttocks present simultaneously. **B,** Frank breech: only the buttocks are born first because the hips are maximally flexed, placing the thighs against the abdomen. **C,** Footling breech: one or both feet appear first.

liveries, is intracranial hemorrhage resulting from excessive and sustained pressure on the head during delivery. In vertex deliveries, the oncoming head may be slowed because of cephalopelvic disporportion. Since labor is still in an early stage, a decision to perform a cesarean section is timely, as well as effective in avoiding head trauma. In breech deliveries, however, difficulty in descent of the head cannot be appreciated early in labor—at least not until the hips and shoulders have already been delivered. It is then too late for a cesarean section, and sustained compression of the head during attempts to extract it often causes trauma and hemorrhage due to torn cerebral veins. The outcome is either lethal or permanent crippling. Spinal cord injury is also more common than in vertex presentations because stretching of the vertebral column occurs as traction is applied to the body during the anxious moments that precede delivery of the head. Hemorrhage into the abdominal viscera may occur, particularly in the adrenals and kidneys, and occasionally in the spleen. It may be due to pressure exerted by the hands of the obstretician while grasping the flanks of the infant's exteriorized body and in an attempt to extract

the head under difficult circumstances. Other injuries include brachial plexus palsy (p. 62), fractures of the humerus and femur (p. 59), and rupture of a distended bladder.

Compression of a prolapsed cord (p. 53) may cause severe asphyxia. This is twenty times more common in complete and footling (incomplete) breech than in vertex deliveries. It is only three times more frequent in frank breech presentations because the buttocks effectively occlude the cervical orifice and the cord is thus prevented from advancing. Placenta previa is an important cause of breech presentation, and in itself often leads to asphyxia. Separation of the placenta well before delivery of the head deprives the fetus of its only source of oxygen.

Persistent hyperextension of the neck in utero is an infrequent association of breech presentation. This unusual position may be detected by abdominal palpation, which reveals the fetal head to be drawn backward, as in opisthotonos. Ultrasound or x-ray examination confirms the suspicion. If hyperextension persists into the onset of labor and vaginal delivery is attempted, 25% of such fetuses will suffer transection of the spinal cord at the cervical level, which results in severe

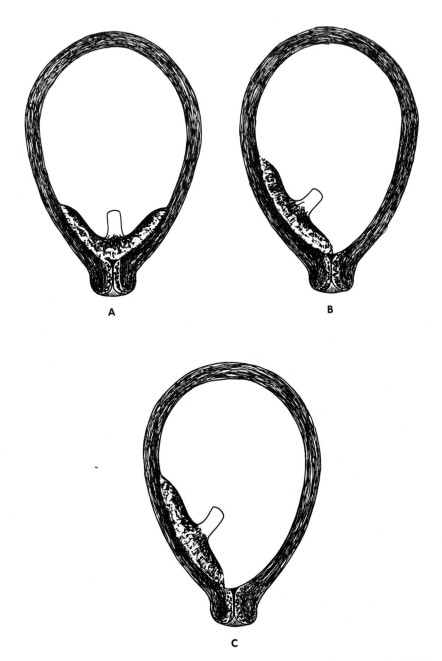

Fig. 2-7. Placenta previa. **A,** Total: the cervical outlet is completely occluded by the placenta, **B,** Partial: the placenta does not completely block the cervical outlet. **C,** Low implantation: the cervical outlet is not obstructed. (Modified from Netter: In Oppenheim, E., editor: Ciba collection of medical illustrations, vol. 2, Reproductive system, 1965.)

permanent disability or in death. Delivery by cesarean section consistently avoids the spinal cord injury.

ABNORMAL PLACENTAL IMPLANTATION AND SEPARATION
Placenta previa

Placenta previa is the result of abnormal implantation of the fertilized egg. Normally implantation is in the thick muscular wall of the upper uterine segment; in placenta previa it is misplaced in the lower uterine segment. Depending on the proximity of the placenta to the cervical os, three types are recognized (Fig. 2-7). Total placenta previa completely covers the cervical orifice. Partial placenta previa occludes the cervical orifice incompletely. In the third type, called low implantation of the placenta, the placental edge barely encroaches on the margin of the cervical aperture. Although these placental positions may impede or totally block fetal passage, the most frequent causes of fetal and neonatal jeopardy are early placental separation and premature onset of labor. In early placental separation, fetal asphyxia occurs because the surface area available for maternofetal gas exchange is dangerously reduced. Even when fetal asphyxia is averted by expert management, perinatal mortality remains high because of the increased incidence of prematurity.

The hemorrhage that follows early placental separation is painless; it may cause maternal shock. Blood loss does not often occur before the end of the second trimester. Hemorrhage may first appear at the onset of labor. Occasionally cleavage also occurs through the fetal side of the placenta, and acute hemorrhage causes fetal shock that is clearly recognizable at birth (p. 276).

The placenta separates early because it is tenuously attached to the thin lower uterine wall. As pregnancy and labor proceed, the wall of the lower segment becomes progressively thinner. The placental attachment is thus easily disrupted before its time; hemorrhage and premature onset of labor are the result.

Placenta previa is effectively identified by ultrasound with 95% accuracy. Other methods are either less accurate or more troublesome.

Abruptio placentae (placental abruption)

Premature separation of a normally implanted placenta is called abruptio placentae. If the placenta separates at its margin, blood drains toward the cervix between the uterine wall and the amniotic membrane, ultimately becoming visible as vaginal bleeding. Approximately 80% of abruptions are of this marginal variety. If separation of the placenta is limited to its central portion while the margin remains intact, a more sinister situation exists because a considerable amount of blood loss may occur before it is recognized. In both instances the major fetal hazards are asphyxia (because of reduced gas exchange surface) and prematurity (because abruptio placentae stimulates early onset of labor). As in placenta previa, separation may cause hemorrhage from the fetal side of the placenta to produce neonatal shock at birth or soon thereafter (p. 276).

IMPAIRED BLOOD FLOW THROUGH THE UMBILICAL CORD

The umbilical vessels may be partially or completely occluded by compression of the cord. Prolapse of the cord involves visible protrusion through the cervical opening in advance of the presenting fetal part. Compression occurs when the cord is trapped between a fetal part and the bony pelvis or the dilated cervix. The same mechanism is operative in occult prolapse, which involves compression by a presenting fetal part but without visible protrusion of the cord through the cervix. Transient compression in utero without prolapse occurs frequently throughout pregnancy and is usually, but not always, innocuous. If fetal heart rate is monitored, these evanescent episodes of compression are marked by periods of deceleration that are unrelated to uterine contractions (variable deceleration). If these episodes are frequent and protracted, the fetus is in danger of severe asphyxia.

Prolapse of the cord, occult or obvious, is a dangerous complication that may cause complete depletion of fetal oxygen within $2^{1}/_{2}$ minutes if the compression is not relieved. Prolapse is most common in breech delivery, multiple gestation, premature rupture of membranes, and transverse lie.

A cord wrapped around the fetal neck or body is generally, but not always, harmless because occlusion of umbilical circulation may occur if the cord is stretched in the extreme.

FETAL ASPHYXIA: RELATIONSHIP TO OBSTETRIC ABNORMALITIES

Fetal distress is often due to diminution in the flow of oxygen from mother to fetus. The factors that inhibit oxygen transfer from mother to fetus simultaneously reduce the transfer of carbon dioxide from fetus to mother. These factors include maternal hypoxia, disrupted uteroplacental circulation, placental dysfunction, impaired blood flow through the umbilical cord, or an intrinsic fetal disorder. The most common cause of fetal asphyxia is impairment of maternal blood flow through the intervillous space.

Biochemical characteristics of asphyxia

Fetal asphyxia implies reduction in P_{O_2} (hypoxia), elevation of P_{CO_2} (hypercarbia), and lowering of blood pH (acidosis). The acidosis is called *mixed* because it is comprised of respiratory and metabolic components (Chapter 7). Respiratory acidosis is characterized by an accumulation of carbon dioxide in the blood that renders it more acid than normal (low pH). Metabolic acidosis refers to a low pH that follows accumulation of organic acids (Chapter 7). In the presence of asphyxia, these acids (principally lactic acid) are the end products of an abnormal process that must produce glucose at low levels of oxygen. This process is called *anaerobic glycolysis* because the breakdown of glycogen (principal source of glucose) transpires in the presence of hypoxia. Hypoxia thus causes metabolic acidosis because it forces anaerobic glycolysis. If the asphyxiated fetus were properly oxygenated by removing the cause of impaired gas exchange, P_{CO_2} would also diminish (eliminating respiratory acidosis), and the production of lactic acid would decline because glycogen breakdown could then proceed aerobically. Thus the concern with suboptimal oxygenation of the fetus is directed not only to the cellular damage caused by lack of oxygen but also to the difficulties of the resultant acidosis.

Signs of fetal asphyxia

Fetal asphyxia is suggested by the presence of meconium in amniotic fluid. It is demonstrable in changes of cardiac rate and by sampling fetal scalp blood. Meconium-stained fluid is observable only when membranes rupture or when amniocentesis is performed. Alterations in heart rate are detectable by fetal heart rate monitoring. Asphyxial blood gas and pH changes are demonstrated by determinations on fetal scalp blood.

Specific maternal abnormalities associated with fetal asphyxia

A number of maternal disorders produce fetal vulnerability to asphyxial episodes. The detection of this vulnerability and the hypoxia that results from it have been discussed in Chapter 1. Maternal disorders that jeopardize the fetus are, with few exceptions, easily identified. The significance of the important ones and the mechanisms by which they endanger the fetus must be understood by all who care for sick neonates. The future of optimal perinatal care will largely depend on the obstetrician's (or perinatologist's) capacity to identify fetal compromise as early in its course as possible. Alertness to fetal hazard will usually depend on identification of maternal difficulty.

Maternal hypoxia deprives the fetus of oxygen by reducing oxygen tension in the blood that perfuses the placenta. The maternofetal P_{O_2} gradient is thus reduced or eliminated, and fetal oxygen deprivation follows. *Maternal vascular disease* may reduce placental blood flow so that the amount of oxygen delivered to the fetus is significantly reduced. Specific conditions that produce maternal hypoxia are (1) acute asthma, (2) severe pneumonia, (3) low environmental oxygen tension at high altitudes, (4) apnea associated with convulsive episodes of idiopathic epilepsy or eclampsia, (5) depressed ventilation caused by oversedation, (6) disturbed oxygen-carrying ability of hemoglobin resulting from carbon monoxide poisoning or hemolytic anemia, (7) diminished blood flow to all maternal organs (including the placenta) that characterizes congestive heart failure, (8) vasoconstrictive states associated with toxemia and essential hypertension, and (9) maternal hypotension from any cause, such as septic shock, traumatic hemorrhage, or the inferior vena cava syndrome (supine hypotension syndrome). The inferior vena cava syndrome results from pressure exerted on the inferior vena cava by the uterus when the mother is supine for long intervals. Venous return to the heart thus is impeded. A change in maternal position removes the obstruction to blood flow. The result of vascular occlusion is diminished perfusion of the intervillous space and reduced fetal oxygen supply. Low maternal blood pressure may also be associated with improperly managed conduction anesthesia (spinal, epidural, caudal, or saddle). Systolic blood pressures below 80 mm Hg impair perfusion of the intervillous space.

As described previously, placenta previa and abruptio placentae reduce placental gas exchange in quite another way. A considerable reduction in the surface area available for oxygen diffusion results from the placental separation that characterizes both of these conditions. Furthermore, considerable maternal blood loss may cause hypotension and impair perfusion of the intact portion of the placenta.

The disorders mentioned above originate on the maternal side of the placenta. On the fetal side, and often unrelated to maternal status, the most frequent cause of fetal oxygen deprivation is compression of the cord, which reduces blood flow to vessels in the chorionic villi. In the extreme the arteries and the vein may be compressed. When less pressure is applied to the cord, the vein may be more occluded than the arteries because venous walls are thinner and more easily collapsed, whereas the thicker walls of the arteries are more resistant to external pressure. Fetal asphyxia also results from cardiac failure in utero (hydrops fetalis of Rh disease) and from fetal hypotension associated with hemorrhage or drugs.

TRAUMA OF LABOR AND DELIVERY

Although trauma to the fetus may be inevitable in certain abnormalities of labor and delivery, skillful obstetric manipulation may often avoid or minimize it. Traumatic lesions of the neonate are listed below. Most of them are mild and transient. Occasionally they cause permanent disability; they rarely cause death.

Mechanical injuries to the fetus

A. Skin, subcutaneous tissue
  1. Caput succedaneum
  2. Cyanosis and edema of buttocks, upper or lower extremities
  3. Diffuse scalp hemorrhage
  4. Subcutaneous fat necrosis (pressure necrosis)
  5. Abrasion of the skin
  6. Petechiae and ecchymoses of the skin
B. Skull
  1. Molding
  2. Fracture (linear or depressed)
  3. Cephalhematoma
C. Long bone fractures
  1. Clavicle
  2. Humerus
  3. Femur
D. Central nervous system
  1. Hemorrhage into brain substance
  2. Subdural hematoma
  3. Spinal cord injury
E. Ocular
  1. Subconjunctival (scleral) hemorrhage
  2. Retinal hemorrhage
  3. Rupture of inner membrane of cornea (Descemet's)
F. Peripheral nerves
  1. Brachial plexus injury
  2. Diaphragmatic paralysis (phrenic nerve injury)
  3. Facial paralysis
G. Hemorrhage into abdominal organs
  1. Liver
  2. Spleen
  3. Kidney
  4. Adrenals
H. Rib fracture

Physical signs of trauma

Skin, subcutaneous tissue. *Caput succedaneum* is a localized edematous swelling of the scalp caused by sustained pressure of the dilating cervix against the presenting part. Venous return from the affected area is thus obstructed, and edema results. The swelling is most pronounced in prolonged labor. It disappears in several days and is of no pathologic significance.

Edema and cyanosis of the buttocks and extremities are produced by obstructed venous return from pressure of the presenting part against the dilating cervix in abnormal presentations. Swelling of the buttocks and genitalia may thus be quite severe in frank breech deliveries. In footling breech the lower extremities are involved (Fig. 2-8); in complete breech the buttocks and lower extremities are simultaneously affected. The upper extremity is involved in shoulder presentation from a transverse lie.

Diffuse scalp hemorrhage is an infrequent occurrence that involves bleeding into the entire scalp or a major portion of it. Loss of blood may be life threatening if a coagulation defect is present. The most severe bleeding is associated with failure to administer vitamin K at birth or with other abnormalities of the clotting process that are unrelated to vitamin K deficiency, such as hemophilia. Hemoglobin levels may fall as low as 3 or 4 grams/100 ml. Immediate simple transfusion is lifesaving. Scalp hemorrhage is cumulative over the first 24 to 48 hours. Tremendous swelling of the scalp extends over the forehead and behind the ears, and a characteristic blue discoloration is seen through the overlying skin. The scalp swelling is not limited by suture lines as in cephalhematoma. The life-threatening nature of this condition requires its early recognition. Swelling of part of the scalp and blue discoloration of the skin are the earliest signs that indicate a need for immediate attention.

Subcutaneous fat necrosis is a localized lesion produced by pressure against the bony pelvis or by forceps. It may also occur if the infant is slapped vigorously in attempts to stimulate the onset of respiration. The area of pressure necrosis varies in size, is sharply limited by distinct margins, and is always firm. The overlying skin remains intact and is occasionally blue or red. Subcutaneous fat necrosis may not be apparent for a number of days after birth. The lesion resolves in a few days to several weeks and is of no pathologic significance. It occurs most often in the face but also over the back and shoulders, arms, thighs, and buttocks.

Abrasion of the skin may be caused by application of forceps, pressure of an involved part against the bony pelvis, or careless handling of the infant after birth. The abraded area may serve as a portal of entry for infection.

Petechiae and ecchymoses of the skin are purple discolorations caused by hemorrhage into the superficial skin layers. By definition, petechiae are pinpoint in size, and ecchymoses are larger areas that resemble the common bruise. These skin lesions may be due to severe systemic infection, but more commonly they are the result of direct injury or of pressure that obstructs the venous return from a pre-

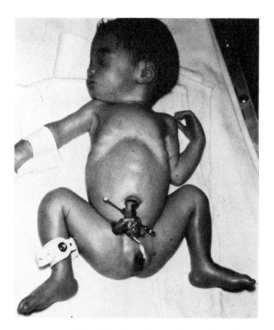

Fig. 2-8. Double footling breech, with edema and cyanosis of legs and feet, considerably more on left than right. Note frog leg position and absence of molding of head.

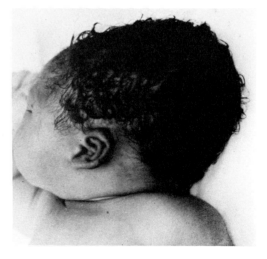

Fig. 2-9. Commonest type of molding, characteristic of vertex presentation.

senting part. The resultant increase in back pressure ruptures capillaries, and skin hemorrhage ensues. Hemorrhage into the skin thus may indicate difficult labor and delivery, severe infection, or a clotting defect. It is also common in small premature infants in whom extensive bruising is evident, presumably as a function of capillary fragility. These small infants regularly develop hyperbilirubinemia from breakdown of extravasated blood.

Skull. *Molding of the head* is usually present to some degree in almost all vertex presentations. The contour of the head may be minimally distorted or grotesquely misshapen. Molding is caused by gradual shaping of the head as it accommodates to the contours of the bony and soft parts of the birth canal during labor. It is more severe in dystocia due to contracted pelvis and in primiparous women. Usually the distortion is characterized by flattening of the anterior half of the head, with gradual rise to an apex at the posterior half, and an abrupt drop at the occiput (Fig. 2-9). Schaffer has described the severely molded head as reminiscent of the drawings of Egyptian queens. The normal spherical shape of the cranium is gradually restored in 2 or 3 days. There is no valid evidence to suggest that subsequent brain dysfunction is associated with molding, but in the most severe cases the suspicion is inescapable.

Skull fractures (Fig. 2-10) may be linear or depressed. Linear fractures are asymptomatic unless the force that produces them also ruptures underlying blood vessels to produce a subdural hematoma. Depressed fractures are often self-correcting, but they may require surgical elevation if the depressed bone compresses underlying brain tissues.

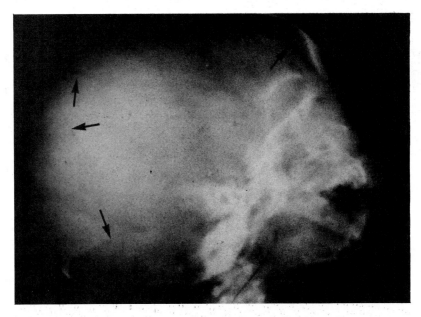

Fig. 2-10. Linear skull fractures (arrows) are straight radiolucent lines as opposed to sutures, which are linear but irregular and sometimes serrated.

These fractures may result from high forceps or midforceps application or from severe contraction of the pelvis, associated with prolonged labor.

Cephalhematoma is a collection of blood from ruptured blood vessels situated between the surface of the parietal bone and its tough, overlying periosteal membrane. It is usually unilateral, but occasionally bilateral (Fig. 2-11). Within 24 to 48 hours an obvious swelling develops beneath the scalp over one or both parietal bones. Rarely, the occipital bone is involved, and even more rarely, the frontal bone is affected. A cephalhematoma is delineated by definite margins. It does not cross suture lines, being limited to an area overlying a single bone. In contrast, the margins of caput succedaneum are indistinct, and the swelling usually crosses suture lines. Cephalhematoma disappears gradually in 2 to 3 weeks, sometimes sooner. In a number of instances x-ray examinations reveal a linear skull fracture beneath it. There are no known abnormal sequelae, whether or not a linear fracture is present. Occasionally, however, and particularly if the lesion is bilateral, hyperbilirubinemia may result from breakdown of the accumulated blood (p. 291).

Long bone fractures. *Fractures of the clavicle and humerus* (Fig. 2-12) are the most common long bone fractures. The clavicle is affected far more frequently than the humerus. Each of these injuries

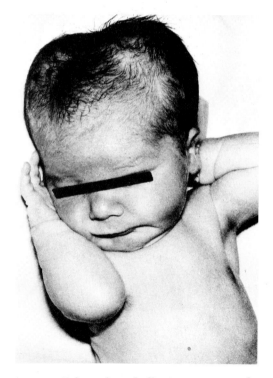

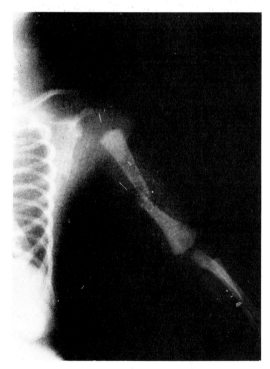

Fig. 2-11. Bilateral cephalhematoma over the parietal bones.

Fig. 2-12. X-ray film of fractured humerus, after difficult breech delivery.

is produced during difficult delivery of a shoulder or upper extremity in vertex or in breech deliveries. The incidence of trauma increases with birth weight. They are thus more frequent among infants who weigh over 4000 grams. Clavicular fracture is usually detectable during movement of the shoulder when a snapping sensation is palpable over the involved bone. Spontaneous movement of the upper extremity may not be restricted, and the Moro response may be normal. Fracture of the humerus is suspected by diminished motion of the extremity, by pain on passive movement, and often by a grossly visible deformity. Attempts to elicit a snap are contraindicated. Spontaneous motion of the involved extremity is diminished, and forced movement is painful. Reduced motion and pain are especially prominent in fractures of the humerus.

Fracture of the femur is an infrequent injury generally associated with breech deliveries. Swelling of the thigh and severely restricted spontaneous motion of the extremity are characteristic findings. Occasionally the involved thigh is blue because of associated hemorrhage into muscle and subcutaneous tissue.

Central nervous system. *Intracranial hemorrhage* is a relatively common event in the sick newborn. It may be caused by trauma or hypoxia. Traumatic hemorrhage occurs into the brain substance or into the subdural space (subdural hematoma). Hemorrhage due to hypoxia occurs in the ventricles of the brain and in the subarachnoid space. Hypoxic hemorrhage is relatively frequent in premature infants and is apparently not associated with trauma. Symptoms are variable. Apneic episodes and other forms of respiratory distress are common. Hypotonia, a tense bulging anterior fontanelle, diminished spontaneous movement, convulsions, coma, and lethargy are the most common neurologic signs.

Subdural hematoma is a life-threatening collection of blood in the subdural space that results from laceration of the dura. The dura is the toughest and most external of the three membranes that envelop the brain (the other two are the arachnoid and the pia mater). Most subdural hematomas are produced by stretching and tearing of large veins in the dural membrane that separates the cerebral hemispheres from the cerebellum (tentorium cerebelli). The resultant collection of blood is usually inaccessible to aspiration by subdural taps. This type of subdural hematoma is caused by compression of the head in the anteroposterior diameter with expansion in the transverse diameter and consequent stretching of the dura. This response can best be visualized by compressing an air-filled balloon on two opposed surfaces and noting the expansion that occurs in the surfaces that are free. The dural membrane that runs parallel to the expanded diameter must also stretch during this broadening process. The danger of compression of the skull is greatest when it is relatively abrupt. Abrupt compression is precisely what occurs during precipitate labor and delivery (less than 3 hours' duration). Occasionally the same type of stress is imposed when high forceps or midforceps are applied inaccurately. Less frequently, subdural hematoma occurs over the surface of the cerebral hemispheres when veins in the subdural space are torn. In this location the collection of blood can be evacuated by subdural taps through the coronal suture. Subdural hematoma increases intracranial pressure, and the resultant telltale signs are separation of the sutures and tense bulging of the anterior fontanelle. Convulsions, coma, and repeated vomiting are frequently noted. Death is not uncommon.

Spinal cord injury is a rare event that is virtually restricted to breech deliveries. It is inflicted by forcible traction applied to the legs during the last phase of breech extraction when the head remains to be delivered. The spinal cord itself is relatively inelastic and does not comply to stretching, whereas the vertebral column is quite compliant. Since the spinal cord is fixed to the vertebral column, stretching of the latter results in tears of the cord or rupture of vessels within it. The type of paralysis that results depends on the level at which the cord is injured. Trauma to the lumbar area is most common, producing paralysis of the lower extremities, bladder, and anal sphincter. Laceration in the cervical region may cause total paralysis below the neck. When injury to the phrenic nerve is included, paralysis of the diaphragm follows, and normal establishment and maintenance of extrauterine respiration is impossible.

Spinal cord injuries present three types of clinical signs. In one, there is stillbirth or death shortly after delivery. In another, survival is only for a short period. These infants are in spinal shock. They have respiratory depression, and the pathologic picture of their lungs simulates hyaline membrane disease. Neurologic abnormalities depend on the level of injury. The intercostal and/or abdominal muscles may be paralyzed; the upper or lower extremities may be similarly involved. The third type is characterized by long-term survival with transient or permanent paralysis, usually of the lower limbs.

Ocular. *Subconjunctival (scleral)* and

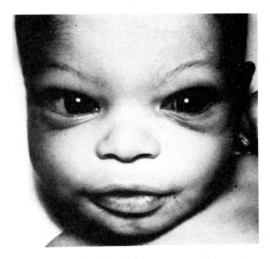

Fig. 2-13. Scleral (subconjunctival) hemorrhage. There were no sequelae.

retinal hemorrhages are due to rupture of capillaries from increased intracranial pressure during the birth process. Ophthalmoscopy reveals flame-shaped and round hemorrhages in the retina. Retinal hemorrhage has been noted in as many as 20% of apparently normal full-term infants. With rare exception, there is no residual visual impairment. The hemorrhages generally disappear by 5 days of age. Subconjunctival hemorrhage (into the sclera) imparts a striking external appearance to the eyes, which in the extreme are bright red except for the iris and pupil (Fig. 2-13). Abnormal sequelae to these lesions have not been documented. They clear within several days after birth.

Rupture of corneal membrane (Descemet's) may be due to forceps injury. The healing process involves formation of a persistent white opacity called a *leukoma*. Edema of cornea occasionally occurs from normal pressure during the birth process. The resultant corneal haziness disappears in several days.

Peripheral nerves. *Brachial plexus palsy* is the result of injury to the brachial plexus, a network of major nerve trunks situated at the base of the neck just above the clavicle. The brachial plexuses are formed by nerves from the fifth cervical through the first thoracic spinal roots (C-5 through T-1). Peripheral nerves that supply the muscles of the upper extremities emanate from the brachial plexuses. Injury thus causes some degree of paralysis of the upper extremity on that side. This rather common occurrence is related to a traumatic delivery. Paralysis of an upper extremity is usually partial, rarely complete. In vertex deliveries, it results from stretch injury to the brachial plexus when the operator laterally flexes the head excessively toward one of the shoulders, thus damaging the brachial plexus on the opposite side. It also occurs during breech deliveries when the extruded body is flexed laterally just prior to delivery of the head. Usually the involved nerve trunks become edematous; this condition resolves within days or weeks, and the paralysis clears. Occasionally paralysis is permanent.

Brachial plexus injury can be suspected at a glance. It occurs in two forms. One type *(Erb's paralysis)* involves the nerve trunks of the brachial plexus that emanate from its *upper spinal roots* (C-5, C-6). It is by far the most common variety, primarily producing variable degrees of paralysis of the shoulder and arm muscles. Spontaneous activity of that extremity is reduced. The arm is held close to the body, and the elbow is straightened, in contrast to that of the opposite, unaffected arm. When the baby is lifted and held in the supine position, the affected extremity is limp whereas the normal one is held in a flexed position. In eliciting of the Moro reflex, the paralyzed arm re-

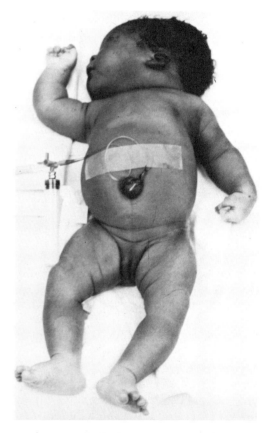

Fig. 2-14. Brachial plexus palsy (Erb's paralysis), left. Diagnosis can be suspected at a glance. See text for complete description.

sponds little or none at all, but the fingers extend almost normally. Involvement is primarily at the shoulder and arm and not in the hand muscles. Fig. 2-14 shows a baby at rest who has Erb's paralysis. The diagnosis can be suspected at a glance. The involved extremity is straight; the opposite one is flexed. Both fists are closed. If the hand muscles of the paralyzed extremity were affected, the fingers would not be fisted. The Moro reflex of such an infant is illustrated in Fig. 2-15. Held supine, the involved left upper extremity is limp; it dangles (Fig. 2-15, *A*).

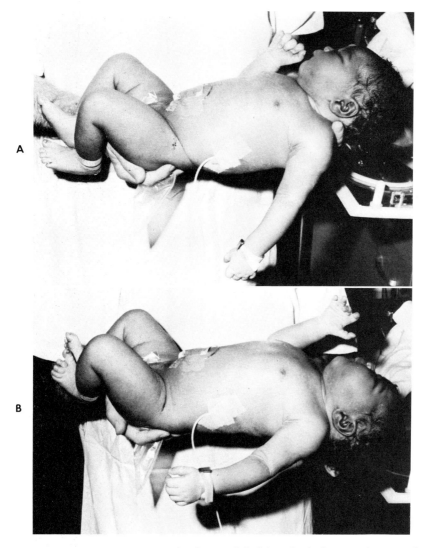

Fig. 2-15. Response to Moro reflex of infant with left brachial plexus palsy. **A,** Baby held supine, with left arm dangling. **B,** When head is dropped, left arm responds weakly, right arm completely. Note the position of fingers before Moro reflex and later.

The Moro reflex is characterized by partial movement of the paralyzed extremity; the baby raises it partially from the original position. The opposite member responds with full motion (Fig. 2-15, *B*). Furthermore, the fingers of the left hand are partially extended. An infant with the

second type of brachial plexus injury, *Klumpke's paralysis,* is shown in Fig. 2-16. This variety involves the nerve trunks that originate from the *lower spinal roots* that supply the brachial plexus (C-7, T-1). Principal clinical involvement is therefore in the hands and forearms. Fig. 2-16

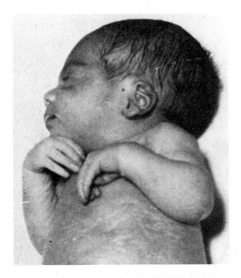

Fig. 2-16. Brachial plexus palsy (Klumpke's paralysis). Note bilateral wrist drop, relaxed fingers.

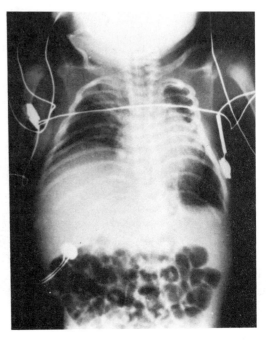

Fig. 2-17. X-ray film of chest showing right diaphragmatic paralysis associated with brachial plexus palsy on same side. Note inordinate height of right diaphragm and partial atelectasis of the upper lobe of the right lung.

shows an unusually affected infant, with bilateral wrist drop. The fingers are relaxed, not fisted as is normal. This baby's Moro reflex was characterized by active motion of the shoulder and arm. The upper extremities extended and abducted normally; the wrists and fingers remained flaccid.

Facial paralysis occurs as frequently in normal deliveries as in traumatic ones. It results from pressure on the facial nerve at a point just posterior to the lower part of the ear lobe, where it lies close to the surface. This pressure is exerted against the maternal bony pelvis during labor or by forceps that are applied inaccurately. Facial paralysis is easily detected when the infant cries. The paralyzed side of the face is immobile, and the palpebral fissure remains open. The muscles on the functional side of the face contract, the eye closes, and the lips deviate toward the normal side. Facial pa-

ralysis usually disappears spontaneously in a few days.

Paralysis of the diaphragm (phrenic nerve palsy) usually occurs in association with brachial plexus injury, rarely by itself. It is caused by the same forces that are implicated in brachial plexus palsy, but with additional involvement of the phrenic nerve at its origin from the cervical portion of the spinal cord. The phrenic nerve receives fibers from the third, fourth, and fifth cervical nerves (C-3 through C-5). Because the phrenic nerve is the only one that innervates the diaphragm, respiratory distress may be severe. The lung on the affected side fails to expand completely, and pneumonia often ensues. In one report, death occured in 20% of affected infants by the third month of life. We have not seen death of any of these infants. The diagnosis of diaphragmatic paralysis is strongly suggested in an infant who has respiratory distress and a paralyzed upper extremity. It is confirmed by x-ray films of the chest in which the paralyzed diaphragm is abnormally high (Fig. 2-17).

Hemorrhage into abdominal organs. The *liver* is more susceptible to injury than any of the abdominal organs. Injury is most likely in the presence of severe liver enlargement (as in Rh disease, congenital nonbacterial infections), particularly in large babies. Most often, the liver parenchyma is focally crushed during the inflicted trauma, and the resultant oozing of blood collects beneath the tough membrane that envelops the liver to form a subcapsular hematoma. Less frequently a laceration involves the capsule and parenchyma simultaneously.

In the case of subcapsular hematoma, blood collects beneath the capsule gradually, over a period of 24 to 72 hours, before illness is apparent. The infant is pale because of the resultant anemia; the liver seems to enlarge progressively, and in some infants a distinct large mass (the hematoma) is palpable. At some point during the accumulation of blood, the liver capsule ruptures abruptly. Now, without containment, hepatic bleeding becomes brisk. Shock and cyanosis appear rapidly, and abdominal distention is severe. Often, the blood in the peritoneal space imparts a bluish hue to the abdominal skin, occasionally also involving the scrotum.

Since affected infants often have a disorder of blood coagulation, this must be identified rapidly. Blood transfusion is lifesaving. Surgical repair of the liver trauma in definitive.

The *spleen* ruptures far less frequently than the liver. In most instances, enlargement of the spleen is present as a consequence of disorders such as syphilis, Rh disease, or one of the nonbacterial intrauterine infections. An enlarged spleen is considerably more fragile than an enlarged liver. Rupture occurs directly from trauma; blood does not accumulate beneath the capsule. Loss of blood into the peritoneal space produces the same clinical signs of hypovolemia that were described for rupture of the liver. Whole blood transfusion must be given immediately. Surgical repair is urgent and definitive.

Small focal hemorrhage in the *adrenals* is asymptomatic, often first perceived months or years later when an x-ray of the abdomen reveals calcifications. Adrenal hemorrhage is most likely to occur in large babies during a dystocic labor when trauma is inflicted. It is probably most common in breech deliveries. These injuries are also more frequent in the presence of syphilis, Rh disease, and neuroblastoma.

Massive adrenal hemorrhage usually produces a flank mass and sometimes also a bluish discoloration of overlying skin. Hemorrhage rarely extends into the peritoneal space because the adrenals are retroperitoneal. Blood may seep downward to surround the kidneys, and they may thus seem to be enlarged to palpation.

Signs of adrenal insufficiency are infrequent. These include vomiting and diarrhea, hypoglycemia, and early hypokalemia soon followed by hypernatremia. In the extreme, shock, seizures, and coma ensue. Without signs of impaired adrenal function, the hemorrhage itself produces pallor and cyanosis, flank masses, and occasionally fever. Surgery may not be necessary unless the blood loss is particularly copious. Restoration of blood volume and treatment of adrenal insufficiency are essential.

MULTIPLE BIRTHS

Perinatal mortality among twins is two or three times greater than among singletons. Therefore the presence of multiple gestation should be detected as early as possible, and the remainder of the pregnancy should be managed with the high risk in mind. The overriding cause of neonatal mortality in twins is prematurity. Other complications of pregnancy, labor, and delivery that occur with increased frequency include placenta previa, premature separation of the placenta, prolapsed cord, and abnormal presentations (especially breech) (Table 2-1). The increased incidence of fetal and neonatal abnormalities is also attributable to congenital malformations, intrauterine growth retardation, (p. 123) fetofetal (twin) transfusion syndrome (p. 124), hypoglycemia (p. 306), and intrauterine bacterial infection.

Approximately one third of all twins born in the United States are identical; the remainder are fraternal. Identical twins originate from a single ovum (monovular, or monozygous), they are thus of the same sex, and they resemble each other very closely. Fraternal twins are derived from the separate fertilization of two ova (biovular, or dizygous). They may not be of the same sex, and they do not necessarily resemble each other. In approximately half the cases, fraternal twins are of like sex. Perinatal mortality is higher among identical twins.

Twinning is more frequent in blacks (approximately one in 70 births) than in whites (one in 80 births). It is least frequent in Orientals. The widely held belief that twin pregnancies are familial applies only to biovular (fraternal) twins. Genetic and ethnic factors do not influence the incidence of identical twins. Multiple gestation appears to increase in frequency as maternal age and parity advance.

REFERENCES

Adamsons, K., and Joelsson, I.: The effects of pharmacologic agents upon the fetus and newborn, Am. J. Obstet. Gynecol. **96:**437, 1966.

Alstalt, L. B.: Transplacental hyponatremia in the newborn infant, J. Pediatr. **66:**985, 1965.

Behrman, R. E.: Neonatal-perinatal medicine: diseases of the fetus and newborn, ed. 2, St. Louis, 1977, The C. V. Mosby Co.

Benirschke, K.: Origin and clinical significance of twinning, Clin. Obstet. Gynecol. **15:**220, 1972.

Bhagwanani, S. G., Price, H. V., Laurence, K. M., and Ginz, B.: Risks and prevention of cervical cord injury in the management of breech presentation with hyperextension of the fetal head, Am. J. Obstet. Gynecol. **115:**1159, 1973.

Bresnan, M. J., and Abroms, I. F.: Neonatal spinal cord transection secondary to intrauterine hyperextension of the neck in breech presentation, J. Pediatr. **84:**734, 1974.

Bronsky, D., Kiamko, R. T., Moncado, R., et al.: Intrauterine hyperparathyroidism secondary to maternal hypoparathyroidism, Pediatrics **42:**606, 1968.

Cannell, D., and Veron, C. P.: Congenital heart disease in pregnancy, Am. J. Obstet. Gynecol. **85:**744, 1969.

Cosmi, E. V.: Drugs, anesthetics and the fetus. In Scarpelli, E. M., and Cosmi, E. V., editors: Reviews in perinatal medicine, Baltimore, 1976, University Park Press.

Desmond, M. M., et al.: The relation of maternal disease to fetal and neonatal disorders, Pediatr. Clin. North Am. **8:**421, 1961.

Ertel, N. H., Reiss, J. S., and Spergel, G.: Hypomagnesium in neonatal tetany associated with maternal hypoparathyroidism, N. Engl. J. Med. **280:**260, 1969.

Goodlin, R. C.: Care of the fetus, New York, 1979, Masson Publishing.

Goodwin, J. W., Godden, J. O., and Chance, G. W., editors: Perinatal medicine, Baltimore, 1976, The Williams & Wilkins Co.

Guillozet, N.: The risks of paracervical anesthesia:

intoxication and neurological injury of the newborn, Pediatrics **55:**533, 1975.

Hutchen, P., and Kessner, D. M.: Neonatal tetany: diagnostic lead to hyperparathyroidism in the mother, Ann. Intern. Med. **61:**1109, 1964.

Jones, K. L., Smith, D. W., Ulleland, C. N., and Streissguth, A. P.: Pattern of malformation in offspring of chronic alcoholic mothers, Lancet **1:**1267, 1973.

Jones, W. S., and Martin, E. B.: Thyroid function in pregnancy, Am. J. Obstet. Gynecol. **101:**898, 1968.

Klein, R. B., Blatman, S., and Little, G. A.: Probable neonatal propoxyphene withdrawal: a case report, Pediatrics **55:**882, 1975.

McKay, R. J., and Lucey, J. F.: Medical progress: neonatology, N. Engl. J. Med. **270:**1231, 1964.

Mizrahi, A., and Gold, A. P.: Neonatal tetany secondary to maternal hyperparathyroidism, J.A.M.A. **190:**155, 1964.

Morgan, J.: Placenta praevia: report on a series of 538 cases, J. Obstet. Gynecol. Br. Commonw. **72:**700, 1965.

Nathenson, G., Cohen, M. I., Litt, I. F., and McNamara, H.: The effect of maternal heroin addiction on neonatal jaundice, J. Pediatr. **81:**899, 1972.

Palmer, R. H., Quellette, E. M., Warner, L., and Leichtman, S. R.: Congenital malformations in offspring of a chronic alcoholic mother, Pediatrics **53:**490, 1974.

Potter, E. L., and Craig, J. M.: Pathology of the fetus and infant, ed. 3, Chicago, 1975, Year Book Medical Publishers, Inc.

Pritchard, J. A., and MacDonald, P. C.: Williams obstetrics, ed. 15, New York, 1976, Appleton-Century-Crofts.

Rumack, B. H., and Walravens, P. A.: Neonatal withdrawal following maternal ingestion of ethchlorvynol (Placidyl), Pediatrics **52:**714, 1973.

Russell, C. S., Taylor, R., and Maddison, R. N.: Some effects of smoking in pregnancy, J. Obstet. Gynaecol. Br. Commonw. **73:**742, 1966.

Seeds, E. A.: Adverse effects of the fetus of acute events in labor, Pediatr. Clin. North Am. **17:**811, 1970.

Sever, J., and White, L. R.: Intrauterine viral infections, Ann. Rev. Med. **19:**471, 1968.

Shearer, W. T., Schreiner, R. L., and Marshall, R. E.: Urinary retention in a neonate secondary to maternal ingestion of nortriptyline, J. Pediatr. **81:**570, 1972.

Soyka, L. F.: Prenatal exposure to stilbestrol and adenocarcinoma of the female genital tract: the pediatrician's responsibility, Pediatrics **55:**455, 1975.

Sutherland, J. M., and Light, I. J.: The effect of drugs on the developing fetus, Pediatr. Clin. North Am. **12:**781, 1965.

Yaffe, S. J., and Catz, C. S.: Drugs and the intrauterine patient. In Aladjem, S., editor: Risk in the practice of modern obstetrics, ed. 2, St. Louis, 1975, The C. V. Mosby Co.

Zelson, C., Lee, S. J., and Pearl, M.: The incidence of skull fractures underlying cephalhematomas in newborn infants, J. Pediatr. **85:**371, 1974.

CHAPTER 3

Evaluation and management of the infant immediately after birth

I have long been convinced that primary evaluation and care of infants at birth should be delegated to an appropriately trained neonatal nurse who can consult a qualified physician when the need arises. Contemporary therapeutic regimens have created a need for skilled personnel to care for infants in the delivery room during the first minutes after birth and in the nursery therafter. Salvage of increasing numbers of jeopardized infants occurs in hospitals that utilize these regimens properly. However, their application has not been sufficiently widespread due to a lack of skilled personnel. The physician performing a delivery is preoccupied with the mother and yet must turn from her to help the distressed baby; or a pediatrician must be summoned, perhaps from some distance, only to arrive after the issue has been resolved unhappily. Obviously, the continuous presence of someone who is adept and knowledgeable is essential for the care of all infants, especially the sick ones; wasted minutes are crucial to survival and to the preservation of intact central nervous system function. The trained neonatal nurse can play a vital role in solving these problems.

EVALUATION: THE APGAR SCORE

In 1952 Dr. Virginia Apgar introduced a simple straightforward scoring system for the clinical evaluation of infants at birth. A total score ranging from 0 to 10 is assigned; the more vigorous the infant, the higher the score. The procedure is best performed by an impartial nurse

Table 3-1. Apgar scoring chart

Sign	Score 0	Score 1	Score 2
Heart rate	Absent	Slow (below 100)	Over 100
Respiratory effort	Absent	Slow, irregular, hypoventilation	Good Crying lustily
Muscle tone	Flaccid	Some flexion of extremities	Active motion, well flexed
Reflex irritability	No response	Cry Some motion	Vigorous cry
Color	Blue, pale	Body pink Hands and feet blue	Completely pink

who is not directly involved with delivery of the infant and is primarily concerned with the postnatal status. This method of evaluation provides a grossly quantitative expression of the infant's condition that is well correlated with prenatal events and the postnatal course.

Procedure for scoring

Table 3-1 presents the components of the Apgar scoring system. A score of 0 to 2 is assigned to each item. The total of the five individual assessments is the Apgar score. A total score of 0 to 3 represents severe distress, 4 to 6 signifies moderate difficulty, and 7 to 10 indicates absence of stress or only the mildest difficulty. Evaluations are ordinarily conducted at 1 and 5 minutes after delivery of the entire body. One minute was chosen as the optimal time for the first score because experience had indicated that maximal depression occurred at that time. The 5-minute score correlates more closely with neurologic status at 1 year of age than does the score at 60 seconds. Most babies score 6 or 7 at 1 minute and 8 to 10 at 5 minutes after birth. If a score of 7 or less is assigned at 5 minutes, assessment should be repeated at 10 minutes. The individual components are evaluated as follows.

The *heart rate* is just as sensitive an in-

dication of hypoxia after birth as it is in utero. A rate below 100 beats per minute is associated with severe asphyxia. The heart rate should be counted for at least 30 seconds. If a stethoscope is not available at the moment, palpation of the umbilical cord at its junction with the skin of the abdomen is also reliable for counting. In fact, pulsations of the cord are normally visible at this location. The heart rate is the most important of the five evaluated items. A score of 2 is assigned if the heart rate exceeds 100, a value of 1 is given if it is below 100, and if no heartbeat is detected, the score is 0. If it is less than 100 beats per minute, an urgent need for resuscitation exists.

Respiratory effort is next in importance to heart rate. Regular respirations and a vigorous cry merit a score of 2. If respirations are irregular, shallow, or gasping, a score of 1 is appropriate, whereas 0 indicates complete absence of any respiratory effort (apnea).

Muscle tone refers to the degree of flexion and the resistance offered to straightening the extremities. The normal infant's elbows are flexed, and his thighs and knees are drawn up toward the abdomen (flexed hips). In addition, some degree of resistance is encountered when one attempts to extend the extremities. This normal muscle tone is assigned a score of 2. At the other extreme, an asphyxiated infant is limp. There is no resistance to straightening of the extremities, nor is there any semblance of flexion at rest. This state of muscle tone is scored 0. Muscle tone that is intermediate between the normal and limp asphyxiated states is given 1 point.

Reflex irritability is judged by the infant's response to flicking the sole of the foot. If he cries, a score of 2 is given. If he only grimaces or cries feebly, a score of 1 is given. If there is no response, the score is 0.

Color evaluation is directed to the presence or absence of pallor and cyanosis. Only a few infants are completely pink; they are assigned 2 points. Most babies are given a score of 1 because normally their hands and feet are blue, whereas the rest of the body is pink (acrocyanosis). Only 15% of all infants score 10 at 1 minute because of the high incidence of acrocyanosis. Pallor and cyanosis over the entire body is scored 0.

Relationship of Apgar scores to arterial pH and clinical depression

Table 3-2 demonstrates the close relationship of the Apgar score to arterial blood pH. As the score declines, pH diminishes. Acidosis is thus more profound, and clinical depression of the infant is increasingly severe. Acid-base status of the infant can be remarkably well estimated from the simple observations of the Apgar evaluation. The scores provide a sound basis for the management of neonates immediately after birth, and the resuscitative procedures that are described later are based on them. There are, however, two notable exceptions to the close relationship between the Apgar score and blood pH: (1) A low score may be associated with a normal or slightly di-

Table 3-2. Relationship of Apgar score to arterial blood pH *

Apgar score	Arterial pH
9 or 10	7.30 to 7.40 (normal)
7 or 8	7.20 to 7.29 (slight acidosis)
5 or 6	7.10 to 7.19 (moderate acidosis)
3 or 4	7.00 to 7.09 (marked acidosis)
0 to 2	Below 7.00 (severe acidosis)

*Modified from Saling, E.: Int. J. Gynecol. Obstet. **10:**211, 1972.

minished pH if the infant is depressed as a consequence of maternal anesthesia; and (2) a relatively high score may be associated with a low pH in small-for-dates infants who have suffered chronic marginal intrauterine hypoxia.

Relationship of Apgar scores to birth weight and neonatal mortality

Systematic observations on thousands of infants have clearly demonstrated a relationship between Apgar scores and birth weight, time of scoring, neonatal mortality, and neurologic status at 1 year of age.

The increased prevalence of stress among low birth weight infants is indicated by the incidence of low scores. In 57% of infants who weigh 1500 grams or less, the 1-minute scores are 0 to 3, whereas these low scores occur in only 5% of infants over 3000 grams. Vigor at birth is far more common among larger babies; scores of 9 and 10 occur in 52% of them, whereas in small infants only 4% score similarly.

The status of most infants improves between the 1- and 5-minute scores. Fewer babies are in a precarious state at 5 minutes than at 1 minute. In the *Collaborative Perinatal Study,* observations on 17,000 infants revealed that at 1 minute

7% scored 0 to 3, and at 5 minutes 2% scored similarly. The same trend toward improvement is indicated by the incidence of higher scores. At 1 minute 79% scored 9 or 10, and at 5 minutes 95% achieved the same scores. Because improvement between 1 and 5 minutes occurs in a substantial number of infants, the later scores are generally more reliable for the prediction of death during the first 28 days of life (neonatal mortality), and of abnormal neurologic status at 1 year.

The risk of death is increased if the 5-minute Apgar score is low. In the absence of an intensive care program, death can be expected during the neonatal period in 50% of all infants with a 5-minute score of 0 or 1, and the vast majority of these babies expire within the first 48 hours of life. Low birth weight enhances this risk considerably. For instance among babies under 2000 grams who score 0 to 3 at 5 minutes, approximately 80% die during the neonatal period, but among infants over 2500 grams with the same scores the mortality is 15%. The vast majority of these deaths occur during the first 2 postnatal days.

These data were compiled in the era that immediately preceded contemporary intensive care of the neonate. Although mortality and morbidity have improved, the relative predictive value of lower scores for more ominous outcomes is probably unchanged. Death of low-scored infants may be up to fifteen times more frequent than in those whose scores are high.

Relationship of Apgar scores to neurologic status at 1 year of age

The link between later brain dysfunction and perinatal distress is also convincingly demonstrated in data from the *Collaborative Perinatal Study.* A close

Table 3-3. Percentage of neurologic abnormality at 1 year according to 5-minute Apgar score and birth weight*

Birth weight (in grams)	5-minute Apgar scores		
	0-3	4-6	7-10
1001 to 2000	18.8%	14.3%	8.8%
2001 to 2500	12.5%	4.6%	4.0%
Over 2500	4.3%	4.2%	1.4%

*Modified from Drage, J. S., and Berendes, H.: Pediatr. Clin. North Am. **13**:635, 1966.

relationship was evident between low birth weight, low Apgar scores at 5 minutes, and an increased incidence of neurologic abnormalities at 1 year of age. That hypoxia around the time of birth may well be lethal can be appreciated from the correlation of low scores with increased neonatal mortality. A low 5-minute score indicates persistence of asphyxia. Thus, if a distressed infant with a low score survives, his chances of brain damage are considerably greater than they would have been if he had scored normally. This is reflected in statistical data that relate birth weight and Apgar scores to 1-year outcomes. Birth weight exerts the same sort of influence on 1-year outcome as on neonatal mortality. Table 3-3 is taken from data compiled by the *Collaborative Perinatal Study.* With identical scores, the frequency of neurologic abnormalities at 1 year increases as birth weight diminishes. At identical birth weights, the frequency of abnormalities increases as the Apgar score declines. Together the effects of weight and score reinforce each other. Thus, of all the groups in the table the smallest infants with the lowest scores are most likely to have brain damage (18.8%), whereas the largest babies with the highest scores are least likely to be affected (1.4%).

The diminished incidence of neurologic deficit among surviving infants that has occurred since the advent of intensive care is well documented. The results described above have thus undoubtedly improved, but the influence of low scores and low birth weight on poor outcome is probably unchanged.

Value of Apgar scores

The quality of neonatal care has improved as a result of the Apgar score. Perhaps the most important contribution of the procedure is that it requires scrutiny of the baby immediately after birth. Thorough evaluation of heart rate, respiration, muscle tone, reflex response, and color was not performed systematically prior to the introduction of scoring. The value of the procedure is so well established that it is unquestionably negligent to omit it. Aside from its predictive value, the score identifies high-risk infants who urgently require resuscitation. It also provides a universally understood quantitative expression of the infant's condition. It further enables statistical assessment of a hospital's perinatal practices and the level of risk in the population it serves. The procedure is simple, but it requires conscientiousness and skill if its purposes are to be fulfilled. The most accurate results are obtained when a knowledgeable nurse executes the scoring.

MANAGEMENT: ROUTINE CARE AND RESUSCITATION OF DISTRESSED INFANTS

Information regarding resuscitative procedures is presented with full awareness that too few nurses have been taught to use them and with the distinct conviction that many infants would be salvaged if more nurses could do so. The procedures cannot be learned from a printed page. These descriptions are like a map; real familiarity with the terrain is gained only after traveling the road, but the itinerary must be known beforehand. Resuscitation and its rationale must first be read about and then performed with proper supervision.

Care of normal infants (Apgar score 7 to 10)

There is often a moment of suspense, sometimes tension, when birth is imminent as the top of the baby's head first becomes visible. *The events that follow birth have their origins in those that preceded it.* If the history is known in detail, and if labor and delivery have been followed closely, many of the infant's potential difficulties can be anticipated, and they have already been discussed in some detail. Although most babies are normal and have no difficulties, they nevertheless must be supported by a few simple procedures.

After delivery of the entire body, the operator holds the head downward as suction is applied to the nostrils and oropharynx with a bulb syringe. The cord is cut and clamped, and the nurse takes the baby in charge. The infant is placed in a 15-degree Trendelenburg position on a table supplied with radiant heat emanating from above. The importance of providing environmental warmth to minimize loss of body heat cannot be overemphasized. Control of body temperature (thermoregulation) is discussed in detail in Chapter 4. At birth, a major cause of heat loss is the evaporation of amniotic fluid that covers the infant's skin. The infant must therefore be dried rapidly, preferably by another individual, while the neonatal nurse removes oropharyngeal secretions with a bulb syringe if they have reaccumulated.

The 1-minute Apgar score should now be performed, and if the result is 7 to 10, resuscitative therapy is unnecessary. The infant should be observed on a warmed table until the 5-minute Apgar score is assigned, and for at least an additional 5 minutes thereafter. During the interval after the 5-minute Apgar score, the nurse should examine the infant. Auscultation of the chest will ascertain proper position of the heart and normal air exchange. The head and body surfaces are scrutinized for trauma and for obvious congenital anomalies. Spontaneous movement of the extremities is observed for indications of weakness or paralysis. The abdomen is palpated for masses and for enlargement of the liver, spleen, or kidneys. The genitalia are examined for normal sexuality. Each of the shoulders is moved while a finger is placed over the clavicle. A crunching sensation (crepitus) betrays a fracture. Normal findings of the physical examination and their variants are presented in detail in Chapter 6.

At some time prior to transfer of the infant to the nursery, the cord is cut again, leaving a stump approximately 1 inch in length to which a clamp is applied. Before the clamp is applied, the cut surface should be examined closely for the normal number of vessels (two arteries and one vein). The presence of only one artery suggests one or more major congenital malformations. The cut edges of the arteries are seen as two white papular structures, which usually stand out slightly from the surface. The vein is larger, often gaping so that the lumen and thin wall are readily discernible (Fig. 1-4). A drop of silver nitrate is now placed in each eye for prophylaxis against gonorrheal infection. The eyes should not be irrigated thereafter. In some communities antibiotic drops are preferred for this purpose, but silver nitrate is the preparation of choice.

A complete record of labor, delivery, and postnatal events must accompany the infant on transfer to the nursery. The condition should be reported verbally to the physician in charge before the nurse leaves the delivery room with the baby. The nursery should have already been notified of the infant's anticipated arrival.

Care of moderately depressed infants (Apgar score 4 to 6)

Moderately depressed infants are limp, cyanotic or dusky, and dyspneic. Respirations may be shallow, irregular, or gasping. The heart rate is normal, however, and there is at least a fair response to flicking of the sole. Management entails the same regimen described for normal infants during the first minute after birth, but if effective spontaneous respiration is not established thereafter, ventilatory support is essential. The urgency for this support is indicated by continued cyanosis and flaccidity. Initially a laryngoscope is inserted. The larynx is visualized, and suction is applied through a catheter attached to a De Lee trap. The De Lee trap is operated by suction from the operator's mouth. This procedure, under direct visualization of the larynx, assures removal of blood clot, particles of meconium and vernix, and thick mucus. The suction catheter is withdrawn, and a curved plastic airway is inserted between the tongue and palate to prevent the base of the tongue from falling backward over the glottic opening of the larynx. Oxygen is then administered through a tightly fitting face mask attached to a hand-operated bag that receives 100% oxygen and delivers it to the infant in high concentrations. At our hospital we have used the Penlon mask-and-bag apparatus with satisfaction. The chest rises with each squeeze of the bag if oxygen is delivered adequately. Further ascertainment is obtainable if an assistant listens to each lung with a stethoscope for the presence of breath sounds. If color and respirations have not improved after 1 minute or the heart rate falls below 100 beats per minute at any time, endotracheal intubation is urgently indicated (see following discussion). If the mask-and-bag procedure is effective, spontaneous respiration begins within 1 minute; cyanosis and hypotonicity should disappear. When the baby begins to breathe, free-flowing oxygen should be supplied.

Care of severely depressed infants (Apgar score 0 to 3)

Gentle swiftness is the essence of resuscitation of profoundly depressed infants. Their woeful state is instantly recognizable. They are blue and limp, and they make little or no attempt to breathe. The heart rate is less than 100 beats per minute, if it is at all present; preliminary suction of the upper airway and a vigorous flick of the sole are of no avail. The Apgar score is 0 to 3. This evaluation should consume no more than a few seconds. The experienced observer recognizes the gravity of the situation without consciously scoring the infant's status. Suction and endotracheal intubation under direct visualization with a laryngoscope are the only procedures that can save an infant in such straits. Generally, once oxygen is delivered to the lungs, the response is gratifying. Improvement may be noted in seconds, although frequently intubation must be maintained for 10 minutes or longer. The heartbeat returns; if it is present initially, the rate quickens and the sounds are louder and sharper.

With the return of more effective cardiac function, the baby becomes pink, and some spontaneous muscle activity may appear. If heart activity is absent after 3 or 4 insufflations, external cardiac massage is mandatory. Occasionally, after cardiac activity is restored, intravenous administration of sodium bicarbonate and dextrose is essential because hypoxia causes metabolic acidosis and it may also produce hypoglycemia as a result of rapid depletion of glycogen store (p. 306). The details of resuscitation follow.

Equipment

1. Laryngoscope (pencil handle with attached Miller size 0 premature or size 1 infant blade). The adequacy of the light source must be ascertained during periodic routine checks of all equipment when not in use.

2. Endotracheal tubes. Some operators prefer Cole endotracheal tubes with metal stylet to prevent kinking. These tubes are tapered at the distal end (sizes 10, 12, or 14). We prefer untapered Portex tubes in sizes ranging from 2.5 mm to 4 mm. We avoid metal stylets because of the trauma they may cause during intubation.

3. De Lee trap. A De Lee trap is preferred for suction, which should be applied by the operator's mouth. Wall suction in delivery rooms is traumatic to neonates because it is far too forceful. If wall suction is used, it must be modulated by a regulator to a level no greater than 120 mm Hg.

4. Bag resuscitator. This bag is attached to the inserted endotracheal tube. It receives 100% oxygen from a wall source or from a tank. Infant masks are usually supplied with this apparatus but are of no value in resuscitation of severely depressed infants.

Procedure for ventilation by tracheal intubation

1. The infant should be supine, with a flattened, rolled towel to support the upper back at the level of the shoulders.

2. The baby's head is held with the right hand; the face looks upward. The laryngoscope is held in the left hand with the blade attachment downward.

3. The blade is slipped past the right corner of the mouth for a distance of approximately 2 cm along the right side of the oral cavity. In so doing, the blade is moved toward the midline, thus displacing the tongue to the left side of the oral cavity.

4. The tip of the blade is advanced slightly so that it comes to rest in a wedge-like space (the vallecula), which is situated between the epiglottis and the base of the tongue (Fig. 3-1). A slight upward tilt of the tip of the blade now exposes the opening of the larynx (glottis). The glottis is more easily seen if slight downward pressure is applied externally to the larynx by the hand that holds the laryngoscope, or by an assistant. As now viewed, the following structures are identifiable from above downward (anterior to posterior): the base of the tongue, the blade placed in the vallecula, the epiglottis, the glottis, the esophageal opening, and the posterior hypopharyngeal wall (Fig. 3-2). The epiglottis is a valuable landmark because it is sometimes visible when the glottis is not. The epiglottis appears as an arched rim of pink tissue, which often tapers to a rounded point so that it resembles a diminutive tongue. If it is visible and the glottis is not, you need only tilt the laryngoscope slightly so that the tip of the blade moves upward. The glottic opening is thus revealed as a black vertical slit. If obstructed by fluid and particulate matter, the slit is discerned with difficulty. Suction is necessary to clear the area and to evacuate unseen material that may fill the trachea as well. The suction catheter should be advanced through the glottis to clear the trachea prior to insertion of an endotracheal tube.

5. If spontaneous respirations do not immediately follow the removal of fluid and particulate matter, an endotracheal tube is introduced through the glottis. If

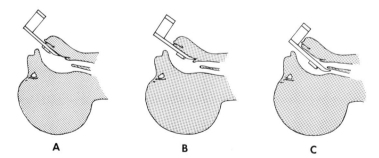

Fig. 3-1. A, Position of laryngoscope blade prior to insertion into the vallecula. **B,** Blade tip resting in vallecula directly above the epiglottis. **C,** Misplaced blade inserted into the esophagus. (Modified from film "Resuscitation of the Newborn," Special Committee on Infant Mortality of the Medical Society of New York, produced by Smith, Kline & French Medical Film Center, Philadelphia.)

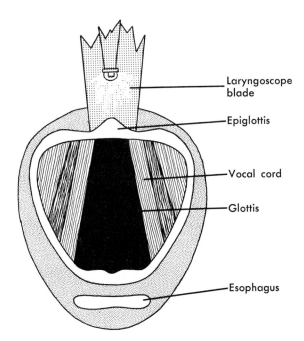

Laryngoscope blade

Epiglottis

Vocal cord

Glottis

Esophagus

Fig. 3-2. Direct view of the glottis and surrounding structures after the blade tip is inserted into the vallecula.

the Cole tube is used, it is advanced until the widened flange of the tube no longer permits passage. If a straight tube such as the Portex is used, insertion past the glottis should not exceed 1 to 1.5 cm. Remove the laryngoscope cautiously while holding the tube in place. Oxygen may now be delivered through a bag (Penlon) attached to the endotracheal tube. The bag is abruptly squeezed and released at a rate approximating 40 times per minute. If the bag is grasped in the palm of the hand and squeezed with all five fingers, pressures in excess of 60 to 70 cm H_2O are delivered, and pneumothorax may ensue. By squeezing with the thumb, index, and middle fingers only, safer and usually effective pressures of 25 to 35 cm H_2O are delivered. Sometimes higher pressures are required initially for adequate lung expansion, necessitating use of the entire hand for bag compression. If the endotracheal tube has been inserted too deeply, it will pass directly into the right main stem bronchus. Delivery of oxygen is therefore confined to the right lung, and insufflation causes expansion in the right chest, with little or no visible excursion on the left. This discrepancy can be determined more accurately by an assistant who listens with a stethoscope. Breath sounds are absent on the left, whereas on the right they are loud and clear. This being the case, the endotracheal tube should be withdrawn slightly until breath sounds are equal on each side of the chest.

External cardiac massage

1. If the heartbeat has not returned after three or four insufflations, external cardiac massage must be instituted immediately. It should be performed by an

assistant, leaving the primary operator free to manage ventilation. When downward pressure is applied at the left margin of the lower sternum, the heart is compressed (systole); when the pressure is released, the heart is dilated (diastole).

2. The index and middle fingers are placed at the appropriate spot and abruptly pressed downward and released. The total downward displacement of the chest wall should not exceed 1 inch. Excessive vigor may cause a laceration of the liver with severe blood loss.

3. It is imperative to maintain cardiac massage and ventilation. This is accomplished by alternating the two maneuvers. The heart is compressed two or three times (at a rate approximating 120 times per minute), after which a breath of oxygen is supplied. The two procedures should never be performed simultaneously, since the pressure applied during cardiac massage may rupture a lung that is simultaneously inflated by artificial ventilation. Pneumothorax and pneumomediastinum may ensue.

4. If cardiac massage is effective, the femoral or temporal artery pulses are palpable in synchrony with depression of the sternum. Cardiac compression should be discontinued every 30 to 60 seconds to detect the presence of spontaneous cardiac activity.

5. When a regular heartbeat is discerned, cardiac massage may be discontinued. Assisted ventilation may be discontinued when spontaneous respiration appears.

Correction of metabolic acidosis

The asphyxiated neonate is by definition, hypoxemic, hypercarbic, and acidotic. Metabolic acidosis is the result of lactic acid accumulation from anaerobic glycolysis during hypoxemia; retention of CO_2 results in respiratory acidosis. To correct acidosis during the resuscitative procedure, the pervasive practice for well over a decade has entailed the administration of sodium bicarbonate by rapid intravenous infusion in the delivery room. Now, well-controlled studies have led to the conclusion that this practice requires revision—the fact is, sodium bicarbonate therapy is only exceptionally necessary and is usually contraindicated for the correction of acidosis during resuscitation. Contemporary evidence also demonstrates that bicarbonate for the acidosis that accompanies hyaline membrane disease is rarely indicated and that it is often dangerous.

Rapid infusion of alkali for resuscitation in the delivery room is, as a rule, contraindicated because:

1. Bicarbonate is changed in the blood to CO_2 and water. Its beneficial effect thus depends on the efficient elimination of CO_2 by the lungs. If bicarbonate is given when the elimination of CO_2 is impaired, the P_{CO_2} rises significantly and the pH actually falls as a result of the bicarbonate therapy.

2. Rapid administration of alkali, particularly if undiluted, may raise serum osmolality to the high levels (over 320 milliosmoles) associated with intraventricular hemorrhage. Hyperosmolar blood causes a shift of interstitial fluid (by osmosis) into blood vessels from the extravascular space. The brain shrinks, and the blood vessels become distended. The stage is set for rupture of capillaries already damaged by asphyxia.

Bicarbonate is also often utilized to reduce the metabolic acidosis that persists after the resuscitative procedure. This generally transpires after admission to the nursery. The data clearly demonstrate that acidosis in these circumstances is not usually corrected and that P_{CO_2} rises. If correction does occur, the process is no more rapid in infants who are given bicarbonate than in infants who receive only dextrose water.

Sodium bicarbonate therapy should thus be a rare event. If it must be utilized, the bicarbonate should be diluted two to five times with water for injection. Addition of five parts of water results in an isotonic solution that can be rapidly injected into an asphyxiated infant. A typical dose would then entail infusion of 10 to 15 ml/ kg, which is quite likely to be effective for the hypotension that is a frequent component of asphyxia. *Sodium bicarbonate is indicated only if there is no response to assisted ventilation. This lack of response is characterized by persistence of bradycardia (less than 100 beats per minute) and hypotension.*

If intravenous medication is an urgent need, rapid access is accomplished by inserting a catheter into the umbilical vein. The catheter is passed into the umbilical vein for distances varying from 5 to 9 cm, depending on the size of the baby. The distal end of the catheter should never be open to room atmosphere because a deep gasp may cause the entry of a significant quantity of air into the heart. A three-way stopcock thus should be attached at the distal end of the fluid-filled catheter for administration of sodium bicarbonate by syringe and for slow infusion of 10% dextrose solution afterward. The umbilical vein should be abandoned as soon as possible in favor of a peripheral vein if continued intravenous administration of fluid is necessary. An infusion pump must be used to maintain the appropriate flow rate.

Maintenance of body heat

Provision of external heat is indispensable if optimal results are to be derived from the resuscitative procedures just described. The implications of low body temperature are discussed in Chapter 4. Evaluation and management of all infants must be performed on a table that is supplied by an overhead source of radiant heat. Without it, the response to resuscitation is delayed, diminished, or absent. The prevention of heat loss is also crucial during transfer of the baby to the nursery. The severely depressed infant should be moved in an incubator that is equipped with a battery-operated heat source and an independent oxygen supply. If this equipment is not available, double-layered plastic bags that are designed to minimize heat loss may be used. These transparent bags fit snugly over the infant. The two layers are separated by large, multiple, self-contained air bubbles. If these bags are unavailable, the baby should be wrapped in a warmed blanket and transferred rapidly.

Errors commonly committed during resuscitation

With so many procedures to be performed and with so little time in which to accomplish them, it is no wonder that errors are sometimes committed even by experienced personnel, not to mention the mistakes of the uninitiated and untrained. Perhaps the most fundamental of all errors is the attempt to resuscitate with little knowledge of rationale and with ignorance of the physiologic processes that have gone awry. The quality of performance increases directly with an understanding of rationale.

Specific errors in technique should be

recognized if they are to be avoided or quickly corrected. The most frequent error during laryngoscopy is passage of the blade beyond the epiglottis into the esophageal opening, which is round or oval rather than slitlike and vertical (Fig. 3-2). At this point one is peering into the esophagus while the glottic slit is concealed above the blade. The blade should be withdrawn slowly while pointing the tip slightly upward. The glottis and the epiglottis soon fall into full view just beneath the laryngoscope blade. If, on the other hand, the blade tip is placed short of its goal, very slight advancement will position it in the vallecula.

Often an operator extends the baby's head in the erroneous assumption that intubation is facilitated, when in fact such positioning virtually precludes success. One frequently observes an operator with one hand on the chin, pulling it backward to extend the head while the laryngoscope is being inserted. The resultant stretching of the neck projects the larynx upward (anteriorly) so that it is hidden by the base of the tongue. It also tends to close the glottis. In these circumstances, the tip of the blade is invariably directed into the esophagus, and even when it is withdrawn gingerly, the larynx will not drop into view while the head is maintained in extension. Rather than pull the chin backward, one should place the head in a neutral position.

Trauma is always a hazard when a metallic instrument is swiftly introduced into soft tissues. Lacerations and bruises of pharyngeal and laryngeal structures may result from rough insertion of the laryngoscope. Injury to the larynx is particularly serious because the airway may be occluded by the resultant edema or hemorrhage.

Another frequently committed error, previously mentioned, is insertion of the endotracheal tube too deeply into the trachea. The bifurcation of the trachea into two main stem bronchi is such that the right bronchus is almost a direct continuation of the trachea, whereas the left one branches from it at a sharper angle. Thus, overinsertion of the tube almost invariably places it in the right main stem bronchus; ventilation is restricted to the right lung, whereas the left lung remains unventilated. Detection and correction of this error have already been described.

In the anxiety of the moment, the operator often inadvertently insufflates at a needlessly rapid rate, sometimes over 100 times per minute. The optimal rate is 40 to 50 times per minute. Also, if a bag-and-tube arrangement is used, the operator should be certain that the bag is connected to a source of oxygen; otherwise only room air (20% oxygen) will be delivered, and although it may sometimes be effective, higher oxygen concentrations are usually an urgent requirement.

Several additional factors require mention. Secretions may accumulate in the pharynx while endotracheal ventilation is in progress. Before removing the tube, suction should be applied to evacuate the secretions. Failure to provide ambient (surrounding) heat is a gross error. Every delivery room must be equipped with a heating apparatus.

The use of central nervous system stimulants such as caffeine, nikethamide (Coramine), and pentylenetetrazol (Metrazol) has no place in modern resuscitative procedures. The latter two drugs are particularly dangerous. The most effective stimulator of respiration is oxygen. Initial efforts to resuscitate the newborn must therefore be concerned exclusively with delivery of oxygen to the lungs. Certain pharmacologic agents are sometimes indicated, but only for purposes other than central nervous excitation. Thus the use of narcotic antagonists is essential in drug-induced respiratory depression due to maternal narcotic overdosage. Naloxone hydrochloride (Narcan) is given if fetal depression from maternal narcosis is due to morphine, meperidine (Demerol), dihydromorphone (Dilaudid), and methadone. If used for respiratory depression due to other causes, the antidotes themselves (except for Narcan) may be depressant. This is especially true if they are used to counteract the effects of barbiturates.

SUMMATION

The extent of resuscitative procedures varies from the simple provision of free-flowing oxygen by mask to insufflation through an endotracheal tube, depending on the severity of depression. The Apgar score is an excellent indication of the infant's status and the type of resuscitation required. All babies need a clear airway and warmth. The establishment of spontaneous respiration is the most important and immediate goal of resuscitation; failure to prevent loss of body heat and to correct acidosis may prolong the time to complete recovery, or preclude it. The ultimate goal of resuscitation is not only immediate survival of the baby but also the prevention of central nervous system dysfunction during the years after birth.

REFERENCES

Apgar, V.: The newborn (Apgar) scoring system, Pediatr. Clin. North Am. 13:645, 1966.

Apgar, V., and James, L. S.: The first sixty seconds of life. In Abramson, H., editor: Resuscitation of the newborn infant, ed. 3, St. Louis, 1973, The C. V. Mosby Co.

Berendes, H., and Drage, J. S.: Apgar scores and outcome of the newborn, Pediatr. Clin. North Am. 13:635, 1966.

Desmond, M. M., Rudolph, A. J., and Philtaksphraiwan, P.: The transitional care nursery, Pediatr. Clin. North Am. 13:651, 1966.

Eidelman, A. I., and Hobbs, J. F.: Bicarbonate therapy revisited—a study in therapeutic revisionism, Am. J. Dis. Child. 132:847, 1978.

James, L. S.: Emergencies in the delivery room. In Behrman, R. E., editor: Neonatal-perinatal medicine: diseases of the fetus and infant, ed. 2, St. Louis, 1977, The C. V. Mosby Co.

James, L. S., and Apgar, V.: Resuscitation procedures in the delivery room. In Abramson, H., editor: Resuscitation of the newborn infant, ed. 3, St. Louis, 1973, The C. V. Mosby Co.

Moya, F., James, L. S., Burnard, E. D., and Hanks, E. C.: Cardiac massage in the newborn infant through the intact chest, Am. J. Obstet. Gynecol. 84:798, 1962.

Shanklin, D. R.: The influence of placental lesions on the newborn infant, Pediatr. Clin. North Am. 17:25, 1970.

CHAPTER 4

Thermoregulation

THERMOREGULATION IN THE NEONATE: IMPORTANCE OF HEAT BALANCE

Maintenance of an optimal thermal environment is one of the most important aspects of effective neonatal care, and without knowledge of the basic principles of thermoregulation, it cannot be provided consistently. However, with the facts at hand, cold stress can be prevented, and many of the riddles that arise daily can be solved. For example, why did a premature infant in our nursery continue to lose body heat even though the air temperature in his incubator constantly registered 33.3° C (92° F) on two thermometers? Why did this same infant fail to gain weight optimally in spite of an adequate caloric intake? The answers: Heat loss occurred because the incubator walls were chilled by a continuous blast of cold air from a window air conditioner that was only inches away. Weight gain was poor because the energy of metabolism was partially diverted to the compensatory production of body heat in preference to the laying down of new tissue. To one of our informed nurses the solution was simple: the baby must be moved across the room in his incubator, away from the air conditioner. The basis for that decision and other aspects of heat balance are discussed in some detail in the following pages.

The association of low body temperature with lower survival rates was observed in 1900 by the French neonatologist Pierre-Constant Budin, who was probably the first such physician on record. In his observation, only 10% of neonates survived if body temperatures were 32.5° to 33.5° C (90.5° to 92.3° F); 77% survived at temperatures between 36° and 37° C (96.8° and 98.6° F). The significance of this early observation was not appreciated until about 40 years later, when modern inquiries began. A voluminous literature continues to accumulate. The complex problem of maintaining an appropriate environment for small, sick neonates is not yet completely solved. However, sufficient data are on hand to permit provision of a thermal environment that minimizes the morbidity and mortality that are directly or indirectly due to cold stress.

The human being is homeothermic (Greek: *homoios* = similar, *thermē* = heat); that is, the organism can maintain its body temperature within narrow limits in spite of gross variations in environmental temperatures. In contrast, animals such as the turtle are poikilothermic (Greek: *poikilos* = variable, *thermē* = heat). Their body temperatures vary widely in response to environmental changes. In man, normal deep-body (core) temperature is maintained within very narrow limits; it does not vary more than 0.3%. This is contrasted to the more variable limits of blood sugar, which may fluctuate 50% normally, and to hydrogen ion concentrations (pH), which vary from 10% to 20% within normal limits.

Heat is produced by the metabolic processes that provide energy. Body heat is thus a by-product of metabolism. Normal temperature is maintained only if there is a balance between the generation of heat and its dissipation. In large animals, body surface is comparatively small for body weight; they therefore dissipate heat at a relatively slow rate. The rate of heat loss is further reduced by a thick layer of subcutaneous fat and a copious coat of fur. The resultant tendency to retain heat is the basis for considerable difficulty in maintaining thermal equilibrium during physical activity, when heat production is markedly increased. These animals are vulnerable to hyperthermia; dissipation of heat is the most important aspect of their thermoregulatory function. On the other hand, in small animals, body surface is disproportionately large for body weight; insulation is meager. In these animals, excessive heat loss is an ongoing threat to the maintenance of normal body temperature; they are thus vulnerable to hypothermia. The most important aspect of their thermoregulatory function is the conservation of heat.

Thermal balance is maintained by regulation of heat loss and heat production. Perhaps the most frequently encountered example of heat imbalance at any age is fever, in which heat is produced in excess of the capacity to dissipate it. Core (rectal) temperature thus rises. In neonates, particularly smaller ones, heat loss is excessive by adult standards in spite of a capacity for reasonably effective heat production. Hypothermia is therefore the principal problem of heat balance in the newborn infant. The tendency to lose heat rapidly at ordinary room temperature is often a threat to survival, particularly for small babies who are ill.

BODY TEMPERATURE OF THE FETUS

A number of direct measurements have demonstrated that, at term, fetal core temperature is 0.5° C (0.9° F) higher than maternal core temperature. Fetal temperature is 37.6° to 37.8° C (99.7° to 100.0° F). It had been previously believed that fetal and maternal temperatures were equal, that the mother's heat maintained the body temperature of the fetus. It is now known that, at term, the fetal metabolic processes produce sufficient heat to maintain the body temperature at a higher level than the mother's. An ongoing need to dissipate fetal heat is thus required. Some is lost through the skin to the amniotic fluid, but the major site of heat loss is the intervillous space in the placenta. Heat is transferred from fetal capillaries in chorionic villi to the slightly cooler maternal blood within the intervillous space. It has been estimated that the total surface area of chorionic villi is greater than the fetus' body surface. In addition, blood is an effective vehicle for heat transfer from the body core to the surface; its rapid flow through the villi delivers a significant quantity of heat to the large villous surface. By this mechanism, the placenta is normally capable of dissipating virtually all the heat produced by fetal metabolism. Normal flow of heat from fetus to mother may be reversed when the mother is febrile. Furthermore, it is quite possible that in the presence of impaired placental perfusion, the fetus may lose heat more slowly.

Based on this thermal relationship between mother and fetus, speculation on two well-known clinical events is in order. The first concerns the extremely poor status of infants at birth whose mothers are severely febrile at the time of delivery. This may be attributable to an increased demand for oxygen in the febrile fetus beyond that which is available. The possibility of brain damage at high body temperatures may also contribute to the infant's stress. The second clinical event is benign. It is not uncommon for a mother to shiver for some time postpartum, beginning immediately after the birth of her baby. The transfer of heat from her fetus has contributed a significant portion of her body heat and she has thus become accustomed to a reduced need to generate her own heat. An important thermal source is eliminated when her infant is born, and she now shivers to rapidly generate heat in response to the abrupt deprivation that follows the baby's birth. It may thus be speculated that her shivering is no different from that which is expected on a very cold day—at a football game, for instance.

HEAT LOSS IN THE NEONATE

Thermal equilibrium is present when the rate of heat generation equals the rate of heat loss. If more heat is produced than is lost, heat storage ensues—body temperature rises. If more heat is lost than is generated, body temperature declines. Thus the normal organism must continuously lose heat to a variable extent, depending on the rate of thermogenesis within the body and the thermal factors outside it (the environment). The heat that is produced by metabolic activity must be transferred from the core of the body to the surface; dissipation then continues from body surface to environment. The difference in temperature between the warmer *body core* and the cooler *body suface* is the *interior thermal gradient* (ITG). The difference in temperature between the *body surface* and the *environment* is the *external thermal gradient* (ETG). Maintenance of normal body temperature is determined by physiologic phenomena and the direction in which they are influenced by thermal factors in the environment.

The internal thermal gradient (the body)

The neonate's anatomy predisposes him to the loss of heat to the environment. Thermal balance is more precarious in newborns than in older individuals, particularly in infants weighing less than 2000 grams. The newborn's normal capacity for heat production in itself presents no problems. The crucial issue is heat loss, which is largely a function of the ratio of body surface to body weight. The larger the surface in relation to body mass, the greater the opportunity to dissipate heat to the environment. At birth the term infant is only 5% of adult body weight; yet his body surface is 15% of the adult's. The neonate has three times more body surface per kilogram of body weight than the adult. The discrepancy between weight and body surface is even greater for low birth weight infants. A larger surface area provides more extensive exposure to the environment, thus promoting more heat loss. Loss of heat per unit of body weight is four times greater in the term newborn and five times greater in a 1500-gram premature infant than in the adult. This loss of heat is the principal source of the neonate's difficulty with maintaining thermal balance.

Another important anatomic handicap to conservation of body heat is the thin layer of subcutaneous fat, especially in infants who weigh less than 2000 grams. Heat is thus more readily transferred from the core of the body to the skin (ITG). Deep body temperature is generally somewhat higher than surface (skin) temperature. Since a gradient exists between the core and the surface, constant transfer of heat occurs in that direction. This transfer is normally impeded in the presence of a substantial layer of subcutaneous fat; it is accelerated if the fat layer is minimal. Therefore, because small infants are poorly insulated, they lose their core body heat to the skin more readily than term infants.

The flow of heat along the ITG is largely a function of blood flow from the core to the subcutaneous tissues. The quantity of heat delivered to the epidermis depends on the amount of blood that flows to the skin and the thickness of the subcutaneous tissues. Fat is a heat-retaining tissue; its capacity to conduct heat (thermal conductivity) is considerably lower than that of other tissues. It is a critical impediment to the transmission of heat to the environment; the thicker the layer of fat, the more effective the insulation. Considerably less heat is lost from blood vessels if they permeate a thick subcutaneous fat layer, as in a term infant. The surface vasculature of a premature baby is prominently visible through the skin because of the virtual absence of subcutaneous fat and the diminished thickness of the epidermis. These blood vessels are immediately beneath the uppermost skin layer and therefore lose heat more readily to the environment.

An infant's posture influences the rate of heat loss. Flexion of the extremities reduces the area exposed to the environment. Normal posture at rest varies with gestational age; the tendency for flexion of the extremities increases as gestational age advances. When thermal balance is concerned, the premature infant is thus at a functional neuromuscular disadvantage as well as an anatomic one.

In summary, the loss of heat from the skin to the environment is increased in low birth weight babies because the skin surface is relatively large; loss of heat from deep body layers to the skin is greater because the insulating layer of fat is thin. Therefore the smaller the infant, the greater the thermal losses to the environment. The difficulties imposed by small body size are not related to gestational age or to age after birth. The well-trained nurse is constantly aware of these factors because they affect survival and the rapidity of recovery from asphyxia, influence the effectiveness of therapy for respiratory distress, and may alter the rate of weight gain.

The external thermal gradient (the environment)

The difference between skin temperature and environmental temperature is the *external thermal gradient*. The physical factors in the environment that determine the extent of this gradient are air temperature and movement of air (velocity), temperature of surrounding surfaces that may be in contact with the body or apart from it, and relative humidity of ambient air. Each of these factors determines the amount of heat that is transferred between the body and the environment by four methods: *convection, radiation, evaporation,* and *conduction.* Although they are discussed in the context of heat loss, the first three methods may also be involved in heat gain.

Convection. Convection involves a flow of heat from the body surface to cooler surrounding air. The rate of loss by convection depends on ambient (surround-ing) temperature and the velocity of air-flow. A rapid flow of air enhances heat loss. Ideal ambient temperature in the incubator reduces convective heat loss only, having no significant effect on the loss of heat by radiation or evaporation (Fig. 4-1).

Radiation. Radiant loss involves transfer of body heat to cooler *solid* surfaces in the environment that are *not in contact* with the baby (incubator walls). Thermal dissipation increases as these solid objects become colder or closer to the body. *Radiant heat loss is independent of ambient temperature in the incubator.* It was by this mechanism that inordinate heat loss occurred in the premature infant mentioned earlier. The incubator wall that was closest to the air conditioner was cold, and as a result the baby continuously lost heat to the wall by radiation in spite of the high temperature of incubator air, which minimized only convective heat loss. Thus, even if the

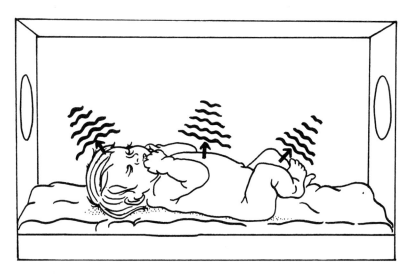

Fig. 4-1. *Convective loss* is indicated here as transfer of heat from body surface to cooler ambient air in the incubator.

temperature of ambient air is high, significant loss may occur by radiation if the incubator walls are inordinately cool. This loss is a common phenomenon at ordinary room temperature, and especially during the winter in inadequately insulated nurseries in which babies are placed close to windows. It is also frequent in air-conditioned nurseries when the vents release concentrated drafts of

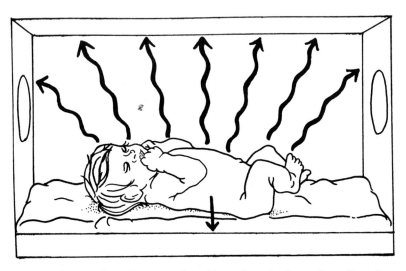

Fig. 4-2. *Radiant loss* is shown as transfer of heat from body surface directly to cooler incubator wall, regardless of the temperature of air within the incubator. *Conductive loss* is shown as heat transfer to mattress in direct contact with body surface.

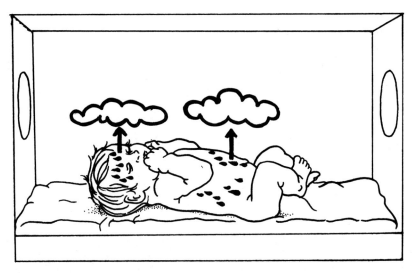

Fig. 4-3. *Evaporative loss* is depicted in the conversion of skin water to vapor. Heat consumed in this process is lost from the body surface.

cool air directly onto incubators (Fig. 4-2).

Evaporation. Evaporative heat loss occurs during conversion of a liquid to a vapor because thermal energy is utilized in the process.

Heat is lost by evaporation of insensible water, visible sweat, and moisture from the respiratory tract mucosa as air is exhaled. Approximately 0.6 calories are lost for each gram of water evaporated. Evaporation, and thus the rate of heat loss, is increased when humidity is low. At birth, a considerable amount of thermal dissipation occurs, especially in air-conditioned delivery rooms with low humidity. Because the infant is covered with amniotic fluid, he loses a considerable amount of heat as the fluid evaporates. This mode of heat loss is readily eliminated when the baby is dried immediately with a warm towel. Another practical consideration in respect to evaporative heat loss is the timing of the first bath after arrival in the nursery. Whether term or premature, neonates should not be bathed until the body temperature is stable at normal levels (Fig. 4-3).

Conduction. Conductive loss of body heat occurs during *direct contact* of the skin with a cooler *solid* object. Placement of a naked infant on a cold table would thus promote conductive heat loss. (Fig. 4-2).

HEAT PRODUCTION: RESPONSE TO COLD STRESS

The homeothermic animal maintains core temperature within a narrow range by virtue of a capacity to produce heat continuously, and, when challenged by a cold environment, to conserve it and increase its production. On the other side of the balanced thermal equation, homeo-thermy also entails a capacity to minimize heat production and to increase the rate of dissipation.

As environmental temperature falls, the homeothermic animal enhances heat production by four mechanisms: (1) voluntary increase in skeletal muscle activity, (2) involuntary rhythmic contractions of skeletal muscle that may be grossly imperceptible but can be demonstrated by electromyograms, (3) involuntary rhythmic contractions that are grossly visible (shivering), and (4) nonshivering thermogenesis.

The human neonate, when exposed to cold, conserves heat by constricting blood vessels in the skin; he attempts to maintain body temperature within a narrow range by increasing the production of heat. Effectiveness of insulation is increased by limiting the flow of blood to the body surface. This neonatal function is as efficient as the adult's, but the neonate's small body size and large ratio of surface to weight make maximal effectiveness impossible.

In a heat-losing environment, newborn infants increase the rate of heat production by increasing metabolic rate. This phenomenon is operative in both term and premature infants, although heat production is augmented somewhat less in the latter. The term infant who is exposed to cold can increase the thermogenic rate two and one-half times over the resting state, to a level that almost equals the adult's.

Heat production is increased in proportion to the fall in environmental temperature. The metabolic response is thus greater, for instance, in a room temperature of 21.1° C (70° F) than in 26.6° C (80° F). Neonates have the capacity to generate heat from the moment of birth, although the response is not as effective during the first 24 hours of life as it is afterward. Of direct clinical interest is the experimental observation that responses to environmental cold occur before there is any drop in core (rectal) temperature. Furthermore, when the environment warms, the rate of heat production diminishes, and this change also occurs prior to a change in core temperature. The infant's thermal activity is therefore increased or decreased with no demonstrable relationship to rectal temperature. Rather, thermogenic activity is stimulated by the response of thermal nerve endings (receptors) in the skin. Heat production becomes elevated when average *skin temperature* declines to 35° to 36° C (95.0° to 96.8° F).

Heat production in the adult who is exposed to cold stress involves involuntary muscle activity (shivering) and increased metabolic rate (nonshivering thermogenesis). In contrast, the nondepressed neonate becomes restless and hyperactive when first exposed to cold, but this form of voluntary muscle activity is not a significant source of heat. This has been shown by the administration of curare (which paralyzes skeletal muscle); the metabolic response to cold stress is not diminished in spite of the resultant absence of muscle activity. The neonate does not shiver when chilled, but in the adult these involuntary tremors are a significant source of heat. Thus nonshivering thermogenesis appears to be the only mechanism available for increasing heat production in the cold-stressed newborn infant.

Nonshivering thermogenesis refers to the heat that is produced by a metabolic rate (and therefore a rate of oxygen consumption) that is minimal in an ideal thermal environment or increased in a cold one. In the neonate, enhancement of

heat production must involve a hypermetabolic state that requires increased oxygen consumption. Obviously a severely depressed hypoxic infant can ill afford the oxygen cost of cold stress. Heat is produced as a by-product of the accelerated chemical reactions that occur at a cellular level when metabolic rate increases. The neonate's brain, liver, and perhaps skeletal muscle are important thermogenic organs. Augmented rates of metabolism at these sites probably contribute in some measure to increased heat production, but the major source of heat that is produced by nonshivering thermogenesis seems to be *brown fat.* Direct evidence for the significant role of this tissue has been derived from animal experiments, but there is also considerable evidence to support its role in human neonates. However, there are presently no data that precisely define quantitatively the contribution of brown fat to the total metabolic response to cold stress (nonshivering thermogenesis). In the newborn rabbit, brown fat is known to account for two thirds of this total response.

In the early 1960s, it became apparent that metabolic activity in brown fat was considerably greater than in white fat. The belief that this tissue was unique to animal hibernators was dispelled by its demonstration in nonhibernating animals, principally in neonates. Its distribution is widespread in the human fetus and neonate. It comprises approximately 1.5% of total body weight. The largest deposits are posterior cervical, axillary, suprailiac, and perirenal. Deposits of intermediate size are found in the interscapular region and in the area around the trapezius and deltoid muscles. Relatively small masses are located in the anterior mediastinum just above and behind the sternum, between the esophagus and trachea, in the intercostal areas and anterior abdomen, and along the aorta. Probably, smaller deposits exist between groups of skeletal muscle fibers throughout the body. Thus brown fat distribution is such that it forms a sort of vest around the thorax (axillary, interscapular, trapezial, deltoid, anterior mediastinal, and intercostal regions) and a collar around the neck (posterior cervical region around the jugular veins and carotid arteries).

The cells of brown fat differ considerably from those of white adipose tissue. The brown fat cell contains a central nucleus; numerous mitochondria and small lipid inclusions are dispersed throughout the cytoplasm. The white fat cell contains a peripheral nucleus and only a single, large, fat globule. The color of brown fat is easily distinguished from white fat distributed throughout the body. The buff to reddish-brown color is imparted by a copious blood supply, dense cellular content, and profusion of nerve endings. Brown fat is densely innervated by sympathetic nerves, which seem to furnish the stimulus for its enhanced metabolism during cold stress by releasing norepinephrine. These nerve endings are seen by electron microscopy to terminate in direct contact with brown fat cell membranes.

Primitive brown fat cells first appear at 26 to 30 weeks of gestation. The tissue mass continues to enlarge as late as the third to the fifth postnatal week, unless significant cold stress intervenes and depletes it. It ordinarily disappears some weeks after birth. Exposure to cold, acutely or over protracted periods, tends to deplete the stores. Tissue from autopsied babies who were clothed and kept in room air at only 21.1° to 26.6° C (70° to 80° F) is considerably depleted in comparison to tissue of infants who were managed in incubators as warm as 33.9° to 35° C (93° to 95° F).

Norepinephrine is released from sympathetic nerve endings. It is currently thought to be the principal mediator of *nonshivering thermogenesis.* When norepinephrine is infused intravenously into the neonate, oxygen consumption increases by 60%, indicating induced hypermetabolism. That enhanced production of norepinephrine occurs in response to cold stress is indicated by its increased excretion in urine at these times. Norepinephrine stimulates fat metabolism in brown adipose tissue. The by-product of this increased chemical activity is a relatively bountiful amount of heat, which is then applied directly to blood that perfuses the tissue mass. Warmer skin temperatures have been recorded over subcutaneous deposits of brown fat during periods of cold stress, suggesting the tissue's thermogenic role in such circumstances.

In summary, the neonate reacts to cold stress by conserving heat (peripheral vasoconstriction) and by generating it in increased quantities on demand. This is accomplished primarily by the enhancement of metabolism; the principal metabolic source of additional heat is brown fat. On the other hand, the neonate responds to excessive warmth by increasing the dissipation of heat. This is accomplished by dilatation of peripheral (skin) vessels and by augmentation of evaporative losses from visible sweat and insensible water. Reactions to thermal challenges in the environment are initiated by thermal receptors in the skin, of which those of the face are the most sensitive and responsive. *Thus, peripheral vasoconstriction and nonshivering thermogenesis (as well as vasodilatation and in-*

creased water loss) become active even though there is no change in core (rectal) temperature. This is the essence of adaptation to changing environmental temperature—peripheral stimulation activates vasomotor and metabolic processes to control the balance of heat, thereby protecting the stability of body temperature at the core.

Impaired response to cold stress

The neonate's capacity to respond to cold stress may be impaired by several factors. Hypoxia is among the most important of these. In babies who suffer from hyaline membrane disease, or hypoxia for any reason, the metabolic response to cold is somewhat limited when arterial P_{O_2} is 45 to 55 mm Hg, and it is abolished at 30 mm Hg. In normal infants, these arterial oxygen tensions are produced by breathing gas mixtures that contain 12% and 8% oxygen, respectively.

Other factors that impair the response to cold include intracranial hemorrhage, severe cerebral malformations, and symptomatic hypoglycemia. Infants in deep sleep, when exposed to cold, at first respond suboptimally until they awaken several minutes later. This observation and the limitation of response that is associated with severe central nervous system abnormalities suggest that the stimulus to heat production depends on intact brain function. Anencephalic infants, for example, do not increase heat production in lowered environmental temperatures; yet their brown fat stores are completely normal. Interference with the response to cold by symptomatic hypoglycemia may thus be rooted in disrupted function of the central nervous system.

Protracted cold stress seems to deplete brown fat stores, and when this depletion is severe, it is hypothesized that effective thermogenic capacity is eliminated. Infants who have died of "neonatal cold injury" were noted to be virtually devoid of brown fat.

HEAT DISSIPATION: RESPONSE TO HYPERTHERMIA

In an inappropriately warm environment, the rate of heat loss must increase; within physiologic limits, the neonate dissipates heat effectively. All infants, regardless of gestational age, respond to external heat by dilatation of peripheral vessels and by enhancement of evaporative heat loss.

The quantity of heat delivered to the skin from deep body tissues depends on vasomotor reactions in the skin itself. Less heat is delivered to the skin (and thus less is lost from the body surface) when external temperatures are low because skin vessels constrict and blood flow is diminished. This vasomotor response is particularly pronounced in the hands and feet. When external temperature is inordinately high, skin vessels dilate, blood flow increases, and more heat is delivered to the skin and lost from the body surface. Vasodilatation is also most pronounced in the hands and feet where more heat is lost per square centimeter of surface than elsewhere. In addition, the neonate dissipates more heat by increasing evaporative losses. This is accomplished by enhanced insensible water loss and by visible perspiration. Visible sweat is first seen at approximately 30 to 32 weeks (conceptional age) when it appears on the forehead and temples. It soon appears on the chest, and by approximately 34 to 46 weeks, sweating also occurs on the lower extremities. The premature infant is less capable of visible perspiration than the term infant; this phenomenon is probably a function of the immaturity of sweat glands.

The factors responsible for the rapid rate of heat loss in neonates (more body surface per gram of weight and minimal subcutaneous fat) also tend to increase the rate of heat gain in excessively warm environments. In the premature infant, the development of hyperthermia is incredibly rapid when equipment is mismanaged or neglected. Core temperature of 41.1° C (106° F) may occur in a very short time; the smaller the infant, the shorter the time. Severe hyperthermia culminates in death or in gross brain damage in the surviving infant.

CONSEQUENCES OF COLD STRESS

The principal difficulties that beset a cold-stressed baby are hypoxemia, metabolic acidosis, rapid depletion of glycogen stores, and reduction of blood glucose levels. The newborn responds to chilling by increasing his metabolic rate, which inherently entails augmented oxygen consumption. Lowered oxygen tension is apparently related to diminished effectiveness of ventilation, which is a consequence of pulmonary vasoconstriction caused by the release of norepinephrine that occurs in response to cold stress. Breakdown of glycogen to glucose now proceeds under hypoxic circumstances, and the alternate chemical pathway (anaerobic glycolysis) that must be utilized dissipates glycogen at approximately twenty times the normal aerobic rate. Hypoglycemia ensues. Furthermore, anaerobic glycolysis generates extra lactic acid, and now metabolic acidosis appears. In babies with intrauterine malnutrition, hypoglycemia is more likely in the presence of cold stress because glycogen stores are already diminished at birth (p. 306). These phenomena are also more pronounced in babies who are inadequately oxygenated because of ventilatory difficulty or as a result of some other disorder. The significance of an optimal thermal environment for such infants is therefore critical. Relentless monitoring is required if normothermia is to be maintained or restored.

Oxygen deprivation itself impairs or abolishes the metabolic response to chilling, thus depriving the infant of the principal source of heat. It may contribute to the abrupt drop in body temperature that occurs in normal infants at birth, since low oxygen saturation is the rule. There is evidence to indicate that thermogenesis is impaired at an arterial P_{O_2} of 45 mm Hg or less. The infant with severe hyaline membrane disease may thus require higher environmental temperatures to maintain body heat, presumably because thermogenesis is handicapped by oxygen deprivation.

During the nursery stay, protracted failure to provide an optimal thermal environment may impair weight gain. This was described in the example cited earlier in this chapter. Experiments with human infants indicate, however, that in most instances increased caloric intake can compensate for energy diverted from the growth process to the production of heat.

THERMAL MANAGEMENT IN THE DELIVERY ROOM

All babies lose body heat to some extent during the moments immediately after birth. Vigorous, full-sized babies usually experience little adversity as a result, but low birth weight infants, depressed or not, are in noteworthy danger. Metabolic acidosis, hypoxemia, and hypoglycemia can be expected in the most severely cold-stressed infants.

Table 4-1. Equivalent centigrade and Fahrenheit temperature reading*

Centigrade degrees	Fahrenheit degrees	Centigrade degrees	Fahrenheit degrees
0	32.0	31	87.8
21	69.8	32	89.6
22	71.6	33	91.4
23	73.4	34	93.2
24	75.2	35	95.0
25	77.0	36	96.8
26	78.8	37	98.6
27	80.6	38	100.4
28	82.4	39	102.2
29	84.2	40	104.0
30	86.0	41	105.8

*For values between centigrade degrees listed, add 0.18° F for each 0.10° C.
EXAMPLE:
   30.5° C = 86.0 plus 5 × 0.18 = 0.9 = 86.90° F.
   35.7° C = 95.0 plus 7 × 0.18 = 1.26 = 96.26° F.

The fall in core (rectal) and skin temperatures is most rapid immediately after birth. In the usual air-conditioned delivery room, if no countermeasures are applied, deep body temperature of the normal term infant falls 0.1° C (0.2° F) per minute; skin temperature declines 0.3° C (0.5° F) per minute. The total drop in deep body temperature may be as great as 2° to 3° C (3.6° to 5.4° F). A dramatic decrease in skin temperature occurs within 10 seconds of exposure to room air. Scalp temperature has been noted to fall from 36° to 34° C (96.8° to 93.2° F) in those few seconds. As other parts of the body are delivered, similarly rapid changes may occur. This high rate of thermal dissipation is largely attributable to the anatomic factors that have been previously described; the relatively large body surface/body weight ratio and the meager deposit of subcutaneous fat are critical. An inappropriately cold environment accentuates the difficulty. The resultant rapid rate of heat loss cannot be fully compensated, even if the infant's metabolic response is unimpaired. In normal infants the metabolic response to cold is somewhat limited during the first few minutes of life because of low arterial oxygen tensions that often persist for 10 or 15 minutes after birth. The observed hypoxemia is comparable to that of an infant who breathes only 15% oxygen. Thermal loss is more accentuated as birth weight declines and as respiratory distress increases. Contemporary standards thus require rational measures to minimize heat loss in normal term babies and especially in those who are small and depressed.

The modalities by which heat is lost in the delivery room, and their relative significance, must be known to all who care for infants during the moments that follow birth. The baby is drenched in amniotic fluid when delivered in a cool room with moderately low humidity. A substantial amount of heat is immediately lost to the cold environment by evaporation. This loss can be minimized by drying the baby with a warm towel or blanket. After drying is done, loss by convection and radiation must be minimized. Thus the baby may be dried and then wrapped in a warm blanket and kept in room air, dried and placed in an incubator, or dried and placed on an open radiant heater. Any of these methods of management is acceptable. If resuscitation is required, the open table is mandatory for adequate accessibility to the infant. There should be one such table in every active delivery room.

In a study that evaluated several methods of thermal management in the delivery room, infants who remained wet in room air experienced a mean decline in rectal temperature of 2.1° C (3.8° F) and a mean fall in skin temperature of 4.6° C (8.3° F) within 30 minutes after birth. In contrast, those who were dried and placed nude under a radiant heater experienced the least fall in core temperature of only 0.7° C (1.3° F) and a decrease in skin temperature of 0.8° C (1.5° F). Wet babies placed under radiant heat had a 60% greater drop in core temperature than those who were dried before being placed under radiant heat. Simply drying and wrapping infants in warm blankets also diminshed their heat loss considerable. Thermal losses were as much as 65% lower in such babies than in those who were not dried and were left nude in room air. Fig. 4-4 is a graphic representation of the decline in skin temperatures after birth according to the various methods of thermal management that were studied. Fig. 4-5 presents the effects of these methods on simultaneously recorded rectal temperatures. During 30 minutes of observation, both skin and rectal temperatures diminished least in those babies who were dried using a warm blanket and placed under radiant heat. The importance of drying and

warming is apparent. Dry babies who were wrapped in blankets had somewhat lower skin and core temperatures than the dry radiated infants, but the drop in skin temperature at 1 minute was followed by an abrupt rise within 5 minutes, presumably after the babies were wiped dry. In these same infants, core temperatures were only slightly lower than in the dried and radiated ones. In normal term babies these decrements in temperature are probably of little clinical significance; they are not a contraindication to family-oriented delivery rooms.

In essence, optimal thermal management requires immediate drying and placement under a radiant heater. Drying and placement in an incubator that is warmed at 32° to 35° C (90° to 95° F) is satisfactory. Simply drying and wrapping in a warm blanket is also acceptable. *Under any circumstances, failure to dry is negligent; allowing a wet, nude baby to remain in room air is callous.*

A certain amount of heat loss is physiologic. Indeed, cold stimuli are probably essential to the initiation of extrauterine respiratory function. Stimuli from thermal skin sensors are transmitted to the reticular formation (respiratory center) in the medulla oblongata, and thence down the phrenic nerve to stimulate contraction of the diaphragm. Experiments with lambs have demonstrated convincingly that delivery into warm fluid, simulating intrauterine conditions, impairs or precludes the onset of respiration. Furthermore, alternate gradual cooling and warming of a water bath in which term newborn lambs are immersed results in stimulation of respiratory activity at the cool temperatures and cessation of respiratory activity at the warm ones. Human infants who are delivered by cesarean

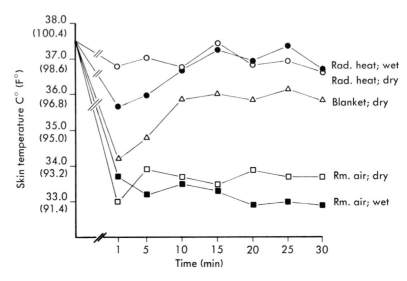

Fig. 4-4. Decline in skin temperature during 30 minutes following birth according to five different methods of thermal management. Babies who were dried and placed on a radiant heat bed maintained their body temperature best. (Modified from Dahm, L. S., and James, L. S.: Pediatrics **49:**504, 1972.)

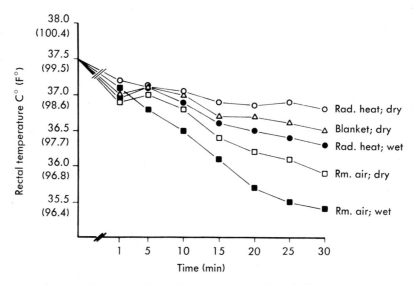

Fig. 4-5. Simultaneously recorded rectal temperatures from babies in the same study as in Fig. 4-4. Note that the decline in rectal temperatures was considerably slower than in skin temperatures shown in Fig. 4-4. See Clinical assessment and management of the infant's thermal status on p. 100, and Heat production on p. 87. (Modified from Dahm, L. S, and James, L. S.: Pediatrics **49:**504, 1972.)

section into a warm bath cease to breathe. Some cold is therefore necessary, but too much is hazardous. Purposeful exaggeration of physiologic cold stimuli cannot be justified by available evidence, nor can delivery into a warm water bath.

Ambient temperature in the delivery room should be 25.5° C (78° F), which is not excessively cool for the infant or uncomfortably warm for the mother. The radiant heater should be utilized only for stressed infants whose accessibility must be assured for effective treatment. The normal term infant can safely be placed prone on the mother's chest immediately after cutting the cord and drying the skin. Skin contact between mother and infant should be assured, but a blanket folded into several layers must cover the baby's back. The skin of the maternal chest is sufficiently warm to provide heat by conduction to her infant; the covering blanket minimizes heat loss by convection and radiation. A radiant heater over mother and baby during the moments of their exciting first contact is thus an unnecessary technologic intrusion.

Radiant heaters effectively prevent excessive heat loss while treatment of a distressed infant is in progress. They are indispensable for the management of asphyxiated babies. A skin sensor for servocontrol of the heat source is not essential during resuscitation.

Transfer of a resuscitated infant to the nursery or to the intensive care unit requires the use of a transport incubator that is heated by power from its own portable battery. A nursery incubator that has no portable power source for the continuous provision of heat is totally inadequate for transport within the hospital. In such incubators, radiant and convective heat losses during transport are sufficient to cause significant cold stress, depending on the ambient temperature of hospital corridors and the duration of transport.

THERMAL MANAGEMENT IN THE NURSERY

By adult standards the neonate's *thermal stability* is restricted, not so much by his inability to produce heat, as by his propensity for losing it. Thermal management in the nursery attempts to provide conditions that are as close as possible to the baby's *neutral thermal environment.* At the very least, the *control range* of environmental temperature must be maintained. Definitions of these terms follow in subsequent paragraphs.

Thermal stability is the capacity to oppose changes in body heat content caused by the loss or gain of heat that results from exchange with the environment. Heat production and heat conservation effected by constriction of surface blood vessels tend to prevent the diminution of core temperature due to dissipation of body heat to the environment. The functions of production and conservation are critical for maintenance of thermal stability in any patient at any age. Thermal stability also requires effective dissipation of heat by vasodilatation, sweating, and rapid breathing to prevent elevation of core temperature due to heat gain from the environment. The net effect of activities that bring about the production and conservation of heat on one hand, and dissipation on the other, is the maintenance of a normal core temperature that is maintained within narrow limits. This is *thermal stability.*

A *neutral thermal environment* provides conditions that permit maintenance of normal core temperature when oxygen consumption in a resting subject is minimal. In the nursery, determination of the components of each infant's neutral thermal environment is not particularly practical; at least four factors are involved: temperature of surrounding air, temperature of surrounding radiant surfaces, velocity of ambient air flow, and relative humidity.

The *control range of environmental temperature* defines the upper and lower limits of environmental temperatures in which the body can effectively regulate heat loss or gain. The lower limit of the control range for nude adults is 0° C (32° F); for the term infant, the lower limit is 20° to 23° C (68° to 73° F). The smaller the infant and the more meager the subcutaneous fat insulation, the narrower the range of environmental temperature (control range) in which heat balance can be maintained.

Provision of a warm microenvironment

Intensive care of neonates almost always requires nudity of the patient. Historically, when the baby was stripped of diapers, shirts, and blankets, monitoring and therapy became feasible as never before. The problems of thermoregulation that resulted, however, have since preoccupied the neonatologist as have few other facets of total infant care.

Since demonstration of the close relationship between abdominal skin temperature and oxygen consumption, it has been the usual practice of intensive care units in this country to automatically adjust the thermal environment in response to changes in skin temperatures as they are registered over the epigastrium. Oxygen consumption (and therefore metabolic rate) is minimal at an abdominal skin temperature of 36.5° C (97.7° F). When skin temperature increases to 37.2° C (98.9° F), oxygen consumption increases by 6%; when skin temperature

declines to 35.9° C (96.6° F), oxygen consumption also increases, but by 10%. Thus the temperature of the skin signals the presence of a metabolic response. It reflects a change in the environment that requires increased metabolic activity to preserve normal core temperature. A drop in skin temperature indicates a heat-losing environment that requires warming. This servocontrol practice is based on data derived from infants in incubators. Similar information is not available for the radiant-heated open beds that are so widely used in special care units.

Normal full-term infants can generally maintain heat balance in an open bassinet when the room temperature is 23.9° to 25.5° C (75° to 78° F) if they are clothed with diaper and shirt, covered with some sort of cotton blanket, and have not been placed in a high velocity of airflow. Sick infants of any size and low birth weight infants in any state of health, especially those below 2000 grams, require a controlled microenvironment for maintenance of normal core temperature. The term infant acquires maximal thermal stability for age several hours after delivery, although the baby's ability to increase metabolic rate in response to cold stress has been demonstrated as early as 15 minutes after birth. Small infants require variable lengths of time for development of a maximal metabolic response, sometimes as long as several weeks. Infants who weigh less than 1500 grams are particularly handicapped because of minimal insulation and a large ratio of body surface to weight.

Incubators. Controlled microenvironments are commonly provided by incubators in which the temperature of circulating air is either manually adjusted or automatically controlled (servocontrolled) in response to signals from a thermal sensor attached to the abdominal skin. Incubators currently available provide heat by convection only. Humidification is provided by passing the heated air over a reservoir of water situated beneath the deck on which the infant lies.

Incubators have several shortcomings. They are constructed of a single-layered plastic wall, which is a major inadequacy. The temperature of these walls is midway between the temperature of room air and that of air within the incubator (Fig. 4-6). The cool walls induce radiant heat loss from the infant. The colder the nursery, the cooler the incubator walls, and consequently the greater the rate of radiant loss. *Heat loss by radiation is independent of the temperature of circulating air in the incubator.* A significant disadvantage of contemporary incubators is their inability to control radiant heat loss, and most of the thermal loss in small babies is by radiation. This deficiency is critical to microenvironmental control for small infants, particularly those below 1250 grams. One solution is to provide an inner plastic heat shield that minimizes radiant losses. The baby is surrounded by an inner removable second wall that serves as the closest (primary) surface to which heat can be lost by radiation. If this surface is warmed by circulating incubator air, radiant losses are far less than to the cool outer wall. The heat shield is shaped like a cylinder that has been cut in half longitudinally (Fig. 4-7). The warmed plastic cylinder is virtually the same temperature as incubator air. Surrounding the baby with a warm primary surface eliminates radiant loss to the cool outer wall.

Another deficiency of incubator design is dependence on a reservoir of water for humidity. Stagnant water is a suitable medium for the growth of "water bugs," most notable of which is *Pseudomonas aeruginosa* (Chapter 12). With a few exceptions involving very small infants weighing less than 1250 grams, humidification of incubator air is not essential; the water reservoir can be eliminated.

Readings from a thermometer located

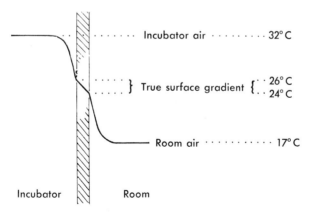

Fig. 4-6. Temperature of incubator wall at 24° to 26° C (75.2° to 78.8° F) is approximately midway between incubator air temperature of 32° C (89.6° F) and nursery air temperature of 17° C (70° F). Radiant loss from body surface increases as temperature of incubator wall decreases as a result of air temperature in the nursery. (Modified from Hey, E. N., and Mount, L. E.: Arch. Dis. Child. **42:**75, 1967.)

in a corner of the incubator are lower than air temperature that immediately surrounds the infant. Better incubator design requires that the thermometer should therefore be located closer to the baby.

Incubator temperature is controlled either by an on-and-off (all-or-none) output of heat or by a gradual (partial) increase or decrease in the output of heat, depending on skin temperature. The set point for activation of the heater is adjustable. A skin temperature of 36.4° C (97.5° F) is usually chosen. In the partial response device, heat output diminishes gradually as skin temperature rises farther above the set point; it increases gradually as skin temperature falls below it. The grad-

ual response eliminates fluctuations in incubator temperature that are characteristic of the all-or-none response mechanism. The partial response mechanism was introduced after abrupt rises and falls in ambient incubator temperature were observed to be associated with an increased incidence of apneic episodes in premature infants. Most of the apneic episodes occurred in relation to sudden rises in incubator temperature.

Cold drafts from air-conditioning vents should not strike directly on incubator walls, nor should incubators be near cold windows. Recurrent or relentless cold stress due to large radiant heat losses can thus be avoided.

Water in reservoirs is required for only

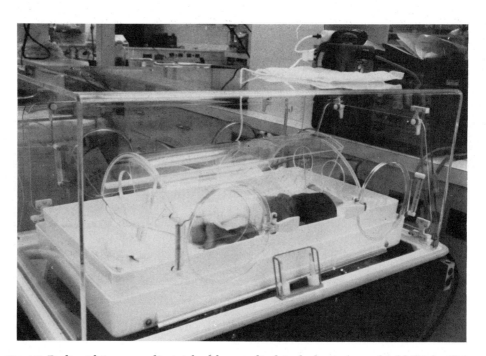

Fig. 4-7. Radiant losses are diminished by a cylindrical plastic heat shield ("igloo") in the incubator. Surrounding air warms igloo walls, thereby minimizing the temperature gradient between body surface and primary radiant surface. Half of the curved wall slides backward over the remaining half to provide convenient accessibility to the baby.

a small number of infants, and if the reservoir is utilized, water should be changed frequently, preferably every 8 hours.

With a heat-sensing probe on the abdomen, the infant should never be prone, since the resultant false registration of high skin temperature diminishes or eliminates activation of the heater. The result may be a very cold baby.

Heat gain is possible from protracted exposure of the incubator to sunlight from a window. Serious elevation of core temperature may ensue. Oxygen consumption increases in response to hyperthermia. The metabolic penalties are similar to those of hypothermia and are often even more dangerous.

Radiant-heated beds. The open bed provides indispensable accessibility for resuscitation during acute emergencies and for sustained treatment of gravely ill infants. Heat emanates from an overhead radiant source that is servocontrolled to abdominal skin temperatures in a like manner as incubators. Heat loss by convection may pose a serious problem for babies on such open tables. Airflow in the nursery often makes if difficult or impossible to maintain normal rectal temperatures, especially in the smallest babies. The skin probe must be covered with a foam plastic pad to prevent spurious registration of high temperatures that are in fact due to the direct effect of radiant heat on the sensor itself. The

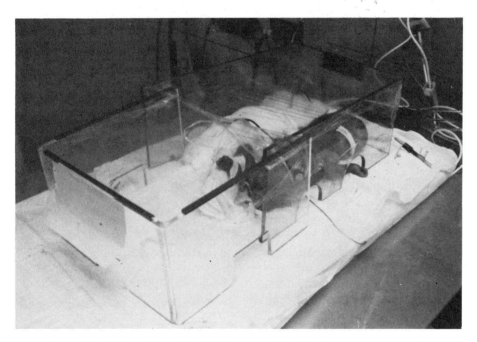

Fig. 4-8. The walls of these "windshields" are 8 inches high. Two separate three-sided structures surround upper and lower halves of the baby for convenient accessibility. They are covered with disposable thin plastic sheets similar to Saran Wrap. Insensible water loss is diminished because normal skin temperature of babies can be maintained using half the quantity of radiant energy required in the absence of these covers.

baby remains hypothermic because the sensor, having been warmed directly by radiant heat rather than by abdominal skin, discontinues the output of heat. In these circumstances, the sensor is heated, but the baby remains cold. We use a foam pad covered with aluminum foil to shield the sensor from the heat source, and it is apparently more effective than the foam pad without an aluminum cover.

The principal disadvantage of the radiant warmer is its well-known effect on insensible water loss (IWL). IWL is considerably greater on a radiant-heated bed than in an incubator. Although the measured quantities of lost water varied from one study to another, greater losses in radiant heat were unequivocally demonstrated in all of them. The amounts of water lost on the radiant bed varies from 25 ml/kg/24 hr to 84 ml/kg/24 hr. Losses are considerably higher in the smallest infants, particularly those who weigh less than 1500 grams. It is necessary therefore, to administer larger quantities of intravenous fluids to infants who are managed on the open beds. Failure to do so will result in severe, life-threatening dehydration.

We have recently found that the use of an inexpensive, specially constructed heat shield (Fig. 4-8) diminishes IWL significantly, thus minimizing the volume of intravenous fluid required for optimal hydration. The shields are easily removed for accessibility; they cause little if any inconvenience in the performance of procedures. Our measurements have demonstrated that infants housed in these shields lose less water because their skin and core temperatures can be maintained with approximately half the amount of radiant energy otherwise required without shields, probably because of diminished convective heat losses. Continuous measurements a few centimeters from the baby revealed, as expected, that ambient temperatures were higher with the shield than without it.

Clinical assessment and management of the infant's thermal status

Traditional recordings of rectal and axillary temperatures for thermal monitoring of sick babies leave much to be desired. *Normal core temperature does not indicate thermal balance in a cold environment.* Axillary temperatures are often falsely high because of subjacent deposits of heated brown fat and because artifactual warmth is created by apposing skin of the inner arm and the upper chest wall.

The major concern in the assessment and management of body temperature is maintenance of normal heat balance at the lowest level of oxygen consumption. Metabolic rate increases rapidly in response to cold stress that is sensed by thermal receptors in the skin, particularly those over the face. The response does not await a drop in core temperature to become activated. Rather, to support core temperature, it is triggered early and rapidly by a change in the environment that is sensed by the skin. Rectal temperature may therefore be normal in the cold-stressed baby because metabolic hyperactivity compensates successfully for thermal losses. (Compare Figs. 4-4 and 4-5.) The increased metabolic rate is triggered by environmental changes that are perceived by thermal receptors in the skin. *When rectal temperature becomes subnormal, the thermal battle is lost; the baby cannot generate enough heat to maintain normal core temperature.*

As previously described, skin temperatures can indicate the state of oxygen consumption. Deviations sufficiently above (hyperthermia) or below (hypothermia) the normal range generally mean that oxygen consumption at the cellular level has increased. Skin temperature also indicates the appropriateness of environmental temperature. If skin temperature drops, cold stress is present; if it rises, hyperthermia exists. Small babies must be managed with abdominal skin temperature readings for variable lengths of time after birth (for over 2 months in the smallest).

Available data unequivocally demonstrate that thermal sensors of the face are more influential in activating increased metabolism than other nerve endings in the skin elsewhere over the body. When the environment is well heated below the neck, a baby whose facial environment is cool will react as if cold stressed. The practical importance of this observation relates to oxygen administration. *It is mandatory that oxygen supplied to a head hood be warmed.* Ambient temperature within the hood should be monitored and maintained at levels equal to the incubator. Furthermore, under no circumstances should oxygen be blasted onto an infant's face through a face mask or tube. The mask is appropriate only for tight application during resuscitation with a manually operated bag.

A significant quantity of heat is lost from the respiratory tract, particularly in infants who are tachypneic. Oxygen must be warmed and humidified, particularly for intubated babies. Dry oxygen causes significant evaporation from the extensive mucosal surface that lines the respiratory tract, and heat loss by this modality can be significant. Furthermore, evaporation may incur significant fluid losses from the respiratory tract.

Whether they are nurses, physicians, or attendants in any capacity, the neonate's best caretakers are his most protective ones. Unflagging attention to the environmental requirements of optimal heat balance is the essence of such protectiveness. In respect to temperament, training, continuous presence, and sphere of activity, no one is better equipped to perform this function than the neonatal nurse. Furthermore, if the nurse fails to perform it, quite likely no one else will.

REFERENCES

Abrams, R. M.: Thermal physiology of the fetus. In Sinclair, J. C., editor: Temperature regulation and energy metabolism in the newborn, New York, 1978, Grune and Stratton, Inc.

Adamsons, K., Jr.: The role of thermal factors in fetal and neonatal life, Pediatr. Clin. North Am. **13**:599, 1966.

Adamsons, K., Jr., and Towell, M. E.: Thermal homeostasis in the fetus and newborn, Anesthesiology **26**:531, 1965.

Adamsons, K., Jr., Gandy, G. M., and James, L. S.: The influence of thermal factors upon oxygen consumption of the newborn human infant, J. Pediatr. **66**:495, 1965.

Anagnostakis, D., Economou-Mavrou, C., Agathopoulas, A., and Matsaniotis, N.: Neonatal cold injury: evidence of defective thermogenesis due to impaired norepinephrine release, Pediatrics **53**:24, 1974.

Anonymous by request: Comment; speed of rewarming after postnatal chilling, J. Pediatr. **85**:551, 1974.

Aynsley-Green, A., Robertson, N. R. C., and Rolfe, P.: Air temperature recordings in infant incubators, Arch. Dis. Child. **50**:215, 1975.

Bruck, K.: Temperature regulation in the newborn infant, Biol. Neonate **3**:65, 1965.

Bruck, K: Heat production and temperature regulation. In Stave, U., editor: Perinatal physiology, New York, 1970, Plenum Publishing Corp.

Cross, K. W., and Stratton, D.: Aural temperature of the newborn infant, Lancet **2**:1179, 1974.

Dahm, L. S., and James, L. S.: Newborn temperature and calculated heat loss in the delivery room, Pediatrics **49**:504, 1972.

Day, R., Curtis, J., and Kelly, M.: Respiratory metabolism in infancy and in childhood, Am. J. Dis. Child. **65**:376, 1943.

Day, R. L., Caliguiri, L., Kamenski, C., et al.: Body temperature and survival of premature infants, Pediatrics **34**:171, 1964.

Fanaroff, A. A., Wald, M., Gruber, H. S., and Klaus, M. H.: Insensible water loss in low birth weight infants, Pediatrics **50**:236, 1972.

Glass, L., Silverman, W. A., and Sinclair, J. C.: Effect of the thermal environment on cold resistance and growth of small infants after the first week of life, Pediatrics **41**:1033, 1968.

Hahn, P., and Skala, J. P.: Nonshivering heat production in the newborn. In Scarpelli, E. M., and Cosmi, E. V., editors: Reviews in perinatal medicine, New York, 1978, Raven Press.

Harned, H. S., Jr., and Ferreiro, J.: Initiation of breathing by cold stimulation: effects of change in ambient temperature on respiratory activity of the full-term fetal lamb, J. Pediatr. **83**:663, 1973.

Hey, E. N.: The relation between environmental temperature and oxygen consumption in the newborn baby, J. Physiol. **200**:589, 1969.

Hey, E. N., and Mount, L.: Temperature control in incubators, Lancet **2**:202, 1966.

Hey, E. N., and Mount, L. E.: Heat losses from babies in incubators, Arch. Dis. Child. **42**:75, 1967.

Hull, D., and Smales, O. R. C.: Heat production in the newborn. In Sinclair, J. C., editor: Temperature regulation and energy metabolism in the newborn, New York, 1978, Grune and Stratton, Inc.

Kajtar, P., Jequier, E., and Prod'hom, L. S.: Heat losses in newborn infants of different body size measured by direct calorimetry in a thermoneutral and a cold environment, Biol. Neonate **30**:55, 1976.

Levison, H., Linsao, L., and Swyer, P. R.: A comparison of infra-red and convective heating for newborn infants, Lancet **2**:1346, 1966.

Mestyan, J., Jarai, I., Bata, G., and Fekete, M.: The significance of facial skin temperature in the chemical heat regulation of premature infants, Biol. Neonate **7**:243, 1964.

Motil, K. J., Blackburn, M. G., and Pleasure, J. R.: The effects of four different radiant warmer temperature set-points used for rewarming neonates, J. Pediatr. **85**:546, 1974.

Oliver, T. K., Jr.: Temperature regulation and heat production in the newborn, Pediatr. Clin. North Am. **12**:765, 1965.

Perlstein, P. H., et al.: Apnea in premature infants and incubator-air-temperature changes, N. Engl. J. Med. **282**:461, 1970.

Perlstein, P. H., Hersh, C., Glueck, C. J., and Sutherland, J. M.: Adaptation to cold in the first three days of life, Pediatrics **54**:411, 1974.

Robinson, R. O., and Jones, R.: Advantages of overhead radiant heaters, Proc. Roy. Soc. Med. **70**:209, 1977.

Scopes, J. W.: Metabolic rate and temperature control in the human baby, Br. Med. Bull. **22**:88, 1966.

Scopes, J. W., and Ahmed, I.: Range of critical temperatures in sick and premature newborn babies, Am. J. Dis. Child. **41**:417, 1966.

Silverman, W. A.: Diagnosis and treatment; use and misuse of temperature and humidity in care of the newborn infant, Pediatrics **33**:276, 1974.

Silverman, W. A., et al.: The oxygen cost of minor changes in heat balance of small newborn infants, Acta Paediatr. Scand. **55**:294, 1966.

Silverman, W. A., and Sinclair, J. C.: Temperature regulation in the newborn infant, N. Engl. J. Med. **274**:146, 1966.

Silverman, W. A., Zamelis, A., Sinclair, J. C., and Agate, F. J.: Warm nape of the newborn, Pediatrics **33**:984, 1964.

Sinclair, J. C.: Heat production and thermoregulation in the small-for-date infant, Pediatr. Clin. North Am. **17**:147, 1970.

Sinclair, J. C.: Metabolic rate and temperature control. In Smith, C. A., and Nelson, N. M., editors: The physiology of the newborn infant, Springfield, Ill., 1976, Charles C Thomas, Publisher.

Stephenson, J. M., Du, J. N., and Oliver, T. K., Jr.: The effect of cooling on blood gas tensions in newborn infants, J. Pediatr. **76**:848, 1970.

Swyer, P. R.: Heat loss after birth. In Sinclair, J. C., editor: Temperature regulation and energy metabolism in the newborn, New York, 1978, Grune and Stratton, Inc.

Williams, P. R., and Oh, W.: Effects of radiant warmer on insensible water loss in newborn infants, Am. J. Dis. Child. **128**:511, 1974.

Wu, P. Y. K., and Hodgman, J. E.: Insensible water loss in preterm infants: changes with postnatal development and non-ionizing radiant energy, Pediatrics **54**:704, 1974.

Yashiro, K., Adams, F. H., Emmanouilides, G. C., and Mickey, M. R.: Preliminary studies on the thermal environment of low-birth-weight infants, J. Pediatr. **82**:991, 1973.

CHAPTER 5

Significance of the relationship of birth weight to gestational age

Until 20 years ago, birth weight was considered the most reliable index of an infant's maturity. If an infant weighed less than 2500 grams, he was assumed to be premature; if his weight exceeded 2500 grams, he was considered mature. This approach implied that intrauterine growth rates were similar for all fetuses and that birth weight could thus be utilized as an accurate expression of gestational age. However, a considerable amount of data have accumulated to demonstrate the inaccuracy of this assump-

103

tion. Regardless of birth weight, an infant is in fact premature if he is born before term. Birth weight less than 2500 grams simply indicates that growth was incomplete, whether due to a short gestational age, impairment of intrauterine growth, or both. These separate considerations of weight (for assessment of growth) and gestational age (for assessment of maturity) have resulted in a more meaningful classification in which important biologic correlates are identifiable.

CLASSIFICATION OF INFANTS BY BIRTH WEIGHT AND GESTATIONAL AGE
Terminology

In 1961 the World Health Organization recommended that babies who weigh less than 2500 grams be designated as "low birth weight" (LBW) infants. This definition eliminated all implications of prematurity. It disregards gestational age. Definitions of gestational age correspondingly disregard any consideration of birth weight. A *premature (preterm)* infant is born before the end of the thirty-seventh week. A *term* infant is born between the beginning of the thirty-eighth week and the completion of the forty-first week. A *postmature (postterm)* baby is born at the onset of the forty-second week or anytime thereafter. Gestational weeks are calculated from the first day of the last menstrual period (LMP). These definitions of fetal age have nothing to do with weight, length, head circumference, or other measurements of fetal size. However, the relationship of these physical attributes to calculated age is of great importance.

The various types of low birth weight infants (under 2500 grams) are as follows:

1. Infants whose rate of intrauterine growth was normal at the moment of birth. They are small only because labor began before the end of 37 weeks. *These premature infants are appropriately grown for gestational age (AGA).*

2. Infants whose rate of intrauterine growth was slowed and who were delivered at or later than term (end of 37 weeks). These term or postterm (postmature) infants are undergrown for gestational age. *They are small-for-dates or small for gestational age (SGA).*

3. Infants whose in utero growth was retarded and who, in addition, were delivered prematurely. These premature infants are small by virtue of both early delivery and impaired intrauterine growth. *They are small-for-dates, premature infants.*

The corollary of 2500 grams for low birth weight is 4000 grams for high birth weight. Optimum weight for the lowest perinatal mortality is between 3500 and 4000 grams. Above the latter level, mortality begins to increase, and on that basis, the weight of 4000 grams serves to delineate high birth weight infants. *Babies are considered large for gestational age (LGA), at any weight, when they fall above the ninetieth percentile on the intrauterine growth curves.*

Intrauterine growth curves

The intrauterine growth chart offers a simple and effective way of assessing growth and maturity of newborn infants. It was derived by plotting birth weights of a large neonatal population against the weeks of gestation to show the range of expected weights for each week. The graph lists birth weights vertically and weeks of gestation horizontally. Data from the Colorado intrauterine growth chart are most widely used for this purpose (Fig. 5-1). They plot birth weights from 400 to 4000 grams against gestational ages from 24 to 43 weeks or more. Five curves are drawn across the charts,

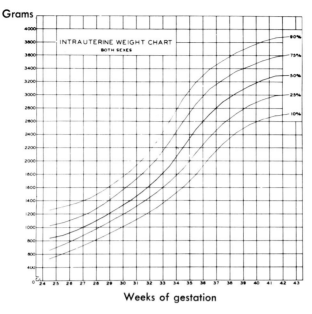

Fig. 5-1. Distribution of birth weights according to gestational age among neonates studied in Denver, Colorado. (From Lubchenco, L. O., Hansman, C., Dressler, M., and Boyd, E.: Pediatrics **32**:793, 1963.)

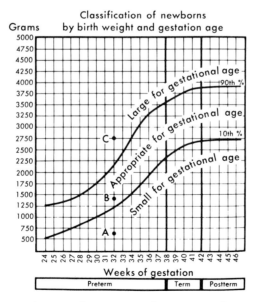

Fig. 5-2. Intrauterine growth status for gestational ages, according to appropriateness of growth. Points *A*, *B*, and *C* (added to original diagram by author) correspond to babies shown in Fig. 5-3. See text for explanation. (From Battaglia, F. C., and Lubchenco, L. O.: J. Pediatr. **71**:159, 1967.)

dividing the population into tenth, twenty-fifth, fiftieth, seventy-fifth, and ninetieth percentiles. Weights below the tenth percentile curve are observed in only 10% of the population for any given gestational age. These infants are considered undergrown (small-for-dates). Weights above the ninetieth percentile curve are higher than the remaining 90% of the population, and these infants are overgrown (large-for-dates). Babies who are categorized between the tenth and ninetieth percentiles are appropriately grown for their gestational age. All infants below 2500 grams, as well as any high-risk baby, regardless of weight, should be evaluated with these or similar graphs soon after admission to the nursery. Consider a neonate you have admitted who weighs 2000 grams at 40 weeks. According to the growth chart this mature infant is well below the tenth percentile, presumably as a consequence of intrauterine growth retardation. He is thus at risk for several disorders that require special measures.

Fig. 5-2 simplifies and extends the graph that is shown in Fig. 5-1 and is generally used instead. It delineates only the tenth and ninetieth percentiles, thereby dividing infants into small, appropriate, or large for gestational age. At the bottom of the chart the weeks of gestation are divided into categories of preterm (through the thirty-seventh week), term (38 through 41 weeks), and postterm (above 42 weeks). Plotting an infant's weight and gestational age on this chart demonstrates that growth is appropriate, excessive, or diminished for age and that the baby is either premature, term, or postmature.

Interpretation of growth curve data

An infant whose weight is appropriate for gestational age has presumably grown at a normal rate in utero, whether the birth was premature, term, or postmature. Preterm babies whose weights are between the tenth and ninetieth percentiles are appropriately grown but small because normal intrauterine growth was interrupted by early onset of labor. If these same premature infants are below the tenth percentile for birth weight, they are small for gestational age as well. Consider, for instance, a 1500-gram infant whose gestational age is 36 weeks. According to the intrauterine growth charts, this infant is below the tenth percentile for birth weight at that age and is thus clearly undergrown. Demeanor, appearance, and course in the nursery will differ considerably from those of an appropriately grown infant of the same size who is born at 31 weeks.

An infant who is small for gestational age (small-for-dates) has presumably grown at a retarded rate in utero, regardless of age at birth. Although this phenomenon may occur at any gestational age, most small-for-dates infants are born at or close to term. Inspection of the intrauterine growth chart reveals that at term most infants who are small for gestational age weigh less than 2500 grams. At first glance these babies may appear prematurely born. At our institution 40% of all low birth weight infants are born at or near term. They are thus mature small-for-dates babies; yet according to the old concept, which interpreted weight and age interchangeably, they would have been considered premature infants. The unique attributes of small-for-dates infants are discussed in more detail later in this chapter.

Infants who are large for gestational age have presumably grown at an accelerated rate during intrauterine life. Less is known about them than the small-for-dates babies. Infants of diabetic mothers

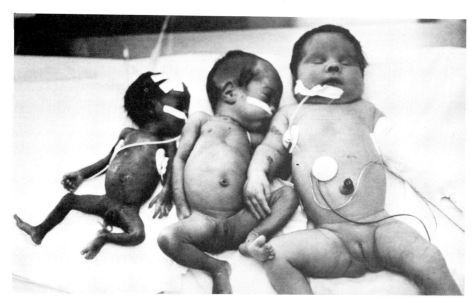

Fig. 5-3. Three babies, same gestational age, weigh 600, 1400, and 2750 grams, respectively, from left to right. They are plotted on Fig. 5-2 at points *A*, *B*, and *C*.

are characteristically large for gestational age (p. 135), but they constitute a minority of all oversized babies. Inaccurately short estimates of gestational age are probably responsible for mistaken classification of many of these infants, although the frequency of these errors has not been documented (p. 135).

Fig. 5-3 shows three infants of different sizes who were born at 32 gestational weeks. From left to right, their birth weights were 600, 1400, and 2750 grams, respectively. The largest baby is the infant of a diabetic mother, and the two small babies are twins delivered of a toxemic mother. On the growth curves in Fig. 5-2, points *A*, *B*, and *C* represent each of the infants on the 32-week line at their respective weights. At the same age, they are, respectively, small *(A)*, appropriate *(B)*, and large *(C)* for gestational age. Their clinical problems vary because their intrauterine growth problems were produced by diverse etiologies.

The smallest baby is grossly malnourished, probably by virtue of impaired placental circulation. The middle baby is small only because of premature delivery. Her growth, which was progressing at a normal rate, was interrupted by her birth. The largest baby was growing more rapidly than normal in utero, as is characteristic of most diabetic pregnancies. These problems in management, as well as the mechanisms by which babies of different size emerge at the same gestational age and by which babies of equal size emerge at different gestational ages, are discussed later in this chapter.

PRENATAL ESTIMATION OF GESTATIONAL AGE
History of pregnancy; maternal examinations

Estimation of gestational age has traditionally involved counting the weeks that have elapsed since the first day of the last menstrual period (LMP); in the majority of instances this procedure is still reasonably reliable. Accuracy of historic data is thus totally dependent on the mother's recall. A valid history is best obtained early in pregnancy, when recall of the LMP is more likely to be accurate. The mother's history should not be underestimated; properly taken, it is valid in at least 75% to 85% of patients. For some women, accurate dating of LMP is virtually impossible. Irregular menses in the nonpregnant state frequently complicate the calculations, or the interval between pregnancies is so short that a normal menstrual pattern has yet to be reestablished. In nursing mothers, menstruation may not resume for months after the end of pregnancy. Another cause of miscalculation is the occurrence of postconceptional bleeding, which is often misinterpreted as a menstrual period, thereby erroneously shortening the calculated gestational age.

The obstetrician utilizes certain physical milestones in pregnancy to estimate fetal age. The height of the uterine fundus above the symphysis pubis provides a good indication of the length of pregnancy. It varies from 25 cm above the symphysis at 26 gestational weeks to approximately 33 cm in the thirty-eighth week. Other useful indications are the first maternal perception of fetal movement at approximately 16 weeks and the perception of fetal heartbeats at approximately 20 weeks. If weekly prenatal visits were scheduled between 18 and 22 weeks (contrary to current practice), the initial appearance of fetal heart tones could be dated more precisely, possibly increasing the accuracy of fetal age calculations.

Prenatal tests for maturity

Estimation of fetal maturity in utero by analysis of amniotic fluid and by other means is important in troubled pregnancies that may require a rapid decision regarding cesarean section. This is particularly true of pregnancies complicated by diabetes and other chronic illnesses in which fetal distress may be indicated by falling maternal levels of urinary estriol (p. 16). In these circumstances the pregnancy must be terminated if fetal survival is in doubt, but on the other hand, the more premature the fetus, the less are the chances of extrauterine survival. Assessment of fetal age is therefore important. Discussion of prenatal evaluation is presented in Chapter 1. It should be reviewed for a better understanding of the application of prenatal data to the postnatal problems discussed in this chapter. In amniotic fluid a creatinine level over 1.8/100 ml generally correlates well with a gestational age of 36 weeks or more (p. 12), assuming that maternal creatinine is normal. High levels in the mother may elevate those of amniotic fluid. L/S ratios are valuable for the estimation of pulmonary maturity and for prediction of subsequent development of hyaline membrane disease (p. 12). At 35 or 36 weeks this ratio rises as lecithin concentration increases. If the L/S ratio is 2 or more, hyaline membrane disease is unlikely to occur after delivery; the fetus is probably more than 35 or 36 weeks of age. The L/S ratio only provides an estimate of lung maturity; it is not a measurement of fetal maturity.

Other means for prenatal estimation of maturity are fully described in Chapter 1. The measurement of biparietal (skull) diameter and circumferences of the trunk by ultrasound is currently the most pervasive. It is probably the most reliable for assessment of gestational age. Enumeration of fat-stained cells from amniotic fluid is also widely used for this purpose.

POSTNATAL ESTIMATION OF GESTATIONAL AGE

In the nursery, examination for certain external characteristics and neuromuscular signs is extremely valuable for assessment of maturity. Once learned, these observations can be made in a few minutes. The neonatal nurse should be familiar with these physical characteristics and neuromuscular responses. The system used in our nursery was reported by Dubowitz and co-workers in 1970. Their study utilized confirmatory observations by three nurses who had no previous experience with these examinations. Once instructed in the procedure, the nurses' appraisals were reliable, correlating well with those of the principal investigator.

Utilizing this system, an estimate of gestational age is usually accurate within

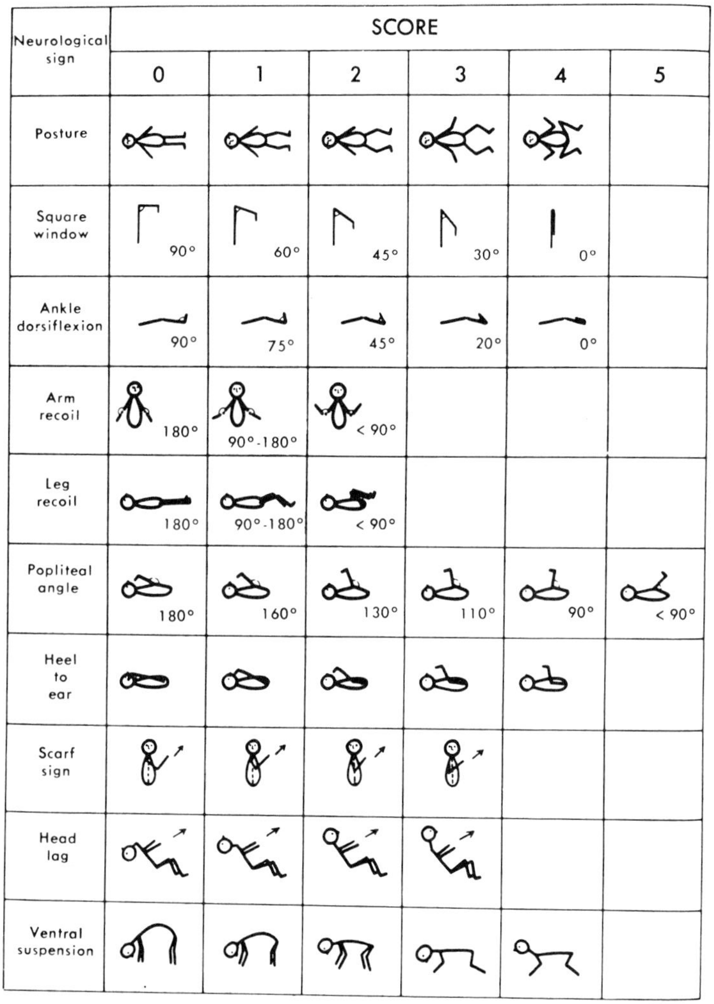

Neurological sign	SCORE					
	0	1	2	3	4	5
Posture						
Square window	90°	60°	45°	30°	0°	
Ankle dorsiflexion	90°	75°	45°	20°	0°	
Arm recoil	180°	90°-180°	< 90°			
Leg recoil	180°	90°-180°	< 90°			
Popliteal angle	180°	160°	130°	110°	90°	< 90°
Heel to ear						
Scarf sign						
Head lag						
Ventral suspension						

Fig. 5-4. Scoring system of neurologic signs for assessment of gestational age. (From Dubowitz, L. M. S., Dubowitz, V., and Goldberg, C.: J. Pediatr. **77**:1, 1970.)

SOME NOTES ON TECHNIQUES OF ASSESSMENT OF NEUROLOGIC CRITERIA
(for use in conjunction with Fig. 5-4 on p. 109)*

Posture: Observed with infant quiet and in supine position. Score 0: Arms and legs extended; 1: Beginning of flexion of hips and knees, arms extended; 2: Stronger flexion of legs, arms extended; 3: Arms slightly flexed, legs flexed and abducted; 4: Full flexion of arms and legs.

Square window: The hand is flexed on the forearm between the thumb and index finger of the examiner. Enough pressure is applied to get as full a flexion as possible, and the angle between the hypothenar eminence and the ventral aspect of the forearm is measured and graded according to diagrams (Fig. 5-4). (Care is taken not to rotate the infant's wrist while doing this maneuver.)

Ankle dorsiflexion: The foot is dorsiflexed onto the anterior aspect of the leg, with the examiner's thumb on the sole of the foot and other fingers behind the leg. Enough pressure is applied to get as full a flexion as possible, and the angle between the dorsum of the foot and the anterior aspect of the leg is measured.

Arm recoil: With the infant in the supine position the forearms are first flexed for 5 seconds, then fully extended by pulling on the hands, and then released. The sign is fully positive if the arms return briskly to full flexion (Score 2). If the arms return to incomplete flexion or the response is sluggish, it is graded as score 1. If they remain extended or are only followed by random movements, the score is 0.

Leg recoil: With the infant supine, the hips and knees are fully flexed for 5 seconds, then extended by traction on the feet, and released. A maximal response is one of full flexion of the hips and knees (Score 2). A partial flexion scores 1, and minimal or no movement scores 0.

Popliteal angle: With the infant supine and his pelvis flat on the examining couch, the thigh is held in the knee-chest position by the examiner's left index finger and thumb supporting the knee. The leg is then extended by gentle pressure from the examiner's right index finger behind the ankle and the popliteal angle is measured.

Heel to ear maneuver: With the baby supine, draw the baby's foot as near to the head as it will go without forcing it. Observe the distance between the foot and the head as well as the degree of extension at the knee. Grade according to diagram. Note that the knee is left free and may draw down alongside the abdomen.

Scarf sign: With the baby supine, take the infant's hand and try to put it around the neck and as far posteriorly as possible around the opposite shoulder. Assist this maneuver by lifting the elbow across the body. See how far the elbow will go across and grade according to illustrations. Score 0: Elbow reaches opposite axillary line; 1: Elbow between midline and opposite axillary line; 2: Elbow reaches midline; 3: Elbow will not reach midline.

Head lag: With the baby lying supine, grasp the hands (or the arms if a very small infant) and pull him slowly toward the sitting position. Observe the position of the head in

*From Dubowitz, L. M. S., Dubowitz, V., and Goldberg, C.: J. Pediatr. **77:**1, 1970.

relation to the trunk and grade accordingly. In a small infant the head may initially be supported by one hand. Score 0: Complete lag; 1: Partial head control; 2: Able to maintain head in line with body; 3: Brings head anterior to body.

Ventral suspension: The infant is suspended in the prone position, with examiner's hand under the infant's chest (one hand in a small infant, two in a large infant): Observe the degree of extension of the back and the amount of flexion of the arms and legs. Also note the relation of the head to the trunk. Grade according to diagrams (Fig. 5-4).

If score differs on the two sides, take the mean.

Table 5-1. Scoring system for external criteria*

External sign	Score†				
	0	1	2	3	4
Edema	Obvious edema of hands and feet; pitting over tibia	No obvious edema of hands and feet; pitting over tibia	No edema		
Skin texture	Very thin, gelatinous	Thin and smooth	Smooth; medium thickness; rash or superficial peeling	Slight thickening; superficial cracking and peeling especially of hands and feet	Thick and parchment-like; superficial or deep cracking
Skin color	Dark red	Uniformly pink	Pale pink; variable over body	Pale; only pink over ears, lips, palms, or soles	
Skin opacity (trunk)	Numerous veins and venules clearly seen, especially over abdomen	Veins and tributaries seen	A few large vessels clearly seen over abdomen	A few large vessels seen indistinctly over abdomen	No blood vessels seen

*From Dubowitz, L. M. S., Dubowitz, V., and Goldberg, C.: J. Pediatr. **77**:1, 1970; modified from Farr, V., et al.: Dev. Med. Child. Neurol. **8**:507, 1966.
†If score differs on two sides, take the mean.   *Continued.*

Table 5-1. Scoring system for external criteria—cont'd

External sign	Score				
	0	1	2	3	4
Lanugo (over back)	No lanugo	Abundant; long and thick over whole back	Hair thinning especially over lower back	Small amount of lanugo and bald areas	At least $1/2$ of back devoid of lanugo
Plantar creases	No skin creases	Faint red marks over anterior half of sole	Definite red marks over > anterior $1/2$; indentations over < anterior $1/3$	Indentations over mt anterior $1/3$	Definite deep indentations over > anterior $1/3$
Nipple formation	Nipple barely visible; no areola	Nipple well defined; areola smooth and flat, diameter < 0.75 cm	Areola stippled, edge not raised, diameter < 0.75 cm	Areola stippled, edge raised, diameter > 0.75 cm	
Breast size	No breast tissue palpable	Breast tissue on one or both sides, < 0.5 cm diameter	Breast tissue both sides; one or both 0.5 to 1.0 cm	Breast tissue both sides; one or both > 1 cm	
Ear form	Pinna flat and shapeless, little or no incurving of edge	Incurving of part of edge of pinna	Partial incurving whole of upper pinna	Well-defined incurving whole of upper pinna	
Ear firmness	Pinna soft, easily folded, no recoil	Pinna soft, easily folded, slow recoil	Cartilage to edge of pinna, but soft in places, ready recoil	Pinna firm, cartilage to edge; instant recoil	
Genitals Male	Neither testis in scrotum	At least one testis high in scrotum	At least one testis right down		
Female (with hips $1/2$ abducted)	Labia majora widely separated, labia minora protruding	Labia majora almost cover labia minora	Labia majora completely cover labia minora		

2 weeks. The accuracy of the method has been confirmed in studies primarily concerned with term infants. Other studies have confirmed accuracy in babies of very low birth weight (less than 1500 grams), large-for-dates and small-for-dates babies, and even in infants with major neurologic malformations. Measurements can be made any time up to 5 days after birth, but because the information is so important in management of sick infants, the examination is best performed within 24 hours after delivery. The accompanying notes on techniques describe the procedures for evaluating postures and primitive reflexes; Fig. 5-4 illustrates responses elicited and the scores assigned to each, and Table 5-1 describes external features and their scores. The scores from all the neuromuscular findings and from all the external characteristics comprise a maximum total of 70. Gestational age may be read from the corresponding score given in Table 5-2. A score of 50 thus corresponds to 37 gestational weeks, and a score of 20 corresponds to 29 weeks. The gestational age and birth weight may now be plotted on the intrauterine growth chart for the classification of an infant according to his growth characteristics and age at birth, as previously described. Proficiency depends on repeated careful performance of this entire procedure. With experience, a nurse can perform it accurately in 5 to 8 minutes.

Having estimated gestational age, the nurse can now plot this information against birth weight on the intrauterine growth chart for assessment of the infant's status as it relates to his age.

Several variations and abbreviations of the Dubowitz method have been reported since publication in 1970. In some instances, examination of external signs

Table 5-2. Dubowitz score/gestational age

Score	Weeks of gestation
0-9	26
10-12	27
13-16	28
17-20	29
21-24	30
25-27	31
28-31	32
32-35	33
36-39	34
40-43	35
44-46	36
47-50	37
51-54	38
55-58	39
59-62	40
63-65	41
66-69	42

alone is asserted to be as accurate as the combination of external and neuromuscular findings that are used in the Dubowitz procedure. Thus, data from an extensive study of 392 babies in England seem to indicate that observation of four external signs is all that is necessary to provide an accurate assessment. This method assigns scores for various gradations in skin texture, skin color, breast size, and ear firmness. However, difficulties arise in scoring the skin color of Asian and African infants. Furthermore, determination of gestational age of less than 30 weeks is not feasible because the essential observations cannot be scored.

More recently, an apparently more balanced system (Ballard score) includes six neuromuscular and six external physical signs (Fig. 5-5) in the assessment. This is in contrast to the ten neuromuscular and eleven external signs that comprise the Dubowitz method. The most useful items of the Dubowitz method are retained, and these are thought to be valid even in the presence of disease. According to the Ballard score, gestational age is assessable from 26 to 44 weeks. Evaluation can be performed any time up to a postnatal age of 42 hours, but peak reliability is at 30 to 42 hours after birth. In this study, the assessments of both scoring methods (Ballard and Dubowitz) are remarkably close to each other.

Simplification of the Dubowitz examination may be feasible. It is indeed tempting to adapt a shorter, time-saving methodology if a reasonable assurance of accuracy can be shown. The Ballard score needs further study and confirmation, however acceptable it may appear at present. A reduction in the number of items would seem to increase the risk of an invalid total score because inaccuracy of a single item then exerts a stronger influence. This is the principal disadvantage of any simplification. In general, the

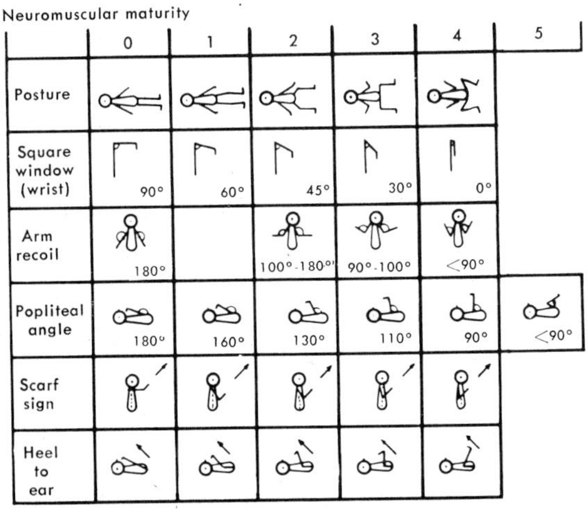

Neuromuscular maturity

	0	1	2	3	4	5
Posture						
Square window (wrist)	90°	60°	45°	30°	0°	
Arm recoil	180°		100°-180°	90°-100°	<90°	
Popliteal angle	180°	160°	130°	110°	90°	<90°
Scarf sign						
Heel to ear						

Physical maturity

Skin	Gelatinous red, transparent	Smooth pink, visible veins	Superficial peeling, &/or rash few veins	Cracking pale area rare veins	Parchment deep cracking no vessels	Leathery cracked wrinkled
Lanugo	None	Abundant	Thinning	Bald areas	Mostly bald	
Plantar creases	No crease	Faint red marks	Anterior transverse crease only	Creases ant. 2/3	Creases cover entire sole	
Breast	Barely percept.	Flat areola no bud	Stippled areola 1-2 mm bud	Raised areola 3-4 mm bud	Full areola 5-10 mm bud	
Ear	Pinna flat, stays folded	Sl. curved pinna; soft c slow recoil	Well-curv. pinna; soft but ready recoil	Formed & firm c instant recoil	Thick cartilage ear stiff	
Genitals ♂	Scrotum empty no rugae		Testes descending, few rugae	Testes down good rugae	Testes pendulous deep rugae	
Genitals ♀	Prominent clitoris & labia minora		Majora & minora equally prominent	Majora large minora small	Clitoris & minora completely covered	

Maturity rating

Score	Wks.
5	26
10	28
15	30
20	32
25	34
30	36
35	38
40	40
45	42
50	44

Fig. 5-5. Ballard Score (see text). (From Ballard, J. L.: J. Pediatr. 95:769, 1979.)

Dubowitz examination has been quite reliable when properly executed. A variety of abnormal infants have been satisfactorily assessed when compared with estimates of gestational age by maternal dates. These satisfactory assessments have involved babies who are undergrown or overgrown in utero, ill or well, with or without major neurologic malformations.

An interesting supplementary method for estimating gestational age entails viewing of the cornea with an ordinary (direct) ophthalmoscope. Pupils should be dilated and the ophthalmoscope should be set at +6 to +12 (black numbers) depending on the examiner's needs. The state of the fetal vascular network over the lens can be seen behind the cornea and can be correlated with gestational age. Fig. 5-6 illustrates the four grades of atrophy of this vasculature.

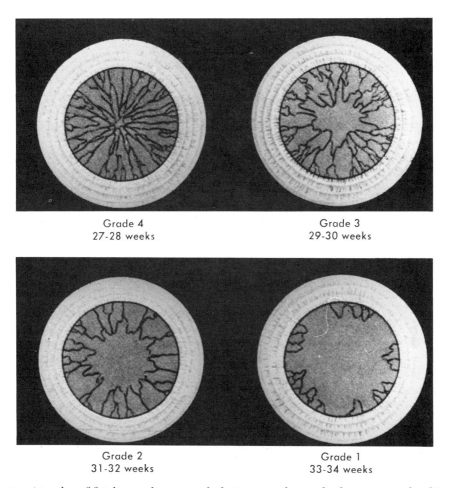

Grade 4
27-28 weeks

Grade 3
29-30 weeks

Grade 2
31-32 weeks

Grade 1
33-34 weeks

Fig. 5-6. Atrophy of fetal vascular network that covers the ocular lens as seen by direct ophthalmoscopy. Disappearance of vascular pattern is correlated with gestational age. (From Hittner, H. M.: J. Pediatr. **91:**455, 1977.)

At 27 to 28 weeks (Grade 4), the vessels cover the entire surface of the lens (as viewed through the cornea and anterior chamber). At 29 to 30 weeks (Grade 3), the peripheral vessels are somewhat less dense and the central portion of the lens is now cleared of them. At 31 to 32 weeks (Grade 2), peripheral thinning and central clearing of vasculature are more extensive. At 33 to 34 weeks (Grade 1), only a few vessels are visible in the periphery. This examination should be performed during the first 48 hours after birth. The vessels may atrophy and disappear in a few days, even those that were Grade 4 at birth. In babies who are less than 27 weeks, the cornea is cloudy and visualization of the anterior chamber is thus precluded. After 34 weeks, the vascular network has disappeared completely; in some infants, only a few remnant strands are observable.

This superficial ophthalmoscopic examination may be useful in infants who are so severely ill that they cannot be evaluated for several days. The ophthalmoscopic method is obviously not intended to replace the more extensive examinations described in preceding paragraphs.

INTRAUTERINE GROWTH RETARDATION
Terminology

Intrauterine growth retardation is also referred to as dysmaturity, small-for-dates, small for gestational age, pseudoprematurity, and fetal or intrauterine malnutrition. We prefer to use the terms *small-for-dates, small for gestational age,* and *intrauterine growth retardation* interchangeably to indicate fetal undergrowth of any etiology. Although the word dysmaturity is used frequently in reference to a small but mature baby, it is not completely accurate; according to its word derivation, it denotes any abnormality of maturity, therefore implying that the baby may be either small or large for his age. The word pseudoprematurity is also unacceptable because it suggests that these small infants appear deceptively premature, which is not the case if they are born at or near term. Fetal, or intrauterine, malnutrition should be reserved for reference to growth retardation due to a deficient supply of nutrient from the mother to her fetus, thus excluding diminished growth that is caused by intrauterine infections such as rubella or that is associated with other congenital malformations (p. 124).

Cellular characteristics of growth-retarded infants

Normal cellular growth. Normal cellular growth progresses through three stages that blend into each other. Overall, growth is characterized by the initial production of nuclei by mitosis, followed by the laying down of cytoplasm. Stated differently, nuclei, and therefore DNA, are first produced, and they are responsible for the early growth of any organ. Organ enlargement that results from cell multiplication is called *hyperplasia.* As growth proceeds, each cell enlarges by the addition of cytoplasm. Organ growth due to cytoplasmic enlargement of existing cells is called *hypertrophy.*

DNA content of any organ can be measured accurately. The amount of DNA in a single nucleus for any given species is uniform. The total number of *cells* in any organ can be calculated by dividing the amount of DNA in a single nucleus into the total DNA determined for that organ. To determine the *average weight per cell,* one need only divide the total weight of the organ by the determined

Table 5-3. Cellular phases of growth

I	*Hyperplasia* (cell multiplication) Increased DNA (nuclei) *maximal* Increased protein (cytoplasm) *minimal*
II	*Hyperplasia* (cell multiplication) *Hypertrophy* (cell enlargement) Increased DNA (nuclei) *moderate* Increased protein (cytoplasm) *moderate*
III	*Hypertrophy* (cell enlargement) Increased protein (cytoplasm) *maximal* Increased DNA (nuclei) *minimal*

number of cells. The weight/DNA ratio varies from one normal stage of growth to the next, as hyperplasia evolves into hypertrophy. It indicates the amount of cytoplasm relative to DNA for each cell and also varies according to the type of growth retardation.

Data from experiments on rats demonstrate a good correlation between weight/DNA ratios and the normal growth stages. Presumably, these same phenomena are applicable to the human growth process. Table 5-3 summarizes the three stages of growth and the role of increments of DNA (new cells) and protein (cytoplasm and cell enlargement) in each.

During the first stage of growth, nuclei proliferate; cytoplasmic mass is minimal, being laid down at approximately the same rate as DNA. During this stage of pure hyperplasia, the weight/DNA ratio is unchanged.

The second stage of growth involves increased production of cytoplasm and decreased proliferation of nuclei (DNA). Existing cells enlarge by addition of cytoplasm, and the rate of cell multiplication declines. Hypertrophy and hyper-

plasia coexist, but the rate of hypertrophy is now greater. Therefore, the weight/DNA ratio increases, indicating an increase in cell size.

The third stage of growth involves increasing hypertrophy and even less hyperplasia. Existing cells continue to enlarge, fewer new cells are produced. Weight/DNA ratio now increases further, indicating that cell size is further increased.

The type of growth inpairment suffered by the embryo or the fetus depends on the stage of growth that is disrupted.

Impaired cellular growth. Mention has already been made of two different types of growth retardation, which may occur separately or simultaneously. The hypoplastic type of impairment involves insult to the embryo early in pregnancy, during the initial stage of growth. Because mitosis is impaired, fewer new cells are formed, organs are small, and organ weight is subnormal. The individual cells usually, but not always, have a normal amount of cytoplasm. The initial stage of growth (hyperplasia) is called the *critical period* because it is during this period that susceptibility to congenital malformations and permanent suboptimal growth is greatest. The period of hyperplasia varies in its schedule from one tissue to another. Fig. 5-7 illustrates the varying rates of hyperplasia among four different tissues. Cell multiplication of the brain is shown to virtually cease in infancy, while skeleton and muscle continue their hyperplasia through adolescence. In contrast, growth failure that begins later in pregnancy is associated with cellular characteristics that are quite different. The total number of cells in affected organs is normal or nearly so, but their size is diminished by virtue of reduced amounts of cytoplasm. Abnormally small

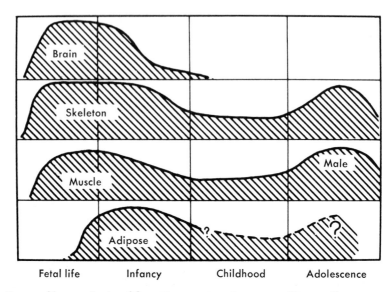

Fig. 5-7. Rates of hyperplasia of four tissues at various ages. New cells cease to appear in the brain during infancy. Note the later hyperplasia of muscle in adolescent males. (From Smith, D. W.: Growth and its disorders, Philadelphia, 1977, W. B. Saunders Co.)

organ size, in this instance, is thus largely the result of decreased cytoplasmic mass, rather than a diminished number of cells as in hypoplasia. Organ weight/DNA ratios correlate well with these anatomic observations. When the weight of an organ is subnormal only because it contains fewer cells (hypoplasia), the ratio of total organ weight to DNA content is similar to that of normally grown tissue if the number of nuclei and the amount of cytoplasm are diminished approximately to the same extent. On the other hand, if an abnormally small organ contains about the same quantity of nuclei (DNA) as a normally grown one, but the cytoplasmic mass is reduced, the ratio of total organ weight to DNA content is lower than normal. Cytoplasm is decreased, whereas the number of cell nuclei (DNA) is not.

Insult during the first stage of growth (hyperplasia) retards the rate of cell division, which results in fewer than normal cells in an organ that is smaller than normal. This type of impairment is not reversible, regardless of attempts to provide optimal nutrition later on. However, if the insult occurs during the hypertrophic stage of growth, individual enlargement of existing cells is impaired. The result is a smaller organ with a normal number of diminutive cells. This impairment is reversible to some extent. With proper nutrition, the cytoplasmic mass becomes normal, and the resultant cellular enlargement ultimately imparts normal size to the involved organ.

In animals (rats, monkeys, dogs, pigs), two types of malnutrition have been produced that are correlated with the distribution of organ involvement rather than with their cellular characteristics. Their significance is in the differing effects they exert on the brain. In one type, ligation of placental blood vessels during the latter third of pregnancy produced an asymmetric type of undergrowth. The overall weight of the rats was reduced by 20%; liver weight was reduced by as much as 50%; brain weight was unaffected. Furthermore, liver cells were devoid of glycogen. The ratio of brain weight to liver weight was inordinately large. *This brain-sparing pattern is characteristic of growth retardation that occurs in fetuses of toxemic women.* In them, uteroplacental vascular insufficiency is thought to contribute fundamentally to fetal undergrowth. The relationship of a relatively large brain to a small, glycogen-deprived liver is thought to be responsible for the high incidence of hypoglycemia in this type of growth retardation. Glucose demands are greater in the brain than in any other organ; glucose supply is principally from the liver. The demand for glucose by a relatively normal-sized brain on a diminutive liver is probably significant in the pathogenesis of hypoglycemia in babies of toxemic mothers.

A second type of malnutrition was produced in these animals. It entailed maternal protein deprivation throughout pregnancy, rather than interference with uteroplacental blood supply late in pregnancy. The resultant pattern of fetal undergrowth involved all organs to an equal extent. The growth failure was symmetric. Weight and DNA content were both reduced. The liver was not affected any more than any other organ and the brain was not spared.

Two types of fetal undergrowth were thus demonstrated in these animals; the one associated with an insult only during the last third of pregnancy was asymmetric, sparing the brain but profoundly affecting the liver and the rest of the body. The other, associated with insult throughout gestation, was symmetric, affecting all organs similarly, including the brain.

The available data demonstrate heterogeneity in the types of fetal undergrowth. These varying types of undergrowth may be responsible for the different outcomes that have been noted in human infants whose growth was retarded in utero. There seem to be two broad categories of intrauterine growth retardation: intrinsic and extrinsic. The intrinsic variety involves reduction of growth caused by factors that are operative within the fetus itself, such as severe chromosomal or genetic disorders, intrauterine infection due to rubella virus or cytomegalovirus, or normal hereditary small stature. The extrinsic variety entails diminution of maternal support to a fetus that otherwise would have been normal. Clincally, diminished maternal support is seen in uteroplacental vascular insufficiency including toxemia, essential hypertension, severe far-advanced diabetes mellitus, chronic renal disease, multiple pregnancy, recurrent bleeding late in pregnancy from a normally implanted placenta, and probably chronic, severe maternal malnutrition throughout gestation.

Data relating malnutrition to general body growth have stimulated an intense interest in the effects of this phenomenon on growth of the brain. Although the issue is far from resolved, evidence from observations in animals, as described previously, indicates that malnutrition during the period of most rapid brain growth is associated with permanent reduction in the total number of cells. In humans this critical period probably begins at about 15 gestational weeks. Estimates of the time of cessation of hyperplasia vary from 8 to 15 months after term. If this critical period does exist in humans, continuous malnutrition from prenatal into postnatal life may reduce cellular quantity irrevocably and thus permanently impair intellectual capacity. Suggestive evidence in support of this assumption was noted in a severely deprived population of low birth weight infants who died of undernutrition during the first few months of life. There was a 60% reduction in the expected number of brain cells. Among infants who were not of low birth weight, but whose lethal malnutrition was apparently confined to the postnatal period, there was only a 15% to 20% reduction in the number of brain cells. In the first group of infants, the combined effects of prenatal and postnatal deprivation may have resulted in a greater reduction of brain cells than in the second group, which suffered only from postnatal malnutrition. That malnutrition sustained in utero and into early infancy can permanently affect brain structure has indeed been well documented in animals. In humans the similarites are suggestive. The public health and socioeconomic implications of these data are awesome to contemplate if one accepts the hypothesis that malnutrition is a pervasive cause of subnormal mentality on the one hand and socially remediable on the other.

Factors associated with intrauterine growth retardation

Intrauterine growth is associated with a variety of disorders in the mother, fetus, and placenta. Most of these known factors are:

I. Maternal factors
    A. Low socioeconomic status
    B. Toxemia
    C. Hypertensive cardiovascular disease
    D. Chronic renal disease
    E. Diabetes (advanced)
    F. Malnutrition
    G. Cigarette smoking
    H. Heroin addiction
    I. Alcohol
    J. High-altitude residence
II. Fetal factors
    A. Multiple gestation
    B. Congenital malformation
    C. Chromosomal abnormality
    D. Chronic intrauterine infection
        1. Rubella
        2. Cytomegalovirus
III. Placental factors
    A. "Placental insufficiency"
    B. Vascular anastomoses (twin to twin)
    C. Single umbilical artery
    D. Abnormal cord insertion
    E. Separation
    F. Massive infarction
    G. ? Vascular anomalies and tumors
    H. ? Site of implantation
    I. Avascular chorionic villi

Maternal factors

Low socioeconomic status. Infant losses, like low birth weight itself, are profoundly influenced by maternal social class, parity, age, and, in particular, maternal height. These factors are interrelated and additive when statistical analysis is undertaken. At the happy end of the spectrum is the well-nourished white woman in her twenties, married to a business or a professional man, who is having her second baby. She is more likely than anyone else to have a well-grown, normal infant who weathers labor, delivery, and the immediate neonatal period with no difficulty. At the unhappiest extreme of the spectrum is a malnourished, short, black, adolescent mother who is unmarried, or perhaps a somewhat older woman who is a grand multipara (more than five previous pregnancies) married to an unskilled, often unemployed laborer. Women from these and similar backgrounds are more likely than anyone else to have low birth weight infants who cannot weather the perinatal experience alive or unscathed.

The association of small stature and poor fetal outcome is undoubtedly an indirect one. Aside from genetically determined short stature in any social class, the repeatedly observed association between height and social class suggests that short stature is in part the result of poor nutrition during the growth period in childhood. It thus follows that short stature merely signifies the many unfavorable circumstances that characterize poverty.

Toxemia. Toxemia of pregnancy (eclampsia, preeclampsia) is a maternal disorder that is frequently cited as a cause of fetal growth retardation. Its clinical attributes include hypertension, proteinuria, and edema. The cause of toxemia and the mechanisms by which the fetus is affected are unknown. There is agreement, however, that toxemia is a generalized vascular disorder in which diminution of uterine and placental blood flow impairs the function of the latter organ. Some evidence suggests that maternal malnutrition predisposes to toxemia. Among infants of toxemic mothers, mortality is increased. The principal abnormality in most babies who die is undergrowth for gestational age. Otherwise, a distinctive pattern of morphologic abnormalities has not been identified. Growth retardation is presumably a function of fetal malnutrition in which cellular abnormalities are characterized by diminished cytoplasmic mass in most organs, particularly the liver and adrenals. The brain is usually less affected than are other organs. The gross and microscopic appearance of tissues in these infants closely resembles that of infants who died during the first year of life from postnatally acquired malnutrition.

Hypertension and chronic renal disease. Hypertension and chronic renal disease exert influences on fetal growth that are similar to those of toxemia.

Diabetes (advanced). Most diabetic women (class A or B; see classification on p. 307) deliver large-for-dates babies who may nevertheless be born prematurely. However, advanced maternal diabetes involves generalized vascular damage that impairs normal placental blood flow. The woman with advanced (early onset) diabetes is more likely to give birth to a small-for-dates infant rather than a large one, particularly if the diabetes has significantly affected her kidneys.

Malnutrition. Evidence for the adverse fetal effects of maternal malnutrition is strongly suggested in a large number of studies. Severe undernutrition in the human female does result in an increased incidence of early abortions or in failure to conceive. The acute shortage of food in Holland during World War II was studied for its effects on birth weight. The average maternal weight gain during pregnancy fell from approximately 25 pounds in normal times to 5 pounds during the period of famine, and the mean birth weight of offspring was reduced by 7%. On the other hand, in circumstances of improved nutrition, there was an approximate 10% increment in birth weight at the end of 20 postwar years in Japan, during which severe poverty was replaced by relative affluence. The studies in Holland and Japan showed changes in mean birth weights, as related to severe changes in economic conditions, but weight is a crude end point compared to sophisticated methodology in which cell quantity and protein/DNA ratios are determined. These and other sensitive procedures may produce more precise data in the future for better definition of the fetal effects of maternal malnutrition. The nature of the consistently positive association between poverty and low birth weight has not been satisfactorily explained. That long-standing maternal malnutrition is the predominant cause of fetal undergrowth in low socioeconomic populations is quite likely. Results of animal experiments strongly suggest a significant role of maternal malnutrition in faulty fetal growth. Maternal undernutrition has been shown to impair cellular growth in the human placenta. As a result, these placentas are smaller than those of normally nourished women. The growth-limiting effect on the placenta is apparently most profound in the villi. It is possible that these anatomic subnormalities exert a functional effect by reducing the total capacity of the placenta to transfer nutrient material to the growing fetus.

Epidemiologic data in humans are strongly suggestive. There is widespread belief that fetal growth is influenced not only by maternal nutritional status during pregnancy, but by prepregnancy status as well. The rate of maternal weight gain during pregnancy seems to be related to infant birth weight and length. Furthermore, in nutritionally deprived populations, enhanced intake during pregnancy is associated with a significant increase in mean birth weight.

Cigarette smoking. Among moderate smokers, the incidence of small-for-dates babies is twice that of nonsmokers; among heavy consumers it is three times as great. The end result is related to the number of cigarettes smoked and the duration of the insult. Birth weight and body length are reduced. At 7 years of age, children of smoking gravidas are shorter than controls and have a higher incidence of educational retardation, regardless of social class, maternal age, or parity. The statistical association of maternal smoking and the incidence of intrauterine growth is among the most direct and unequivocal of all the maternal factors thus far scrutinized for this purpose. There is evidence that fetal undergrowth does not occur if the mother ceases smoking at the onset of pregnancy. There is also evidence that consumption of as few as five cigarettes a day may impair fetal growth. The mechanism by which smoking impairs fetal growth has not been unequivocally demonstrated, although several have been suggested. The blood level of carbon monoxide is elevated in affected infants at birth, and therefore carboxyhemoglobin concentration is higher than normal because carbon monoxide has a high affinity for hemoglobin. Less hemoglobin is available for oxygen transport; it is thus possible that affected fetuses are chronically hypoxic. This could account for an impaired rate of intrauterine growth. It has also been suggested that placental vasospasm reduces blood flow, thereby interfering with the transmission of nutrients. The transplacental passage of toxic products of cigarettes has also been proposed as an important consideration. Some authors have concluded that suppression of the smoking mother's appetite exerts the most significant negative influence on fetal growth.

Heroin addiction. In some urban hospitals the incidence of addicted babies from maternal addiction is as high as one in fifty deliveries. The threats to survival of the fetus and neonate are multiple, particularly when one considers the daily life most addicts must resort to if their drug need is to be met. Generally, about half the babies born of maternal addicts are low birth weight infants; 40% of these infants are small-for-dates, and 60% are appropriately grown premature infants. Undergrown offspring of addicted mothers are small by virtue of reduced numbers of organ cells, indicating early growth impairment of the hypoplastic variety. The effect of heroin and morphine is probably independent of the malnutrition that is so frequent among addicts. Intrauterine growth deficiency has been observed among ex-addicts and has been demonstrated in animal experiments. The effect of narcotics therefore seems to persist beyond the period of addiction. The incidence of fetal undergrowth among heroin addicts has been shown to be reduced somewhat by the administration of methadone instead.

Alcohol. Maternal alcohol consumption causes acute effects in the infant immediately after birth; it also causes the chronic effects of fetal undergrowth and malformations (fetal alcohol syndrome). *Acute toxicity* consists of withdrawal symptoms (agitation, hyperactivity, tremors, seizures) up to 72 hours in duration, followed by lethargy for 24 to 48 hours. Subsequently the infant is normal. Alcohol is often detected in the infant's breath soon after birth. Acute symptoms occur in the infant because alcohol freely crosses the placenta. Chronic maternal alcoholism is associated with the *fetal alcohol syndrome.* In addition to fetal wastage, maternal alcoholism causes severe growth deficiency and a constellation of characteristic structural defects. These consist of microcephaly, short palpebral fissures and microphthalmia, epicanthal folds, micrognathia, malformed and immobile joints, dislocation of the hips, cardiac malformations, and malformation of the brain. Severe or mild mental retarda-

tion occurs in almost half the infants. Less profound effects have been reported in babies who are apparently only growth retarded. Perinatal mortality is approximately 20%.

High altitude. Residence at high altitudes may be related to lower birth weight of offspring, presumably as a function of lower oxygen tension. There is some reason to doubt this relationship, since adults adjust satisfactorily to high altitudes by increasing the oxygen-carrying capacity of blood. Furthermore, large changes in maternal arterial P_{O_2} cause only small ones in the fetus. Nevertheless, at least a superficial association between altitude and birth weight at term has been demonstrated. The median birth weight at term in Lake County, Colorado (altitude 10,000 feet), was 3.07 kg. Approximately 30% of babies in this community were 2500 grams or less at birth, whereas the national average for low birth weight was 10%. In Denver, at 5000 feet, the median birth weight was 3.29 kg, and in Baltimore, virtually at sea level, it was 3.32 kg. These figures suggest a relationship between high altitude and retarded fetal growth.

Fetal factors

Multiple gestation. Most twins have a subnormal rate of growth late in gestation. This pattern is not unlike the decelerated growth rate in normal singletons, which begins at 36 to 38 weeks and is sustained for several days after birth. This effect is more pronounced in twins, and it begins earlier, at approximately 35 weeks. In either case the slowed rater of growth has been attributed to progressive diminution in the effective transfer of nutrient substances across the placenta, perhaps as a function of placental aging. Tissue abnormalities in twins seem to correlate with the prevalent impression that nutritional deficiency late in pregnancy is responsible for their small size. Subnormal organ weights are primarily a function of diminished cytoplasmic mass. The slowed growth rate of twins has also been ascribed to a lack of intrauterine space for both fetuses. The resultant small placentas can only support small fetuses. In the instance of discordant twins (large discrepency in birth weight and other body measurements), the smaller twin is nurtured by the smaller placenta. Ordinarily, fetal growth retardation is seen in twins if they are delivered after 35 weeks because, until then, their intrauterine growth parallels that of singletons.

Congenital malformations and chromosomal abnormalities. Anencephalic babies, infants with congenital heart disease, and infants with chromosomal abnormalities are small-for-dates as a result of hypoplasia. This variety of growth retardation originates early in pregnancy, when cell multiplication (hyperplasia) is the predominant factor in the growth process. Mitotic activity is impaired, and the number of cells is reduced. The incidence of a variety of major congenital anomalies is increased severalfold in small-for-dates infants compared with those who are appropriately grown for their age.

Chronic intrauterine infections. Impairment of growth is virtually a hallmark of fetal infections that begin early in pregnancy, particularly during the first trimester. Rubella is the best known example of this phenomenon; infections due to cytomegalovirus are similarly implicated. Hypoplastic growth retardation is identical to that described for congenital malformations. The details of these and other infections are discussed in Chapter 12.

Placental factors

General considerations. A great deal of mystery surrounds the role of placental pathology as an original cause of fetal undergrowth. When a placental lesion is identified, the question arises whether it is a manifestation of intrauterine growth retardation or whether it is the original source of fetal difficulty. Vascular anomalies, tumors, infarctions, and abnormal implantation sites have all been observed in association with isolated instances of fetal malnutrition, but apparently they are not responsible for a significant number of growth-retarded babies.

Placental insufficiency. Placental insufficiency is a conceptual term that is frequently invoked to explain the occurence of fetal malnutrition. It implies impaired exchange between mother and fetus, particularly suboptimal delivery of nutrient material and hormones to the fetus. A number of well-defined pathologic lesions in the placenta seem to be associated with placental insufficiency, but these lesions occur in only a few cases. They include extensive fibrosis, occlusion of fetal vessels in the villi, large hemangiomas, and early separation. Clinical entities such as advanced diabetes and toxemia are apparently associated with insufficiency of placental function. However, in most instances, dysfunction is not associated with morphologic abnormalities, and quite often there are no apparent maternal disorders. In any case, retarded fetal growth seems to be the end result of placental insufficiency, which is a concept that requires better definition than is presently available.

Intrauterine parabiotic syndrome (twin transfusion). The intrauterine parabiotic syndrome occurs in a small percentage of identical twins. It is a direct result of placental arteriovenous anastomoses that connect the circulations of both fetuses. Blood is transferred from artery to vein (twin to twin) when there is a connection between the arteries of one fetus and veins of the other. The discrepancy in blood volume between the two infants at birth may or may not be associated with weight differences in other body organs, depending on the duration and extent of fetofetal blood transfer. At birth the twin who received the blood (the "venous" twin) is intensely red because of polycythemia, whereas the donor twin (the "arterial" twin) is pale as a consequence of anemia. Increased blood volume in the polycythemic twin may cause congestive heart failure due to cardiac overload, and hyperbilirubinemia often occurs because there are more red cells available for breakdown (p. 281). The anemic twin may be in shock at birth if blood loss to his sibling was acute. A dramatic discrepancy in birth weight is usually but not always noted. Weight of the recipient twin may exceed that of the donor by as much as 50%, but in many instances a difference in size is less obvious. Polyhydramnios is often present in the recipient baby, whereas oligohydramnios is observed in the donor. The most important inital observation that the nurse can make is the difference in color between the twins. This is sometimes an urgent situation that requires immediate withdrawal of blood from the overloaded baby and a transfusion for shock in the anemic one.

Single umbilical artery. Presence of only one umbilical artery is often associated with a variety of major congenital anomalies, most commonly in the urinary tract. A number of investigators have reported single umbilical artery in 0.2% to 2% of all births. Among such infants, 20% to 65% have congenital anomalies. In the delivery room or in the nursery, the nurse should inspect the cut surface of the umbilical cord to ascertain the presence of two arteries and one vein. Observation of a single artery may lead to the early identification of major congenital malformations.

Physical findings of intrauterine growth retardation

On first inspection of many small-for-dates infants, several obvious physical characteristics immediately suggest the presence of impaired intrauterine growth. One is struck by the seemingly large head, but head circumference is actually normal or nearly so; it is the chest and abdominal circumferences that are reduced. The head merely appears large for the body. Apparently the brain was spared or less affected by the intrauterine insult, which probably had its inception relatively late in pregnancy. Since the ratio of brain mass to liver mass is large, hypoglycemia is likely to be present in such infants. It was largely the hypertrophic (third) stage of growth that was impaired; one would expect a normal number of cells (nuclei) and diminished cytoplasm in most organs. The weight/DNA ratio would be smaller than normal. Diminution of subcutaneous fat and loose, dry skin are prominent (Fig. 5-8). Even though the skin appears pale, half of these babies are polycythemic; their venous hematocrit may be greater than 60 vol %. In the extreme, muscle mass over the buttocks, thighs, and cheeks is also wanting. Since body length is not as diminished as subcutaneous fat, these infants often appear thin and long.

Fraternal twins are shown in Fig. 5-9; the longer is minimally undergrown, and the smaller is poorly grown. The paucity of subcutaneous fat in the small baby imparts a relatively long and thin appearance, whereas the head gives the illusion of being large. Longitudinal skin creases in the thighs indicate severe subcutaneous fat depletion, in contrast to the horizontal thigh creases of the larger baby, whose nutritional state is far better. Note the sparse hair of the small twin and the normal hair in the large one. The smaller baby is wide-eyed, presumably as a result of chronic hypoxia in utero. He appears alert compared with his sleepy sibling. The abdomen is sunken (scaphoid), rather than rounded as in the better-nourished baby. At birth the umbilical cord is thin, slightly yellow, dull, and dry in con-

trast to the normal cord, which is rotund, gray, glistening, and moist. Because all cords wither progressively after birth, their condition after 24 hours of age is of little diagnostic significance. The cords of small-for-dates babies wither more rapidly. Scalp hair is typically sparse; heavy hair growth is exceptional in growth-retarded babies, except in those who are postmature (p. 134). Skull sutures are frequently wide as a result of impaired bone growth. The anterior fontanelle, although large, is soft or sunken, thereby ruling out increased intracranial pressure as a cause of the widened su-

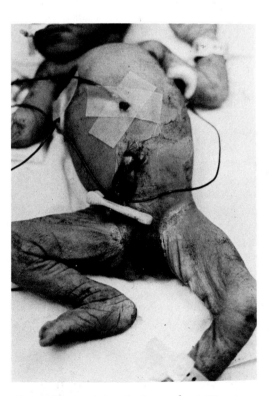

Fig. 5-8. Severe intrauterine malnutrition in a postterm baby. Diminished subcutaneous fat is in dramatic evidence at lower extremities. Cord is stained, thin, and dull. Body is thin and appears long, although length was normal.

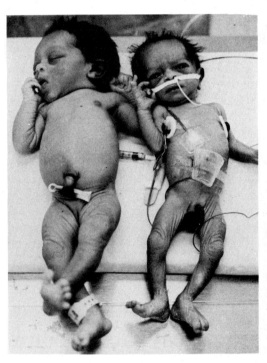

Fig. 5-9. Fraternal twins. The smaller infant is typically malnourished. Thin body gives a large appearance to head, longitudinal skin creases in thighs are characteristic of diminished subcutaneous fat, and hair is sparse. Alert appearance is in contrast to sleepy sibling; the wide-eyed look indicates chronic intrauterine hypoxia.

tures. Ossification centers at the distal femur and proximal tibia are frequently absent in term babies who are undergrown (Fig. 1-17). Most of these infants are more active than expected for their low weight. The vigor of their cry may be particularly impressive. Often, an alert, wide-eyed facial expression is combined with repetitive tongue thrusts that simulate a sucking motion. The overall impression of vigor and well-being is misguided, for these are signs of chronic marginal hypoxia in utero. Many of these babies convulse 6 to 18 hours later, particularly those whose anterior fontanelle is firm due to cerebral edema from intrauterine hypoxia. On the other hand, when perinatal asphyxia is severe, the baby is depressed, appearing flaccid and lethargic. Hypoglycemia produces similar symptoms.

Another type of growth retardation is seen in small-for-dates infants whose appearance is quite different from that just described. These babies, whose insult probably began early and was sustained throughout gestation, do not appear wasted. They are diminutive, but body members are of proportionate size. The head does not appear large for the trunk. The skin is not redundant, but it is thicker (the subcutaneous vascular pattern is obscure or absent) than expected for infants of the same size who are appropriately grown for their gestational age. They are generally quite vigorous and are much less likely to be hypoglycemic or polycythemic. These are hypoplastic babies in whom major malformations are present or in whom an early intrauterine infection occurred (rubella or cytomegalic inclusion disease). Their weight/DNA ratio is probably normal, although absolute weight is subnormal.

Two general types of fetal undergrowth are thus identifiable by body measurement and by reference to intrauterine growth curves (Table 5-4). In one type, the most common one, the insult seems to begin during the last trimester. These babies have a head circumference and body length within the normal percentiles, generally between the twenty-fifth and fiftieth, but their body weight is below the tenth percentile. *These infants are hypotrophic.* Associated maternal factors most frequently include toxemia, chronic hypertension, and chronic renal

Table 5-4. Clinical differences of hypoplastic and hypotrophic intrauterine growth retardation

Hypoplastic	Hypotrophic
Universal, proportionate diminution in size and weight; percentiles of head, length, and weight are similar	Selective, disproportionate diminution in size and weight; percentiles of head and length normal, for weight below tenth percentile
Subcutaneous fat appropriate for size; skin taut	Subcutaneous fat diminished for size; skin redundant
Congenital malformation frequent	Congenital malformation infrequent
Intrauterine, nonbacterial infection frequent	Intrauterine, nonbacterial infection rare
Hematocrit usually normal	Hematocrit often elevated
Hypoglycemia, hypoproteinemia uncommon	Hypoglycemia, hypoproteinemia common

disease. The second type probably begins early in pregnancy. It is characterized by equally distributed reduction in head circumference, body length, and weight. All these measurements fall below the tenth percentile. *These infants are hypoplastic.* Associated factors include intrauterine virus infection, chromosomal disorders, major congenital malformations, genetically small but otherwise well infants, and probably maternal malnutrition.

Predisposition to neonatal illness in small-for-dates babies

Thus far this chapter has been concerned with the fundamental characteristics, classification, and causes of fetal growth retardation. The diagnosis and treatment of certain neonatal illnesses are greatly facilitated by early identification of abnormal growth status. Clinical application of the concepts that have been discussed should reduce neonatal morbidity and mortality significantly, particularly when one considers that in low socioeconomic groups as many as 7% of all term infants are growth retarded. The incidence of undergrowth in premature infants is not known. At our facility this percentage represents more than 400 babies annually who must be identified to ensure proper management. The illnesses to which small-for-dates infants are vulnerable are discussed in the following paragraphs.

Perinatal asphyxia. Growth-retarded fetuses are often chronically hypoxic for variable periods prior to the onset of labor. Whereas healthy fetuses can withstand the asphyxia of normal birth and are well equipped to compensate for it after delivery, those who are chronically distressed can ill afford the insult. They are thus severely disturbed by normal labor, and at birth recovery is difficult or impossible without proper therapy. Apgar scores at 1 and 5 minutes reflect their depressed state. Appropriate management of these infants in the delivery room is often crucial to their survival. The details of resuscitation at birth are described in Chapter 3. Evaluation before the onset of labor with the oxytocin challenge test predicts the inability of the fetus to withstand labor. Later, fetal heart monitoring during labor demonstrates the presence of stress. Even if this information is not available, identification of high-risk historic factors are a valuable aid in identifying these infants in advance of their birth. From the maternal history the neonatal nurse can often anticipate the arrival of babies at risk even before the onset of labor. The most common antecedent conditions are toxemia, cigarette smoking, low socioeconomic status, multiple gestation, previously diagnosed infections during pregnancy (such as rubella), and advanced diabetes.

Meconium aspiration. Aspiration of meconium may occur in utero before the onset of labor or during the birth process. Small-for-dates infants are more likely to be affected than others because intrauterine hypoxia occurs so frequently among them. The aspiration of meconium is apparently mediated by the fetal response to hypoxia—the release of meconium into amniotic fluid by increased intestinal peristalsis and reflex relaxation of the anal sphincter plus reflex gasping movements that suck the released meconium particles into the bronchial tree. Much of the material in the respiratory tract is aspirated more deeply into terminal bronchioles and alveoli after birth. Respiratory distress thus occurs at birth, and a normal rapid recovery from intrauterine asphyxia is precluded. The extrauterine asphyxial state should be viewed as a continuation of events that have transpired in utero. The meconium aspiration syndrome can be clearly distinguished from hyaline membrane disease by the distinctive radiologic appearance of the lungs in each of these disorders. Diagnosis is also aided by accurate estimation of gestational age; hyaline membrane disease is unlikely to occur in term infants. The prognosis for the baby with syndromes due to aspiration or fluid retention is generally better than for the infant with hyaline membrane disease. These disorders and their complications are discussed in Chapter 8.

Hypoglycemia. Hypoglycemia is characterized by an abnormally low concentration of blood glucose. In full-sized infants at term, blood glucose levels below 30 mg/100 ml are considered abnormal during the first 72 hours of life, whereas levels below 40 mg/100 ml are abnormal thereafter. The corresponding abnormally low values for *serum* glucose are 40 and 50 mg/100 ml, respectively. In low birth weight infants, blood glucose concentrations below 20 mg/100 ml (25 mg/100 ml in *serum*) are thought to indicate hypoglycemia. Hypoglycemia is frequent among small-for-dates infants, whether they are born at term or before. The incidence may be as high as 40% among the most severely underweight and wasted infants. Babies of toxemic mothers and the smaller of twins are particularly vulnerable if birth weight is below 2000 grams. Untreated symptomatic babies with low blood sugar have a higher incidence of neurologic abnormality and a lower mean IQ level later in childhood than normal controls. Because of this suboptimal outcome in later life and because survival may be endangered during the early neonatal period, hypoglycemia must be identified and treated at the earliest possible moment. Infants who are below the tenth percentile on

the intrauterine growth chart must be monitored periodically for blood glucose concentrations during the first 3 or 4 days of life. Most small-for-dates infants first become hypoglycemic after 12 to 24 hours of age, but we have encountered this disorder much earlier is severely undernourished premature infants. Although a central laboratory can perform blood sugar determinations several times daily, nurses should screen frequently for low blood sugar with Dextrostix. *Optimal management requires that they do so according to their own judgment, without need for physicians' orders.* The details of hypoglycemic syndromes—their pathogenesis, symptoms, and treatment—are presented in Chapter 11.

Heat loss. Compared to their full-sized contemporaries, small-for-dates infants are ill equipped to conserve body heat because of their disproportionately large surface area. The problems of thermoregulation in the neonate are discussed in Chapter 4. Chilling must be avoided in the delivery room and nursery because it delays recovery from birth asphyxia; depletes the stores of glycogen, which are already sparse in undernourished babies; and increases the risk of hypoglycemia.

Cerebral edema. Cerebral edema is an infrequent complication in malnourished infants, but it occurs in any term infant who suffers severe fetal asphyxia. It may occur more frequently in undergrown infants because they are subject to intrauterine asphyxia because of placental dysfunction. Cerebral edema may be noted within 24 hours after delivery, at which time convulsions often occur. The skull sutures are abnormally wide; the increased intracranial pressure caused by cerebral edema is indicated by tightness and bulging of the anterior fontanelles. Anticonvulsant drugs are adminstered for control of seizures.

Polycythemia. Abnormally high hematocrit values (greater than 60 vol %) have been reported in as many as 50% of small-for-dates infants. Symptomatic babies whose difficulties were attributed to polycythemia have regularly had capillary or venous hematocrits in excess of 60 vol %. *However, the hematocrit in capilliary blood is generally higher than that of venous or arterial blood.* We therefore insist on central blood samples, since capillary samples yield misleadingly high results. Contrary to reported experiences, we have not encountered symptoms attributable to polycythemia in babies whose hematocrits were less than 70 vol %. In fact, most infants with these high values do not have detectable clinical abnormalities.

The symptoms associated with polycythemia are most commonly those of respiratory distress (trachypnea, retractions, grunting). They are probably the result of diminished lung compliance in polycythemic babies. Hyperbilirubinemia due to the breakdown of erythrocytes is also common. Less frequently, convulsions appear. Cardiac failure, pleural effusion, edema of the scrotum, and priapism have also been reported. A more detailed discussion of symptomatic polycythemia may be found in Chapter 9.

Outcome of small-for-dates infants

Neonatal mortality is a crude but critical measure of the risk imposed by intrauterine growth retardation. The consequences to central nervous system function later in childhood are equally sensitive.

Neonatal mortality. The differing rates of mortality and their relation to birth weight and gestational age have been clearly but crudely demonstrated by designating five general categories: infants over 2500 grams who are above and below 37 gestational weeks, respectively; infants between 1500 and 2500 grams who are similarly divided according to gestational age; and a fifth category that includes infants under 1500 grams regardless of their age at birth. Table 5-5 lists these groups and the percentage of neonatal mortality for each from records of single live births in New York City over a period of 3 years. The increased risks are indicated in the last column as a multiple of the mortality percentage in group I, which is the lowest-risk category. The column entitled "weight for age" characterizes the majority of infants in each group. Most growth-retarded infants are in group III. In comparison to the appropriately grown term infants in group I, neonatal mortality is increased

Table 5-5. Relationship of percentage of neonatal mortality to birth weight and gestational age*

Group	Weight (grams)	Gestational age (weeks)	Weight for age	Percentage of mortality	Increase over group I
I	Over 2500	37 or over	Appropriate term	0.5	—
II	Over 2500	Less than 37	Large-for-dates, preterm	1.4	×2.8
II	1501 to 2500	37 or over	Small-for-dates, term	3.2	×6.4
IV	1501 to 2500	Less than 37	Appropriate, preterm	10.5	×21.0
V	1500 or less	All	Preterm	70.7	×141.0

*Modified from Yerushalmy, J.: J. Pediatr. **71:**164, 1967.

sevenfold. Additional perspective is gained by comparing the mortality of small-for-dates term babies in group III to premature infants in group IV. Although the outlook for undergrown infants is considerably worse than for those who are normal and at term, it is not as grim as in premature infants of group IV. The gravest prognosis prevails among group V babies who weigh less than 1500 grams, over 90% of whom are preterm. Their mortality rate is 141 times greater than that of normal term infants in group I. Little is known about the babies in group II who are large for gestational age, but increased neonatal mortality rates have been noted by a number of investigators. Infants of diabetic mothers, who are at comparatively great risk, usually fall into this category, but they comprise only a minority of the babies in group II.

Assessment of neonatal mortality must be considered in finer detail than by means of the statistical associations just described. The variations and disagreements between numbers of published inquiries are no doubt largely due to the heterogeneous nature of infants who are categorically labeled "small-for-dates." Immediate outcomes vary among infants with major malformations, those whose insult began early in pregnancy, and those whose insult began later on; yet in all three categories, the babies are simply labeled small-for-dates. Heterogeneity is even more significant when one attempts to analyze long-term status in regard to stature and central nervous system function.

Postneonatal outcome. Any analysis that seeks to relate fetal growth to stature, weight, and IQ in later childhood must consider the heterogeneity of small-for-dates babies—that is, the magnitude and type of in utero insult, and the time of its inception. Furthermore, the postnatal environmental influences exerted by socioeconomic level must also be assessed in the light of the long-term outcome. Intrauterine growth retardation is most common among poor families, and the socioeconomic factors that influence impaired growth in utero are likely to be operative after birth as well. Thus an abnormal outcome may not be due solely to intrauterine events. The IQ is a case in point. A study in Scotland has revealed that infants who were undergrown at birth had lower IQ scores at 10 to 12 years of age than those who were appropriately grown at the same gestational age, but this phenomenon was noted only in poor homes. On the other hand, in superior homes, IQ scores were virtually identical in both groups. According to these data, fetal malnutrition exerts an influence on intellectual status, but primarily in low socioeconomic familes. Apparently the low IQ of children in poor homes cannot be attributed solely to intrauterine growth retardation, unless there exists one type of undergrowth among the poor and yet another among the more favored socioeconomic groups.

There seems little doubt that fetal undergrowth plays a significant role in later subnormal central nervous system function. What remains in doubt are the specific variety or varieties of fetal insult that are implicated and the extent of that implication. It is obvious from years of published studies that not all undergrown neonates fare poorly. Babies who are small by virtue of intrauterine virus infection (rubella, cytomegalovirus) are profoundly affected from direct invasion of the brain by the offending virus, and babies who are small-for-dates by virtue of a chromosomal disorder or some major anomaly are similarly affected. The data are straightforward and uncontested. However, infants who are small for no other reason than that their well-nourished parents are small are not afflicted later in life. The data on these infants are also unequivocal. Between these categories is a heterogeneous group of babies whose fetal growth was impeded by an adverse social environment, such as maternal malnutrition, as well as by disorders of pregnancy itself regardless of social class. Any inquiry that does not limit its data and conclusions to specific etiologic categories of fetal undergrowth, insofar as these categories can be determined, will produce invalid results. This failure to establish specific categories is probably the fundamental reason for the differing literature on this subject. An attempt to assess the severity of in utero insult was made in a well-controlled study of approximately 500 babies. It indicates that low birth weight babies (1500 to 2500 grams) whose gestational age is at term (40 weeks) are most likely to be smallest in weight and height at 10 years of age compared with babies of similar birth weight but shorter gestational age (34 to 38 weeks). Stated differently, infants of equal weight in whom intrauterine growth was slowest (born after the longest gestations, 40 weeks) were the most deeply insulted group and experienced the worst outcome at 10 years of age. Similar assessment of IQ was not made.

The difficulties that beset a follow-up study of sick infants who are managed in an intensive care facility are clearly exemplified in a report from Toronto. Of 71 small-for-dates infants who were evaluated at 2 years of age, 49% had major developmental handicaps. The authors emphasized that these results bore no direct relationship to the degree of fetal undergrowth. Rather, the *handicaps were strongly associated with central nervous system depression at the time of admission,* which in turn was related to perinatal asphyxia and to postnatal management prior to the transfer of infants to their tertiary care facility. The study infants, all of whom were transferred from other hospitals, were in poor condition on admission. Thus in this report, the evaluation of the long-term effects of intrauterine growth retardation was complicated by a high incidence of perinatal asphyxia (63% were affected) and by transfer from hospitals of birth to the tertiary care unit. Studies that evaluate long-term outcomes of impaired intrauterine growth must therefore also consider a variety of perinatal misadventures that later contribute to subnormality. The issue of inborn versus outborn births is frequently neglected, yet it is critical in the assessment of outcomes.

It now appears that if one excludes intrauterine infections, chromosomal disorders, and major congenital malformations, small-for-dates term infants have a low incidence of severe mental and neurologic handicaps. However, less profound impairments that cause learning difficulties and behavior problems are probably quite common. From various studies, these impairments include minimal cerebral dysfunction characterized by hyperactivity, short attention span, and poor fine coordination. Neurologic abnormalities of a mild, diffuse nature are common. Speech defects featuring immature reception and expression are also rather frequent. Furthermore, the stimulating postnatal environment and optimal nutrition in preschool years that are so essential for all children are probably more urgently required for those who were poorly grown in utero.

The incidence of severe central nervous system handicaps such as mental retardation and cerebral palsy seems to be more clearly a function of gestational age. Premature low birth weight infants have a higher incidence of these unfortunate results, and the more premature the birth, the higher the incidence of abnormality. In terms of central nervous system function, growth impairment in babies born at or near term may result only in some diminution of intellectual capacity, rather than in the severe disabilities that characterize cerebral palsy. Generally the immediate prognosis for survival and the long-term outlook for normal function seem to be better in small-for-dates infants born at or near term than in those who are premature and normally grown for gestational age; yet neither group fares as well as the normal-sized term infant. In most categories of abnormality, the application of contemporary intensive care techniques has substantially reduced the incidence of neonatal mortality and brain damage among survivors.

PREMATURITY

As discussed at the beginning of this chapter, premature births occur before the end of the thirty-seventh gestational week, regardless of birth weight. The majority of babies who weigh less than 2500 grams and almost all infants below 1500 grams are born prematurely. Most of them are appropriately grown; some are small-for-dates. On the other hand, many premature infants of diabetic mothers weigh over 2500 grams at birth.

Prenatal factors

In the past, most studies of the maternal factors associated with prematurity were based on birth weight as the sole criterion of premature birth. Among the so-called premature babies who were studied, a substantial number of low

birth weight infants were actually born at term. In spite of this difficulty, a number of factors have been shown to be clearly associated with prematurity, although definitive causes are demonstrable in only a minority of affected mothers. The obstetric conditions that play a role in the initiation of premature labor include chronic hypertensive disease, toxemia, placenta previa, abruptio placentae, multiple gestation, and cervical incompetence. Other factors that have been implicated are low socioeconomic status, short maternal stature, absence of prenatal care, malnutrition, and a history of previous premature delivery. The difficulty in evaluating any of the latter group of conditions singly is that they usually occur in some sort of combination with each other. Thus mothers of short stature are often malnourished, do not receive prenatal care, and are the same women who deliver premature infants repeatedly. Furthermore, these particular factors are inseparable from poverty, of which they are the essence. In spite of remarkable advances in perinatal medicine, our persistent ignorance of the causes of prematurity remains a major disappointment.

Mortality and morbidity

Mortality rates are highest among premature infants, and these rates increase as birth weight and gestational age decrease. Premature infants are poorly equipped to withstand the stresses of extrauterine life. The lungs may not be ready for air exchange; the digestive tract fails to absorb 20% to 40% of the fat contained in milk feedings. Defenses against infections are relatively ineffective, and an increased rate of heat loss creates serious thermoregulatory problems. The capillaries are relatively sparse so that perfusion of tissues is at best marginal. Increased capillary fragility predisposes to hemorrhage, especially in the ventricles of the brain. The most common disorders to which premature babies are predisposed are hyaline membrane disease, intracranial hemorrhage, infections, and fetal asphyxia. Retrolental fibroplasia (p. 219), which often culminates in blindness, occurs almost exclusively in preterm infants in response to inappropriately high concentrations of ambient oxygen. Anemia of prematurity occurs at 4 to 8 weeks, when hemoglobin levels may be as low as 6 or 7 grams/100 ml.

Postneonatal outcome

Premature infants have a relatively high incidence of mental retardation and abnormal neurologic signs. Microcephaly, spastic diplegia, convulsive disorders, and abnormal electroencephalograms are the most frequently encountered signs of brain disorder. The incidence of neurologic abnormality has diminished substantially since the advent of intensive care techniques. Approximately 70% to 90% of very low birth weight infants who survive are neurologically intact. Blindness due to retrolental fibroplasia was quite common between 1940 and 1955, and it was shown to be caused by excessive ambient oxygen concentrations. It was particularly frequent among infants whose birth weights were less than 1500 grams. Restriction of oxygen administration resulted in a significantly decreased incidence of the disease. Sophisticated therapeutic regimens requiring high concentrations of oxygen have diminished mortality rates impressively, but there has also been a resurgence in the incidence of retrolental fibroplasia.

POSTMATURITY

Prolonged gestation is dated from the beginning of the forty-second week; infants born afterward are said to be post-mature. By this definition, approximately 12% of all pregnancies are prolonged. Postmature infants may be appropriately sized for gestational age; yet quite often they are small-for-dates by virtue of a progressive increase in placental dysfunction. In such circumstances the infant may be considerably wasted.

Abnormal physical signs of wasting are observed in 4% to 12% of infants who are born in the forty-third week of gestation or later. The incidence of affected infants varies among populations. In the United States, 5% of postmature white infants and 8% of black infants have physical signs of postmature placental dysfunction. In Sweden and Germany, the incidences are 12% and 7%, respectively. There is a higher incidence of Apgar scores below 7 among affected infants, and their hematocrits are more frequently greater than 65%. The physical appearance of a wasted postmature baby differs in several respects from the appearance of his earlier born counterpart of equal size. Changes in the skin, nails, hair, subcutaneous tissue, and body contour are the obvious differences. Vernix caseosa is characteristically absent in postmature babies, except in the deepest skin folds at the axillae and groin, whereas at term the skin of malnourished infants is well covered with this cheese-like material. In postmature babies the skin becomes dry and cracked quite soon after birth, imparting a parchmentlike texture to it. The nails are often lengthened. Scalp hair is profuse, in contrast to earlier born malnourished infants, whose hair is quite sparse. Wasting involves depletion of previously deposited subcutaneous tissue; as a consequence, skin is loose, and fat layers are almost nonexistent (Fig. 5-4). The body appears thin and long. Meconium staining occurs frequently, coloring the skin, nails, and cord in shades ranging from green to golden yellow. Release of meconium in response to intruterine hypoxic stress may occur just before delivery or about 10 to 14 days before. Typically, these infants appear alert and wide-eyed, an attractive but misleading feature that is ominous because it may indicate chronic intrauterine hypoxia.

Perinatal mortality is higher in postmature infants than in term infants, particularly in pregnancies that progress into the forty-third week and beyond. In these infants, mortality is two or three times greater than in term babies. Approximately 75% to 85% of all deaths among postmature babies occur during labor. This is not particularly surprising when one considers that fetal oxygenation is marginal or depressed for days prior to the onset of labor. The subsequent stresses of labor are poorly tolerated, and intrauterine demise or severe depression at birth ensues.

Postneonatal outcomes have differed among various studies. In one such study, black infants were no different than their controls in weight, height, neurologic function, and psychologic performance. These parameters were observed on several occasions up to 7 years of age. Weight and height attainment and neurologic and psychologic functions were all normal. Among similarly affected infants in Sweden, IQ score and weight were significantly lower than control infants.

INTRAUTERINE GROWTH ACCELERATION (BABIES LARGE FOR GESTATIONAL AGE; MACROSOMIA)

The highest birth weight recorded in medical literature is 11,350 grams (25 pounds), a stillborn infant who was delivered in 1916. The *Guinness Book of* *World Records* (1979) reports the heaviest normal neonate weighed 10,795 grams (23 pounds 12 ounces); a baby weighing 13,381 grams (29 pounds 8 ounces), who lived only 2 hours, was born in 1939. Five percent of infants weigh over 4000 grams at birth, and from 0.4% to 0.9% weigh over 4500 grams. Whereas low birth weight is delineated below 2500 grams for any gestational age, high birth weight is above 4000 grams. The same variations in weight for age at birth that were described for small infants are applicable to large ones. An infant who is plotted above the ninetieth percentile on the intrauterine growth curve (at any week of gestation) is large for gestational age (LGA).

Large babies are characteristic of diabetic mothers, except for those mothers with advanced disease. However, only a minority of all large infants are born of diabetic mothers. Excessive birth weight (over 4000 grams) often reflects the genetic predisposition of the fetus. It has been found to be proportional to prepregnancy weight and to weight gain during pregnancy. Large mothers have large babies. Large infants are born to multiparous mothers three times as often as to primiparous ones; male infants have long been known to be heavier at birth than females. The small number of infants who have transposition of the great vessels are usually overgrown.

Categorization of babies as large for gestational age has been found, in the majority of instances, to be due to miscalculation of dates. The source of error, difficult to avert, appears to be postconceptional bleeding, a spurious menstrual episode after fertilization.

In diabetic women, birth weight over 4000 grams is four times more frequent than in nondiabetic women. The discrepancy is of greater magnitude for babies over 4500 grams: they are fourteen to twenty-eight times more frequent among diabetic women than in the general population.

The mortality rate for large babies born at or near term is higher than for average-sized neonates. The obvious mechanical difficulties posed by delivery of an over-sized baby are significant. The need for midforceps and cesarean section is considerably increased. Cesarean section is usually necessary because of cephalo-pelvic (fetopelvic) disproportion. Shoulder dystocia has been noted in 10% of large babies delivered per vaginam. Fractured clavicle, depressed skull fracture, brachial plexus palsy, and facial paralysis are all increased in frequency, together occurring in 15% of oversized infants. Low Apgar scores occur more frequently in overgrown infants.

Large babies have received relatively scanty attention compared with those who are undergrown. Prenatal identification of overgrown fetuses would seem to be as necessary as the identification of those who are undergrown. Abnormal and traumatic labor and delivery could thus often be averted.

SUMMATION

Expert care of newborn patients requires, among other things, an understanding of the abnormalities of intrauterine growth patterns as they relate to gestational age. An infant's course in the nursery is in large measure determined by these factors, and the illnesses that develop postnatally are often peculiar to a particular type of aberrant intrauterine growth pattern. Thus hyaline membrane disease, for all practical purposes, is confined to preterm babies, whereas hypoglycemia is a frequent hazard in small-for-dates infants. With knowledge of ma-ternal factors and with the ability to categorize babies in terms of growth status, the nurse can readily recognize a large number of high-risk infants and plan their management accordingly.

REFERENCES

Ballard, J. L., Novak, K. K., and Driver, M.: A simplified score for assessment of fetal maturation of newly born infants, J. Pediatr. **95:**769, 1979.

Battaglia, F. C., and Lubchenco, L. O.: A practical classification of newborn infants by weight and gestational age, J. Pediatr. **71:**159, 1967.

Beck, G. J., and van den Berg, B. J.: The relationship of the rate of intrauterine growth of low-birth-weight infants to later growth, J. Pediatr. **86:**504, 1975.

Campbell, S.: Fetal growth, Clin. Obstet. Gynecol. **1:**41, 1974.

Clifford, S. H.: Postmaturity with placental dysfunction: clinical syndrome and pathologic findings, J. Pediatr. **44:**1, 1954.

Commey, J. O. O., and Fitzhardinge, P. M.: Handicap in the preterm small-for-gestational age, J. Pediatr. **94:**779, 1979.

Cornblath, M., and Schwartz, R.: Disorders of carbohydrate metabolism in infancy, Philadelphia, 1976, W. B. Saunders Co.

Drillien, C. M.: Prenatal and perinatal factors in etiology and outcome of low birth weight, Clin. Perinatol. **1:**197, 1974.

Dubowitz, L. M. S., and Dubowitz, V.: Gestational age of the newborn, Reading, Mass., 1977, Addison-Wesley Publishing Co.

Dubowitz, L. M. S., Dubowitz, V., and Goldberg, C.: Clinical assessment of gestational age in the newborn infant, J. Pediatr. **77:**1, 1970.

Fitzhardinge, P. M., and Steven, E. M: The small-for-date infant. II. Neurological and intellectual sequelae, Pediatrics **50:**50, 1972.

Gluck, L., Kulovich, M. V., Borer, R. C., Jr., and others: The diagnosis of the respiratory distress syndrome (RDS) by anmiocentesis, Am. J. Obstet. Gynecol. **109:**440, 1971.

Gruenwald, P.: The fetus in prolonged pregnancy, Am. J. Obstet. Gynecol. **89:**503, 1964.

Gruenwald, P.: Growth of the human fetus. I. Normal growth and its variation, Am. J. Obstet. Gynecol. **94:**1112, 1966.

Hittner, H. M., Hirsch, N. J., and Rudolph, A. J.: Assessment of gestational age by examination of the anterior vascular capsule of the lens, J. Pediatr. **91:**455, 1977.

Horger, E. O., III, Miller, C., III, and Conner, E. D.: Relations of large birthweight to maternal diabetes mellitus, Obstet. Gynecol. **45:**150, 1975.

Humbert, J. R., Abelson, H., Hathaway, W. E., and Battaglia, F. C.: Polycythemia in small for gestational age infants, J. Pediatr. **75:**812, 1969.

Iffy, L., Chatterton, R. T., and Jakobovits, A.: The "high weight for dates" fetus, Am. J. Obstet. Gynecol. **115:**238, 1973.

Jones, K. L., and Chernoff, G. F.: Drugs and chemicals associated with intrauterine growth deficiency, J. Repro. Med. **21:**365, 1978.

Koenigsberger, M. R.: Judgment of fetal age. I. Neurologic evaluation, Pediatr. Clin. North Am. **13:**823, 1966.

Low, J. A., and Galbraith, R. S.: Pregnancy characteristics of intrauterine growth retardation, Obstet. Gynecol. **44:**122, 1974.

Lubchenco, L. O.: The high risk infant, Philadelphia, 1976, W. B. Saunders Co.

Lubchenco, L. O., Hansman, C., and Boyd, E.: Intrauterine growth in length and head circumference as estimated from live births at gestational ages from 26 to 42 weeks, Pediatrics **37:**403, 1966.

Lubchenco, L. O., Hansman, C., Dressler, M., and Boyd, E.: Intrauterine growth as estimated from liveborn birth-weight data at 24 to 42 weeks of gestation, Pediatrics **32:**793, 1963.

Lubchenco, L. O., Searls, D. T., and Brazie, J. V.: Neonatal mortality rate: relationship to birthweight and gestational age, J. Pediatr. **81:**814, 1972.

Malan, A. F., and Higgs, S. C.: Gestational age assessment in infants of very low birth-weight, Arch. Dis. Child. **50:**322, 1975.

Naeye, R. L.: Human intrauterine parabiotic syndrome and its complications, N. Engl. J. Med. **268:**804, 1963.

Naeye, R. L.: Unsuspected organ abnormalities associated with congenital heart disease, Am. J. Pathol. **47:**905, 1965.

Naeye, R. L.: Abnormalities in infants of mothers with toxemia of pregnancy, Am J. Obstet. Gynecol. **95:**276, 1966.

Naeye, R. L., Bernirschke, K., Hagstrom, J. W. C., and Marcus, C. C.: Intrauterine growth of twins as estimated from liveborn birth-weight data, Pediatrics **37:**409, 1966.

Parkin, J. M., Hey, E. N., and Clowes, J. S.: Rapid assessment of gestational age at birth, Arch. Dis. Child. **51:**259, 1976.

Robinson, J. S.: Growth of the fetus, Br. Med. Bull. **35:**137, 1979.

Rosso, P., Wasserman, M., Rozovski, S., and Velasco, E.: Effects of maternal undernutrition on placental metabolism and function. In Young, D. S., and Hicks, J. M., editors: The neonate, New York, 1976, John Wiley & Sons, Inc.

Scott, K. E., and Usher, R.: Epiphyseal development in fetal malnutrition syndrome, N. Engl. J. Med. **270:**822, 1964.

Shanklin, D. R.: The influence of placental lesions on the newborn infant, Pediatr. Clin. North Am. **17:**25, 1970.

Silverman, W. A.; Dunham's premature infants, New York, 1961, Paul B. Hoeber, Medical Division, Harper & Row, Publishers.

Silverman, W. A., and Sinclair, J. C.: Infants of low birth weight, N. Engl. J. Med. **274:**448, 1966.

Sinclair, J. C.: Temperature regulation and energy metabolism in the newborn, New York, 1978, Grune & Stratton, Inc.

Smith, C. A.: Effects of maternal undernutrition upon the newborn infant in Holland, J. Pediatr. **71:**390, 1967.

Smith, D. W.: Growth and its disorders, Philadelphia, 1977, W. B. Saunders Co.

Ting, R. Y., Wang, M. H., and Scott, T. F. Mc.: The dysmature infant, J. Pediatr. **90:**943, 1977.

Winick, M.: Cellular growth of human placenta. III. Intrauterine growth failure, J. Pediatr. **71:**390, 1967.

Winick, M.: Cellular growth in intrauterine malnutrition, Pediatr. Clin. North Am. **17:**69, 1970

Winick, M.: Malnutrition and brain development, New York, 1976, Oxford University Press.

Winick, M., Brasel, J. A., and Velasco, E. G.: Effects of prenatal nutrition upon pregnancy risk, Clin. Obstet. Gynecol. **16:**184, 1973.

Yerushalmy, J.: The classification of newborn infants by birth weight and gestational age, J. Pediatr. **71:**164, 1967.

CHAPTER 6

Physical examination of the newborn infant

The physical findings associated with birth trauma are described in Chapter 3.

The nurse who learns to evaluate physical signs in the neonate can contribute substantially to his proper management. Contemporary expansion of nursing skills involves many new functions, one of which is the competent performance of a physical examination. Physical findings in the newborn will thus be presented in considerable detail, with emphasis on normal characteristics and their variations, most of which require no therapy. *Some pathologic findings will be described, but they are usually dis-cussed more completely in chapters devoted to the specific diseases in which they occur.*

The initial physical examination should be performed as soon as possible after arrival in the nursery. Its purpose is to identify existing abnormalities and to provide a basis on which future changes can be assessed. After the admission examination a number of observations must be made during the nursery stay. The first passage of stool and the first urination should be noted. Sucking behavior and performance during feedings are extremely important observations. The appearance of jaundice, cyanosis, pallor, excessive salivation, abdominal distention, abnormal stools, respiratory distress, and a number of other events must all be sought in a systematic fashion.

The purpose of the neonatal physical examination is to identify and record evidence of stress, trauma, malformations, and disease during the first days of life. Physical assessment is only one component of the total evaluation. A well-considered chronologic account of antecedent events must be known prior to examination. Laboratory and other procedural data are usually acquired afterward.

SEQUENCE OF EXAMINATION

The sequence in which the various features of the examination are assessed is a

138

matter of personal preference. All examiners eventually develop their own individual approach. Regardless of the system used, it is best to order observations in reference to the amount of disturbance they produce. I prefer to first make assessments that cause the least disturbance, particularly those that require a quiet baby. It seems advisable to then proceed to the more disturbing maneuvers that are not so dependent on the resting state for accurate interpretation.

Inspection without contact. A tremendous amount of information is available by simply looking at a baby, without touching him. The examiner should not, when first confronting an infant, abruptly place a stethoscope on the chest before doing anything else. This maneuver betrays a sad lack of sensitivity to the neonate's reactions and a total lack of perspective regarding the relative importance of the individual observations that comprise the physical examination.

The infant's overall size and contour are immediately apparent, as is the relative size of the head, extremities, and trunk. Microcephaly or cranial enlarge-

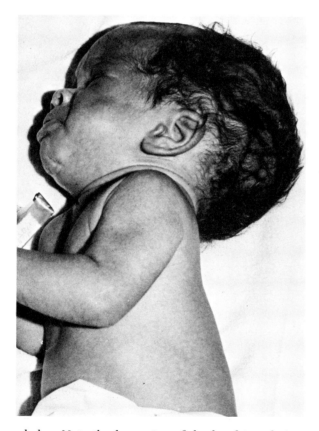

Fig. 6-1. Hydrocephalus. Note the large size of the head in relation to the face. The occiput is prominent, the forehead less prominent than usual. This infant also had severe chorioretinitis. The diagnosis was toxoplasmosis.

ment are obvious. If hydrocephalus is present, the forehead is often prominently protrusive (bossing). The cranial vault is always large in relation to the face (Fig. 6-1). The amount of subcutaneous fat is assessable at a glance. A thin trunk often causes a normal head to appear enlarged. The abdomen is either distended, flat, or sunken (scaphoid), or it may bulge on one side because of a massively enlarged kidney (hydronephrosis, Fig. 6-2).

The baby's *posture* is informative. Normal flexion of the extremities indicates good muscle tone. Lack of flexion is associated with hypotonicity (flaccidity), whereas excessive flexion usually suggests hypertonicity (spasticity). Both these findings are evident in the baby in Fig. 6-3, who had flaccid upper extremities and spastic lower ones. If only one arm is straight instead of flexed, it is probably paralyzed to some extent. This paralysis suggests brachial plexus palsy, which is described on p. 62 and is illustrated in Figs. 2-14 and 2-15. Breech presentations can be identified by the characteristic positions of the lower extremities. These positions are described later in this chapter. The absence of molding plus the position of the lower extremities should suggest a breech delivery. Retraction of the head with relatively normal vertebral posture indicates a face presentation.

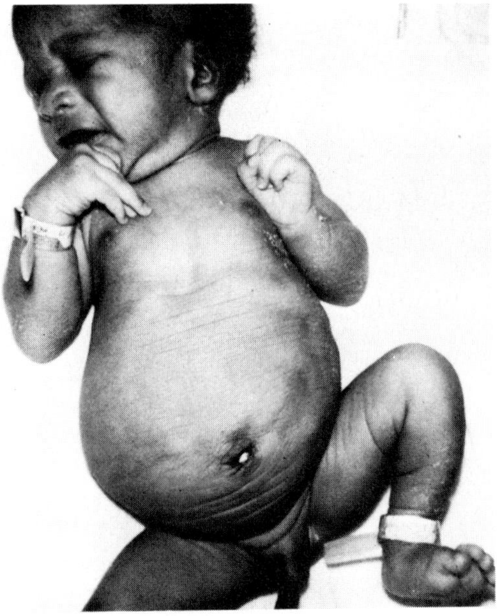

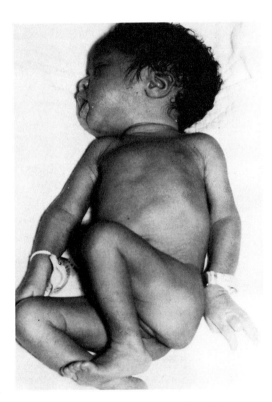

Fig. 6-2. Abdominal distention due to unilateral hydronephrosis. Bulging of the right side is immediately apparent.

Fig. 6-3. Upper extremities are flaccid, as seen in the relaxed fingers and elbows. Lower extremities are spastic, and their flexed posture is exaggerated. Note the congenitally amputated finger on the left hand.

A number of features of the *skin* are immediately obvious. If cyanosis is present, its distribution is of great importance because distribution relates to the significance of cyanosis (generalized cyanosis) or lack of it (acrocyanosis). Jaundice, pallor, rash, and evidence of trauma are all there to be discerned by those who will look.

The *face* is informative. Abnormal facies must be appreciated. The alert, wide-eyed baby who appears to be sucking is really agitated as a result of intrauterine hypoxic insult to the brain (Fig. 5-9). Facial paralysis may be evident at rest, or it may not be apparent until the baby cries (p. 64).

Spontaneous movements can be evaluated only if the infant is not disturbed. At rest, sporadic, well-coordinated movements are the rule. If no movement is noted, significant depression is probably the cause, whether from hypoxia in utero, maternal anesthesia, hypoglycemia, or any other of a large number of etiologies.

The baby who moves little or not at all is usually flaccid as well. Repetitive, rhythmic motions of one or more extremities are convulsive movements. Facial and eyelid twitches are also convulsive phenomena. Absent or diminished movement of one extremity (or two), while the others are used normally, is indicative of paresis or paralysis.

Much information is obtainable for the evaluation of *respiration* by simple inspection. Retractions are obvious (Fig. 6-4); grunting and stridor are audible. Increased anteroposterior diameter of the chest (barrel chest) usually indicates overexpanded lungs (massive aspiration, respiratory distress syndrome type 2). If one side of the chest appears larger than the other, pneumothorax, chylothorax, or diaphragmatic hernia are possible causes. If the left chest is larger, cardiomegaly associated with congenital heart disease is an additional possibility.

Several *scattered observations* by inspection are also of value. The under-

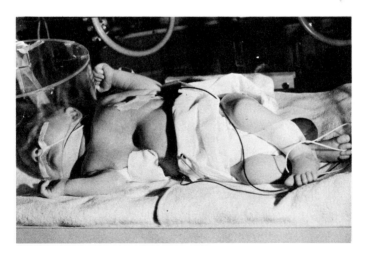

Fig. 6-4. Severe retraction during inspiration. The lower end of the sternum and the subcostal margins are severely indrawn. The upper anterior thorax is somewhat expanded. Electrodes to the chest are connected to apnea and heart rate monitors.

grown term or preterm infant's hair is sparse (Fig. 5-9), whereas the postmature baby's hair is dense. The cord is thin in mature infants who are small-for-dates, and it may be the only part of the body that is meconium stained, if meconium release occurs immediately before delivery. Fingernails are long in postmature infants.

These diverse signs are described here to emphasize the value of purposeful inspection without touching. This inspection accomplished, one may then proceed to the more manipulative aspects of the physical examination.

Auscultation, palpation, and other manipulations. With the baby supine, I prefer to palpate the abdomen immediately after the initial inspection. If the infant is disturbed by manipulations beforehand, an adequate evaluation of the abdomen is difficult or temporarily impossible. The fingertips must be gently placed on the abdomen while not exerting any downward pressure. Deep palpation should then proceed gradually. Sudden plunging of the examining hand into the abdomen is thoughtless; it produces discomfort and precludes a successful examination. The neonate is easily agitated by abrupt manipulations. Auscultation of the anterior chest should follow abdominal palpations. In conjunction with cardiac evaluation, gently palpate the femoral and brachial pulses. Now palpate the extremities by enveloping them with your hand and then move the joints gingerly. This maneuver completed, take the wrists and pull the infant into the sitting position to evaluate head lag. The baby may now be turned to the prone position. Crying caused by the disturbance is of little concern because the resultant deep inspirations and the noise of crying are helpful in auscultation of the lungs.

Now move the index finger over the vertebrae down to the sacrum to ascertain the absence of gross anomalies such as agenesis of the sacrum. Separate the buttocks and look at the anus for position and presence. The infant, who is probably crying now, is then returned to the supine position. Manipulate the hip joints to rule out congenital dislocation. The head, neck, and face are next to be examined. With one hand holding a flashlight, gently separate the eyelids with the index finger and thumb. Shine the light tangentially into the eyes to rule out corneal lesions and large cataracts. Now proceed to the neurologic evaluation (p. 162). Examination of the mouth and throat is performed as the last maneuver of the physical evaluation. It is the most agitating. After completing the physical examination, hold the baby in your arms for a few moments. Both of you will feel better.

PHYSICAL FINDINGS
Contour, proportions, and postures

The body of a normal newborn is essentially cylindric; the head circumference slightly exceeds that of the chest. For the term baby, average circumference of the head is 33 to 35 cm (13 to 14 inches), whereas for the chest it is 30 to 33 cm (12 to 13 inches). Sitting height may be measured from crown to rump, and it is approximately equal to head circumference. These values may vary somewhat, but their relationship to each other is normally constant. For example, if the head circumference is significantly smaller than the chest, microcephaly is suspect; if it is larger than expected, hydrocephalus must be considered. During the first 24 hours, because of molding, the head may be equal to or slightly smaller than the chest. On the second and third days a normal contour replaces the molded one, and the head circumference increases by 1 or 2 cm as a result. If the head is over 4 cm larger than the chest, and this has been verified by repeated measurements on several successive days, abnormal enlargement due to increased intracranial pressure is suspect. In these circumstances, additional signs of increased intracranial pressure are ordinarily detectable. These signs are described later in this chapter. A word of caution is in order regarding the relative sizes of head and chest when one is considering abnormal enlargement of the cranial vault. A discrepancy between the two measurements may be exaggerated in a malnourished baby if the chest circum-

ference is diminished by virtue of depleted subcutaneous tissue. If this is the case, other signs of malnutrition are evident, and the head size itself is in the range of normal, even though the chest size is not.

During the first few days of life, posture is largely the result of position in utero. Placed on the side, the normal infant who was delivered from a vertex presentation tends to keep the head flexed, with the chin close to the chest. The arms are close to the trunk, the elbows are flexed so that the forearms rest on the chest to some degree, and the hands are held in a fisted position. The back is somewhat bent, and the hips are flexed so that the thighs are drawn on the abdomen. Flexion is also maintained at the knees, and the feet are dorsiflexed onto the anterior aspects of the legs. This fetal position is often assumed to some extent by adults and older children while they sleep. During the first days of life, it is the position of comfort for the baby. Frequently he may be quieted during crying episodes by taking him up from the crib and gently curling him into this described position.

Other postures are associated with more unusual fetal positions. After a footling breech presentation, the thighs are abducted in the so-called frog-leg position (Fig. 2-8). Some babies born in the frank breech position tend to keep their knees straightened. After a brow or face delivery, the head is extended and the neck appears elongated.

These postures depend on normal muscle tone, which is strikingly diminished in hypoxic babies. Thus affected, they make no attempt to assume previous intrauterine postures but remain in almost any position imposed on them by the examiner. The extremities lie flat on

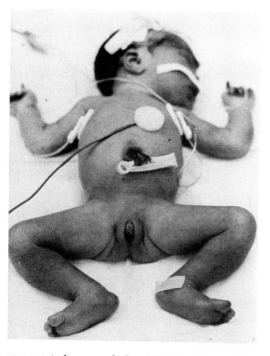

Fig. 6-5. A depressed, flaccid baby delivered in breech position. Extremities lie flat on table, and head remains turned to one side. Note traumatic cyanosis of lower half of body, a result of breech delivery.

the table surface, and the head turns to one side, depending on the position in which it is placed (Fig. 6-5).

Skin and subcutaneous tissue

At birth the skin is covered extensively with *vernix caseosa*, a gray-white substance with a cheeselike consistency. If not removed, it dries and disappears within 24 hours. For the first day of life the skin is blush red and smooth; toward the second or third days it becomes dry, somewhat flaky, and pink.

In approximately half of all normal newborn infants, *jaundice* is visible during the second or third days of life and disappears between the fifth and seventh days. This is physiologic jaundice; the mechanism of its development is described in Chapter 10. Jaundice in the first 24 hours is abnormal and requires extensive diagnostic evaluation. Icteric skin may be difficult to detect when redness is prominent, but blanching readily demonstrates the underlying yellow discoloration. Jaundice is best demonstrated by blanching the skin over the nasal bridge. Place one thumb on each side of the nose and stretch the skin over the nasal bridge by pressing firmly as each finger is moved a few centimeters laterally. A relatively large area of skin is thereby blanched. Early jaundice is more easily detected on the face than anywhere else.

The subcutaneous tissue may be moderately *edematous* for several days. Edema is most noticeable about the eyes, legs, and dorsal aspects of the hands and feet.

Peripheral cyanosis (acrocyanosis) involves the hands, feet, and circumoral area (around the lips). It is evident in most infants at birth and for a short time thereafter. If limited to the extremities in an otherwise normal infant, it is due to venous stasis and in innocuous. Localized cyanosis may occur in presenting parts, particularly in association with abnormal presentations. In breech presentations, the buttocks or the feet and legs are blue as a result of venous stasis and are edematous (Fig. 2-8); in a transverse lie, a prolapsed arm may be similarly discolored because of obstructed venous re-

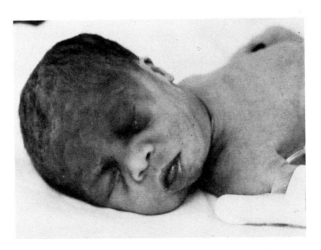

Fig. 6-6. Traumatic cyanosis, with bruising of forehead and scalp. Vertex delivery of a premature infant.

turn. Occasionally a circular area of edema and cyanosis in the scalp is present at the top of the head as a result of pressure against a dilated cervix (caput succedaneum). Sometimes the forehead and scalp (or even the entire head above the neck) are cyanotic (Fig. 6-6).

Pallor usually accompanies other signs of distress except in anemic babies in whom there has been fetomaternal bleeding across the placenta over a protracted period (chronic hemorrhage in utero; see Chapter 9). Such infants are in no distress even though their pallor may be extreme. Pallor is more commonly a sign of anemia, hypoxia, poor peripheral perfusion due to hypotension (shock), and infection. Subcutaneous edema sometimes imparts a pale appearance, even though blood pressure and hematocrit are normal, because increased water content of subcutaneous tissue impairs transmission of the color of blood. Some postmature infants are pale because they have *parchment skin,* which also transmits less color from blood because it is thicker than normal.

Ecchymoses appear as bruises of varying size anywhere over the body, sometimes involving extensive areas. They are most frequently due to trauma during difficult labor or to brisk handling of the infant during or after delivery. Occasionally they indicate serious infection or a bleeding diathesis. When the extravasated blood in an ecchymosis is broken down, the resultant elevated serum bilirubin levels may occasionally reach dangerous heights. The pathogenesis of hyperbilirubinemia and the role of extraneous blood are discussed in Chapter 10.

Petechiae are pinpoint hemorrhagic areas that occur in a number of disease states involving infection and thrombocytopenia. Occasionally, however, scattered petechiae are noted over the upper trunk or the face as a result of increased intravascular pressure, which causes capillaries to rupture during delivery. These petechiae fade within 24 to 48 hours, and fresh lesions do not appear subsequently. Identification of petechiae may be verified by blanching the skin. Both index fingers are held next to each other, and while maintaining pressure, they are separated to reveal the area in question. Petechiae and ecchymoses do not disappear when the skin is blanched, since blood is fixed in the tissue. Red rashes involving local vascular engorgement disappear completely when the skin is blanched, since blood is emptied from the engorged vessels. The same maneuver reveals underlying jaundice that would otherwise be masked by flushed skin that is suffused with blood.

Mongolian spots are irregular areas of blue-gray pigmentation over the sacrum and buttocks, but they may be so extensive as to cover the back and sometimes the extensor surfaces of the extremities as well. They are common in black infants and in babies of Asian and southern European lineage. These harmless discolorations are caused by pigmented cells in the deep layer of the skin. They disappear by 4 years of age and often much sooner.

Hemangiomas may appear as isolated lesions in otherwise normal infants, or they may be a component of several serious generalized disorders. Microscopically, hemangiomas of the skin are *capillary* or *cavernous. Capillary hemangiomas* are comprised of a mass of dilated capillaries. They are usually found in the superficial skin. *Port wine nevi* (nervus flammeus) are dense concentrations of such dilated capillaries. They may be small and single, or multiple and sparse; they may also involve large areas of skin, even as much as half the body surface. Their color varies from pink to deep purple; in the neonate their surfaces are continuous with that of adjacent normal skin. Edges are clearly delineated. As a rule, they are permanent, but those that are pale may largely disappear. Port wine nevi over the face may indicate Sturge-Weber syndrome (cerebral calcification and glaucoma on the same side as the lesions and hemiparesis on the opposite side) and several other serious generalized disorders as well. *Telangiectatic nevi (stork bites)* are flat, red, localized areas of capillary dilatation seen in almost all neonates. Microscopically the dilated capillaries are considerably less dense than those seen in port wine nevi. They can be eradicated by blanching the skin. They are most commonly situated at the back of the neck, the lower occiput, the upper eyelids, and the nasal bridge. They disappear by 2 years of age, but in many children they often reappear during crying episodes. *Strawberry hemangiomas* are not seen in normal term infants during the nursery stay because they generally appear in the second or third week of life. As a result, they are seen in premature infants who are hospitalized for protracted periods and in term babies after discharge. They are first evident as bright red, flat spots, 1 to 3 mm in diameter, which blanch easily. Subsequently they grow in all directions, protruding prominently from the skin surface. They may not reach their fullest size for 1 to 3 months or more. There is a great temptation to remove these lesions, but it should be resisted because they invariably resolve spontaneously several weeks or months after reaching peak growth. *The cosmetic effect is best when they are allowed to resolve.* Resolution is her-

alded by a pale purple or gray spot on the surface of the lesion, which grows as the hemangioma shrinks. Appearance of the pale spot indicates spontaneous sclerosis, and thus obliteration, of the capillaries that comprise the lesion. *Cavernous hemangiomas* are in the subepidermal layer. They tend to be more diffuse and less sharply demarcated than capillary hemangiomas. Color of the overlying skin may be normal, or bluish as a result of the transmission of color from subjacent blood. Cavernous hemangiomas are usually spongy when touched, but on occasion they are tight cystic masses. Generally these localized lesions have no other significance. They grow at first (like strawberry hemangiomas) and then often resolve spontaneously in a few months or 1 to 2 years. They may be situated so that during their growth they seriously impair the function of an adjacent organ such as

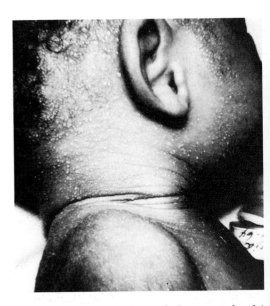

Fig. 6-7. Sudamina (distended sweat glands) appear vesicular. They disappear spontaneously.

the trachea, esophagus, or eye. Cavernous hemangiomas may also be associated with serious thrombocytopenia (Kasabach-Merritt syndrome). *Mixed hemangiomas* are common. They are composed of a superficial strawberry lesion that is continuous with a deeper cavernous one.

Subcutaneous fat necrosis (p. 57) is due to trauma. These lesions are sharply demarcated, firm masses of varying size that are located in subcutaneous tissue and are fixed to overlying skin. Occasionally a pale purple discoloration is in evidence at the surface of these lesions.

Harlequin color change is a rare, peculiar discrepancy in color between the two longitudinal halves of the body, extending from the forehead to the symphysis pubis. A curiosity of no known pathologic significance, it is elicited by placing the baby on his side for several minutes. The dependent half of the body turns pink while the upper half remains pale. The colors are reversed when the infant is turned onto the opposite side. The same phenomenon may occur in the supine position.

Lanugo is fine hair, sometimes barely visible, that is characteristic of the newborn period. It is more noticeable in premature infants and is most easily seen over the shoulders, back, forehead, and cheeks.

Milia are minute, white papules on the chin, nose, cheeks, and forehead. They represent distended sebaceous glands that disappear spontaneously in several days or weeks. *Sudamina* are tiny vesi-

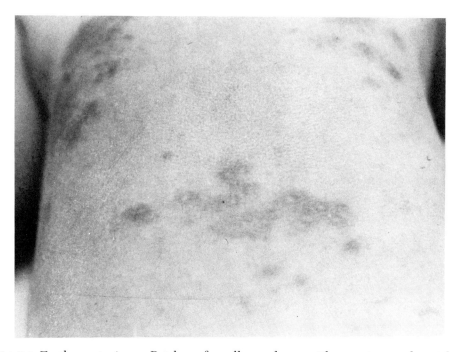

Fig. 6-8. Erythema toxicum. Patches of swollen redness with superimposed vesicles, often mistaken for staphylococcal lesions. Lesions in this instance are distributed over the abdomen and thorax.

cles over the face and neck that are formed by distention of sweat glands (Fig. 6-7).

Erythema toxicum is a pink papular rash on which vesicles are often superimposed (Fig. 6-8). The vesicles frequently appear purulent and are sometimes confused with the lesions characteristic of staphylococcal pyoderma. They appear anywhere over the body within 24 to 48 hours after birth and resolve spontaneously after several days. The vesicles contain eosinophils that are demonstrable on a smear prepared with Wright's stain. The rash is innocuous, and its etiology is unknown.

Sclerema is hardening of the skin and subcutaneous tissue associated with life-threatening disorders such as septicemia, shock, and severe cold stress. As a rule, the cheeks and buttocks are first involved, then the calves and thighs, and eventually perhaps the entire body. The skin is so hard it feels wooden. Sclerema should not be confused with subcutaneous fat necrosis, which is confined to small areas and is usually present in babies who are otherwise well.

Café au lait spots are so named be-cause their color resembles coffee to which milk has been added. In black babies they may be a darker brown color. They are irregularly shaped oval lesions of varying size and distribution, which are not elevated above the skin surface. If six or more of these spots are present, suspicion of neurofibromatosis (an autosomal dominant neurocutaneous syndrome) is appropriate.

Puncture wounds are the result of the attachment of electrodes from fetal monitors. In breech presentations they are incurred on the buttocks or thighs. Rarely, electrodes are accidently applied to eyelids and other parts of the face. Occasionally, these puncture wounds become infected.

Head

After vaginal deliveries from the vertex position, molding of the head is apparent to some degree in virtually all neonates as a result of pressures exerted during the birth process. The change in shape is more pronounced in first-born infants and in those whose heads are engaged for prolonged periods. Pressure during the

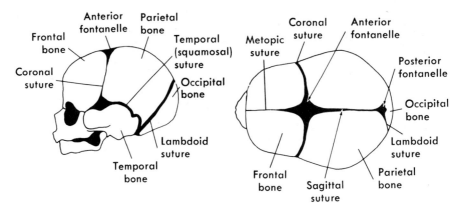

Fig. 6-9. Neonatal cranial bones, sutures, and fontanelles from lateral view and from above. (Modified from Crelin, E. S.: Anatomy of the newborn, an atlas, Philadelphia, 1969, Lea & Febiger.)

usual vertex delivery causes flattening of the forehead with a gradual rise to an apex posteriorly and an abrupt drop at the occiput (Fig. 2-9). In brow presentations the forehead may be unusually prominent, rather than flattened as in vertex deliveries. When the forces of the birth process are not exerted on the cranium, its spherical contour is undisturbed. Thus the head is characteristically spherical in an infant born from the breech position or delivered by cesarean section. These modes of delivery can be presumed from inspection of the cranial contour. Molding generally disappears by the end of the first or second day of life.

The *cranium* comprises six bones (Fig. 6-9): the frontal, occipital, two parietals, and two temporals. The *frontal bone* runs the width of the cranium at its anterior third. The *occipital bone* occupies the width of the cranium at its posterior third, whereas the two *parietal bones* are situated in the middle third between the frontal and occipital bones. The *temporal bones* are the most lateral and inferior of the cranial bones. They are adjacent to the parietals.

The *sutures* and *fontanelles* of the cranium are extremely important landmarks (Fig. 6-9). They are bands of connective tissue that separate the six major cranial bones. Sutures are palpable as cracks; fontanelles are broader "soft spots" at specific locations. The *coronal suture* runs from one side of the cranium to the other, separating the frontal bone (the forehead) from the two parietal bones posterior to it. In some infants a *metopic suture* bisects the frontal bone into right and left halves. It extends from the frontmost angle of the anterior fontanelle downward toward the nasal bridge. It is usually as wide as the other normal sutures, sometimes wider. The *lambdoid*

suture, situated toward the posterior third of the skull, runs from one side to the other, separating the occipital bone from the two parietal bones anterior to it. The *sagittal suture* runs in an anteroposterior direction in the midline, terminating anteriorly at the coronal suture and posteriorly at the lambdoid suture. It separates the two parietal bones. The *squamosal (temporal) sutures* also run in an anteroposterior direction, but they are situated just at the level of the earlobes. They, like the sagittal suture, terminate at the coronal and lambdoid sutures.

The *fontanelles* are relatively wide, soft areas at the junctions of each of the sutures. The *anterior fontanelle* is at the junction of the sagittal and coronal sutures. It is diamond shaped and variable in size. It may be small as a result of

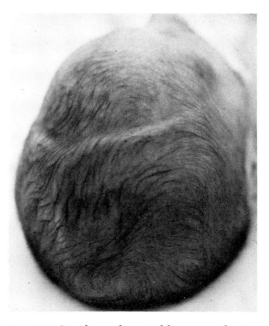

Fig. 6-10. Overlapped cranial bones producing visible ridge in a small premature infant. Easily visible overlapping does not often occur in term infants.

molding, but it enlarges as the molding disappears. At its widest point it may measure up to 5 cm. The *posterior fontanelle* is triangular; it measures 1 cm or less in width and is situated at the junction of the sagittal and lambdoid sutures. Four other fontanelles are of less clinical significance. They are at the junctions formed by the squamosal sutures with the coronal and lambdoid sutures.

Appraisal of the head by external examination depends on an appreciation of the contours that are expected as a result of various presentations and on the status of sutures and fontanelles, particularly the anterior fontanelle. At birth and for a day or two afterward, as a result of molding, the edges of the cranial bones may overlap, obliterating the sutures. The lines of overlap seem to be ridges when palpated, and the fontanelles are small (Fig. 6-10). Later, as the shape of the cranium becomes more normal, the bones separate and the sutures can be felt as cracks several millimeters in width. The anterior fontanelle now expands to its full size. In premature infants the overlapping is often easily seen (Fig. 6-10). It may persist for weeks in the smallest infants. In malnourished infants the sutures may be wide at birth, perhaps over 1 cm, because of impaired growth of the cranial bones. The anterior fontanelle is large for the same reason, but it is also flat and soft. Inordinately large, flat, anterior fontanelles and wide sutures also suggest the presence of hypothyroidism, osteogenesis imperfecta, and cleidocranial dysostosis. Unusually *small anterior fontanelles* are the rule in very small premature infants as the result of severe molding during vertex deliveries, in microcephaly of any etiology, and in craniosynostosis. On the other hand, an abnormal increase in intracranial pressure

actually separates the cranial bones, expanding suture lines and fontanelles. Rather than being flat and soft, the anterior fontanelle is firm and bulging as a function of high intracranial pressure. These signs, especially those in the anterior fontanelle, are present in babies with hydrocephalus (Fig. 6-1), meningitis, subdural hematoma, and cerebral edema. If there is doubt concerning the firmness and fullness of the anterior fontanelle, the baby should be taken from the crib and held erect in one arm while the fontanelle is palpated. A pathologically bulging fontanelle does not soften and flatten.

Eyes

Eyelids are frequently edematous during the first 2 days after delivery, and the infant rarely opens them. Separation of lids must be accomplished gently because forceful traction easily everts them, thus precluding an adequate view of the eyes.

Instillation of silver nitrate drops into the eyes at birth may cause *chemical conjunctivitis* to appear within an hour or soon thereafter. The resultant purulent discharge disappears without treatment in 1 or 2 days with no residual difficulty.

Purulent conjunctival exudate is also a sign of *conjunctivitis* due to infection (p. 329). Most commonly, these infections are caused by staphylococci and by a variety of gram-negative rods. Gonorrheal infection, which may also involve the eye itself, occasionally occurs in spite of the application of silver nitrate drops that are ordinarily effective in preventing it.

Subconjunctival hemorrhages are frequent. They result from pressure on the fetal head during delivery, with resultant impairment of venous return and rupture of capillaries in the sclera. They can be

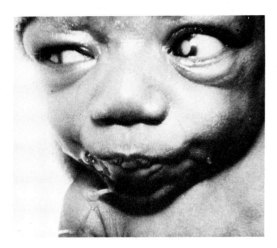

Fig. 6-11. Bilateral cataracts. Note white pupils. Entire lenses were involved. Infant had congenital rubella.

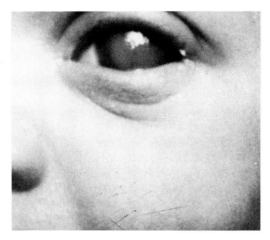

Fig. 6-12. Corneal opacity, unilateral. Cornea is white, its surface rough; overall appearance is that of ground glass. This baby had congenital glaucoma due to intrauterine rubella infection. The cornea is thus abnormally large.

seen in the sclerae and are of no pathologic significance, even when the entire sclera is reddened by extravasated blood (Fig. 2-13). *Retinal hemorrhages* are produced by the same mechanism, and they may occur in as many as 10% of normal neonates. They are flame shaped or round and are thought to be harmless. However, extensive hemorrhage over a large segment of the retina usually indicates the presence of a subdural hematoma.

Cataracts, if present, must be identified at the time of the first examination. Cataracts are opacities of the lens that can vary from pinpoint size to involvement of the entire lens. Occasionally they develop several days or weeks after birth. If the entire lens is affected, they are usually seen easily by shining a light into each eye, with the light source held to one side. If the opacity is small, it can be identified only with an ophthalmoscope. Bilateral cataracts involving the entire lens are illustrated in Fig. 6-11. In this picture the pupils are white because the

opacified lens behind them reflects the light, which is applied close to the eyes from the side of the face. White pupils may also be seen in the presence of lesions deeper in the eye, such as retinoblastoma. Normally the pupils appear black to the bare eye of the examiner when light is directed at them. Cataracts are usually bilateral, but they are sometimes unilateral. They are a major manifestation of intrauterine rubella infection (p. 331) and are occasionally seen in cytomegalovirus infection (p. 332). They may be hereditary, being transmitted as a dominant trait from an affected parent. In congenital galactosemia, cataracts sometimes appear several weeks after birth.

Corneal opacities are also discerned by directing light to the eyes (Fig. 6-12). They occur after trauma, in association with congenital glaucoma, and as a result of infection such as herpesvirus and congenital rubella. Compare the illustrations of the cataracts (Fig. 6-11) and the corneal opacity (Fig. 6-12). The two lesions are clearly distinguishable from each other. In the presence of a cataract, the iris can be seen because the affected structure (the lens) is behind it. The cornea is smooth and clear. The corneal opacity involves the eye's outside window (the cornea), and the underlying iris is thus obscure. Furthermore, the surface of the involved cornea is rough, much like ground glass.

Iris coloboma is one of the most common congenital malformations of the eye. The defect varies from a small notch at the inner iris margin to segmental absence, usually at the inferior portion. It is generally limited to the iris and is thus not associated with visual difficulty. Infrequently, the defect involves deeper eye structures such as the retina, macula, and optic nerve, thus impairing normal vision. Rarely, colobomas are associated with serious generalized malformation syndromes.

Nose

Neonates must breathe through the nose; they cannot ordinarily breathe through the mouth. Any obstruction to the nasal passages thus causes some degree of respiratory distress. Partial or complete occlusion may be caused by mucus secretion that has not been removed or by choanal atresia or stenosis. The latter are congenital anomalies of the posterior nares, which may be life threatening (p. 256).

Mouth and throat

Complete visualization of the mouth and pharynx is difficult when the tongue is depressed; such attempts are usually met with strong reflex protrusion of the depressed tongue. However, an excellent view is obtained by stimulating a cry be-

fore gently depressing the tongue. Examination of the mouth is extremely important for the identification of a cleft palate, which often occurs in the absence of a cleft lip. Cleft palate may involve either the hard or soft palates or both. Occasionally only the uvula is cleft.

Precocious teeth occur infrequently. They are most often situated at the lower central incisor positions (Fig. 6-13). When covered with membranous tissue, they are pink rather than white. If detachment is imminent, they should be removed to prevent aspiration.

Epstein's pearls are small, white papular structures, one on each side of the midline of the hard palate. They are insignificant and usually disappear within a few weeks after birth.

The *frenulum* of the tongue is a sharp, thin ridge of tissue that arises in the midline from the base of the tongue and attaches to its undersurface for varying distances toward the tip. When the attachment extends far forward, a concav-

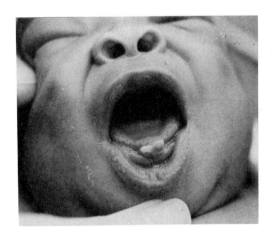

Fig. 6-13. Precocious teeth in the usual location. Teeth were sufficiently loose to threaten spontaneous detachment and aspiration, and they were removed.

ity (or a groove) is evident at the tip of the tongue on its upper surface. This condition is referred to as tongue-tie. It rarely if ever interferes with feeding, not does it produce a speech impediment in childhood. "Clipping of the tongue" by incising the frenulum is therefore rarely indicated, especially since there is some danger of severing a rather large vein in the area of the frenulum. Furthermore, the procedure creates a portal of entry for infection.

Neck

The neonate's neck is characteristically short; abnormalities are infrequent. A *webbed neck* in females is seen in Turner's syndrome. Webbing is characterized by redundance of skin that extends bilaterally from the posterolateral aspect of the neck, down to the medial portions of the shoulders along the superior margins of the underlying trapezius muscles. *Branchial cleft cysts* may be evident on the lateral aspects of the neck, along the anterior margin of the sternomastoid muscle. They are generally firm, 1 cm or less in diameter, and are covered by normal skin. More commonly, and in the same areas, dimples are evident. These are *branchial cleft sinuses*. *Branchial cleft cysts or sinuses* are rarely of clinical significance, unless they become infected. They are inherited autosomal dominant traits. *Thyroglossal cysts* are superficially evident as subcutaneous structures in the midline of the anterior neck at the level of the larynx above it. They indicate the presence of a *thyroglossal duct*, which is an abnormal remnant of thyroid gland formation during embryogenesis. The duct extends deeply into the neck, often opening at its deep end onto the surface of the tongue at its base (root). The duct may contain thyroid

tissue. Later surgical excision is generally indicated. *Goiter* (enlargement of the thyroid gland) is a visible, easily palpated mass in the midline of the anterior neck immediately inferior to, and partially overlying, the larynx. Goiters are generally the result of thyroid medication used in treatment of maternal thyroid disorders. Goiters are not often functional; rarely, however, they are associated with *neonatal hyperthyroidism.*

Thorax

The ribs are flexible; slight sternal retraction is sometimes evident during normal respiration. The *xiphoid cartilage* is at the lower end of the sternum. It may curve anteriorly to produce a prominent pointed protrusion beneath the skin that disappears in several weeks.

Rib fracture may be present in the neonate. Fig. 6-14 depicts the fracture of two

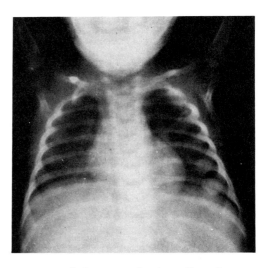

Fig. 6-14. Rib fractures, healing. Round opacities in the ribs to the left of cardiac apex are sites of callus formation during healing process. They were palpated as round, bony masses.

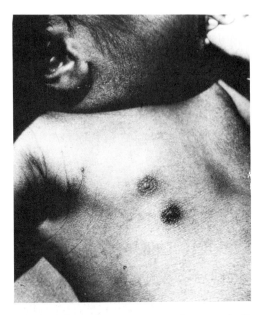

Fig. 6-15. Supernumerary nipple, unusually well developed. The upper nipple is the supernumerary one. Above and lateral to it, near the axilla, is a small spot that is another rudimentary extra nipple.

ribs that were palpable as rounded, bony masses. They are seen as two opaque, white nodules in the lower left chest that are not present in the lower right chest. Resuscitation was attempted by the ineffective and dangerous method of squeezing the thoracic cage. Vigorous application of this useless procedure resulted in fracture of the anterior portion of the fourth and fifth ribs.

Supernumerary nipples (Fig. 6-15) are occasionally noted inferior and medial to the normal ones, less often they occur superior and lateral to the normal nipples. They are harmless pink or pigmented spots that vary from a few millimeters in diameter to the size of normal nipples, but they do not contain glandular tissue.

Breast enlargement may occur in some

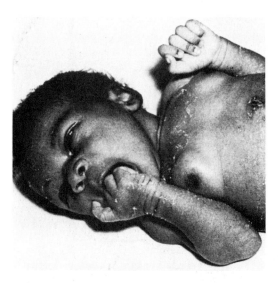

Fig. 6-16. Breast hypertrophy.

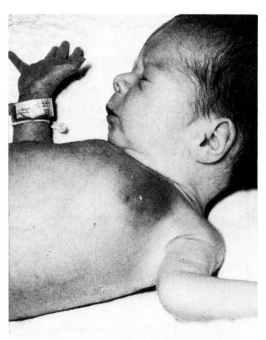

Fig. 6-17. Breast abscess. Note purulent drainage just superior to nipple.

infants (Fig. 6-16). It appears on the third day, and toward the end of the first week a milklike substance ("witch's milk") may be evident. Massaging such breasts with various preparations is a common lay practice that often produces breast abscess. Breast hypertrophy should not be confused with *breast abscess* (Fig. 6-17), which involves asymmetric swelling around the areola and severe erythema of the skin. Pus, usually yellow or blood tinged, may exude from the nipple or through inflamed skin; it should not be confused with "witch's milk," which is blank white.

Lungs

Physical examination of the lungs is only a first step, but an indispensable one, in the identification of respiratory disorders. Radiologic and blood gas studies should follow if the suspicion of a respiratory disorder is aroused by positive physical findings. The respiratory pattern should be observed before the infant is disturbed. Normal neonates breathe at rates varying between 40 and 60 respirations per minute. Rapid rates are likely to be present for the first few hours after birth. Fluctuations of respiratory rates are the rule, and for this reason several assessments may be necessary before one can conclude that an abnormality exists. *Periodic breathing,* a frequent normal finding in premature infants that requires no therapy, is characterized by sporadic episodes in which respirations cease for up to 10 seconds. Periodic breathing is not associated with cyanosis or bradycardia, and it is rare during the first 24 hours of life. It should not be confused with apneic episodes, which are of longer duration, often cause generalized cyanosis, and may occur at any time.

In the normal neonate, respiratory movements are predominantly diaphragmatic. The thoracic cage remains relatively immobile while the abdomen rises and falls with inspiration and expiration. Occasionally the immobile chest gives the false appearance of being drawn inward as the abdomen protrudes with each inspiration. This should not be confused with the retractions that characterize abnormal respiration.

Respiratory difficulties can be identified by simply observing the infant. A number of abnormal signs are clearly indicative of distress, generalized cyanosis being the most obvious and serious. A sustained rate in excess of 60 respirations per minute *(tachypnea)* after 3 or 4 hours of age is abnormal, but this condition should be ascertained by obtaining several counts of no less than 30 seconds' duration. Irregular respirations associated with repeated *apneic episodes* are often the result of depressed central nervous system function caused by severe hypoxia or intracranial hemorrhage. *Retractions* indicate obstruction to airflow at any level of the respiratory tract from the nose to the alveoli. They are visible with each inspiration and are characterized by indrawing of the thoracic wall at the sternum between the ribs, above the clavicles, and below the inferior costal margins (Fig. 6-4). The *respiratory grunt* is an unequivocal sign of difficulty. It is a fascinating compensatory mechanism by which an infant attempts to retain air to increase arterial P_{O_2} (p. 208). An audible sigh during each expiration is a variant of the respiratory grunt that serves the same purpose. Air hunger is commonly associated with *flaring of the nostrils* (alae nasi) during each inspiration. As a rule, an infant in respiratory distress has more than one of the abnormal signs just described.

No matter how accurate and well phrased they may be, descriptions of *auscultatory findings* cannot replace experience with the stethoscope. Nevertheless, several introductory remarks may serve to properly orient the examiner. Auscultatory signs in the lungs are of less value in the neonate than in any other pediatric age group. The chest is so small that localization of findings is often impossible. The diminutive lung effectively transmits breath sounds from one region to another. The absence of breath sounds in one part of the lung may not be appreciated because the sounds from the unaffected areas are transmitted from a distance. With experience, diminution of air exchange can be confidently detected, particularly when there is a discrepancy between the two lungs. Diminished breath sounds occur in hyaline membrane disease, atelectasis, emphysema, pneumothorax, and as a function of shallow respirations from any cause. Fine *rales* are produced in terminal bronchioles and alveoli by the rush of air through fluid within them. These rales are classically described as crackling in character. They can be reproduced with some degree of accuracy by rubbing your own hair between two fingers as close to your ear as possible. Rales are heard in some infants with hyaline membrane disease, pneumonia, and pulmonary edema, and occasionally in normal babies immediately after birth. They are sometimes audible only after deep inspiration, which must be induced by stimulating a cry. *Rhonchi* are coarse sounds that resemble snoring. They emanate from large bronchi as air rushes through fluid contained within them. Rhonchi are most frequently present after aspiration of oral secretions or feedings.

Heart

Inspection occasionally reveals a localized pulsation on the chest wall at about the fifth intercostal space in the midclavicular line, toward the lateral half of the left hemithorax. The pulsations are more evident in small babies with thin chest walls. If pulsations are prominent in the epigastrium, the heart is probably enlarged considerably.

By *palpation*, the normal apical impulse can be identified at the fifth intercostal space. Ascertainment of cardiac position is particularly important in dyspneic infants. Detection of an abnormal position early in the examination is an important initial step in establishing a correct diagnosis. A shift in the mediastinum caused by pneumothorax, for example, moves the apical impulse away from the affected side of the chest (p. 249). Pneumothorax in the right chest thus causes a shift of the mediastinum to the left; the apical impulse can be felt farther toward the left lateral chest wall than is normal. On the other hand, if the left chest is affected, the apical beat is palpable closer to the midline of the chest or sometimes to the right of it. Such cardiac displacements also occur in diaphragmatic hernia, which usually affects the left chest (p. 260). In the rare occurrence of bilateral pneumothorax, the point of maximal cardiac impulse is displaced downward toward the epigastrium. Abnormal apical location also occurs in dextrocardia, which is a mirror image reversal of cardiac position; the apex is in the right chest. If abdominal organs are also reversed, the anomalous position of the heart may or may not be significant in terms of abnormal cardiovascular function. However, if the abdominal viscera are normally placed and the position of the heart is reversed, cardiac anomalies are more likely. The normal locations of abdominal organs are described on p. 158.

Auscultation is the most informative component of the physical examination of the heart. The ability to perceive abnormalities by evaluating heart sounds depends on continuous, thoughtful practice. The first and second heart sounds are normally clear and well defined. In the neonate they acoustically resemble the syllables toc-tic. The second sound is somewhat higher in pitch and sharper than the first. Heart rates normally fluctuate between 120 and 160 beats/min. In agitated states a rate of 200 beats/min may occur transiently. The heart rate of premature infants is usually between 130 and 170 beats/min, and during occasional episodes of bradycardia it may slow to 70 beats/min or less. *Murmurs* are erroneously considered to be regularly indicative of congenital cardiac malformations, when in fact over 90% of those detected during the neonatal period are not associated with anomalies. Many murmurs are transient. Conversely, murmurs are sometimes absent in seriously malformed hearts. Most murmurs are systolic; they occur after the first sound and end at or before the second sound. Continuous murmurs extend beyond the second sound into diastole. According to their intensity, murmurs are Grade I (softest) to Grade VI (loudest). Murmurs heard very soon after birth are quite likely to indicate cardiac malformations. The appearance of a murmur at any time requires an evaluation of several additional parameters such as the peripheral pulses, blood pressure, the size and consistency of liver, and the size and contour of the heart as revealed by a chest film.

The state of the *peripheral pulses* is important. Brachial, radial, and femoral pulses are the most easily evaluated. Normal pulses are readily discernible, but the examiner's capacity to assess abnormal weakness and fullness depends on careful and experienced observations in normal neonates. Weakness of all pulses is indicative of a diminished cardiac output. This occurs in "hypoplastic left heart syndrome," in the hypoxic myocardium of an asphyxiated baby or in cardiac failure from other causes, and in septic or hemorrhagic shock. Excessively full pulses ("bounding pulses") generally appear several days after birth in premature infants who have developed a large left-to-right shunt from the aorta to the pulmonary artery through a patent ductus arteriosus (see Chapter 8). Another group of malformations is indicated by a strong right radial pulse and a weak left one. This suggests obstruction to blood flow along the aortic arch due to a coarctation that is proximal to (above) the entry of the ductus arteriosus into the aorta. On the other hand, weak femoral pulses and strong radial pulses suggest coarctation distal to (below) the ductus arteriosus. Most aortic coarctations are preductal (proximal to the entry of the ductus). The presence of a murmur also requires assessment of *liver size and consistency.* In babies with right-sided congestive heart failure, the liver enlarges; its inferior edge is palpable 5 to 6 cm below the right costal margin. The enlarged liver is quite firm because it is tightly distended by blood that has not progressed through the failing heart. Its inferior margin is thus easily palpated. A chest film is indispensable for initial assessment of *cardiac size and contour. Blood pressure* is simply and accurately measured with a Doppler apparatus and an ordinary blood pressure cuff. Some types of Doppler equipment provide systolic and diastolic readings; other less expensive types are adequate even though they are limited to systolic readings. The cuff should be no wider than 1 inch; in larger babies a 2-inch cuff may be essential. Blood pressure readings are usually obtained more easily at the popliteal space with the cuff around the thigh. A loose cuff may result in spuriously high readings; an excessively tight cuff may yield falsely low readings. If the peripheral pulses are weak, the baby may be hypotensive. If the pulse is stronger in one extremity than in another, widely discrepent blood pressures may be demonstrated and the presence of a coarctation is quite likely.

Abdomen

Inspection. The contour of the abdomen should be noted before it is palpated. It is ordinarily cylindric, sometimes protruding slightly in normal term infants. Several gross abnormalities are apparent on inspection. *Distention* in its most severe form is characterized by tightly drawn skin through which engorged subcutaneous vessels are easily seen. *Localized bulging* at one or both flanks suggests enlarged kidneys, usually hydronephrosis (Fig. 6-2). A grotesque abnormality of contour characterizes the rare malformation known as congenital absence of abdominal musculature ("prune belly" syndrome), in which severe renal anomalies are also present. The anterior aspect of the abdomen is sunken, or perhaps slightly protuberant, whereas the intestines, which are covered only by skin and a thin layer of subcutaneous tissue, bulge pendulously from the flanks (Fig. 6-18).

Palpation. With rare exceptions the edge of the *liver* is normally palpable be-

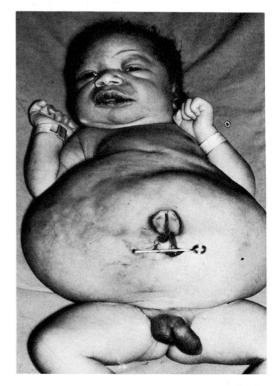

Fig. 6-18. Congenital absence of abdominal muscle ("prune belly" syndrome). Massive bilateral hydronephrosis and hydroureter were present.

low the right costal margin, often as far as 3 cm inferior to it. The tip of the spleen can sometimes be felt in normal infants. Examination of the abdomen must include palpation of each *kidney*, and this is most easily accomplished immediately after birth, when the intestines are not yet distended with air. With the infant supine, a finger is placed at the posterior flank (costovertebral angle) to maintain upward pressure while the other hand presses downward toward the posteriorly placed finger. The kidney can be felt as an oval structure between the finger and hand. The lower poles of each kidney are normally situated approximately 1 or 2 cm above the level of the umbilicus. If enlargement is present, they are below this level. By simple palpation, the astute examiner can identify approximately 90% of gross renal anomalies. *Bladder distention* should be sought in the suprapubic region. If present, a firm globular mass is palpable. If it persists to any degree after voiding, the bladder is incompletely emptied, and an obstruction may be present at the outlet. *Masses* that are perceptible elsewhere in the abdomen are usually of intestinal origin.

Diastasis recti is an inconsequential longitudinal gap in the abdominal midline between the two rectus muscles. It can be palpated from the epigastrium to the umbilicus as a linear absence of abdominal wall musculature approximately 1 cm in width. When the infant cries, thereby raising intraabdominal pressure, a bulge is visible through the linear gap in musculature. Diastasis recti disappears within a few weeks.

The normal *umbilical cord* is blue-white and moist at birth. Within 24 hours, it begins to dry and becomes dull and yellow-brown. Later it turns black-brown and shrivels considerably. In this gangrenous state it sloughs from its attachment at approximately 1 week of age. After birth, the cut section of the cord reveals three blood vessels (two arteries and one vein). A diagram of the cut surface can be seen on p. 4. The arteries appear to be smaller, round, papular protrusions from the cut surface; the vein is larger and oval. The arterial walls are thick; their lumens are obliterated by vasospasm. In contrast, the venous wall is thin and relaxed; the lumen is thus easily discerned. On the cut surface, the relative positions of the three vessels vary considerably, depending on the level at which the cord is cut, because the vessels

pursue a spiral course along the entire length of the cord. A *single umbilical artery* is reason for an assiduous search for congenital malformations of any type. In some reports, a significant number of these infants have major congenital anomalies. Other reports assert that there is not a higher incidence of anomalies in surviving infants with a single umbilical artery; the higher incidence of malformations only occurs in babies who do not survive.

If meconium has not been passed by the end of the first day of life, *patency of the anus* should be ascertained by inserting the tip of a thermometer or a plastic feeding tube for a distance not in excess of 1 cm.

Inguinal hernias occur most frequently in males and in a large number of low birth weight babies as well. They are readily discernible when the characteristic swelling is present in the inguinal canal; they are usually unilateral, occasionally bilateral. The swelling in males may extend into the scrotum. Sometimes, the hernia is not perceptible until the infant cries. The hernias contain intestine, but in females the ovary and fallopian tubes are also occasionally present. The ovary is palpable as a movable nodular mass in the inguinal canal that is not unlike a swollen lymph node. Surgical correction is required. Infrequently, intestinal contents are trapped (incarcerated) in the inguinal canal and cannot be returned (reduced) into the abdomen. Vomiting and progressive abdominal distention appear, and immediate surgical intervention is necessary.

Male genitalia

The *prepuce* covers the entire *glans penis* so that the external meatus is not visible. The prepuce is not retractable in the neonate and sometimes cannot be displaced until 4 to 6 months of age. It thus should never be forcibly retracted. This condition is not phimosis, and it is not an indication for circumcision. The trauma of forceful retraction is thought by some to be responsible for phimosis later on. According to a statement by the American Academy of Pediatrics, *"there is no absolute medical indication for routine circumcision of the newborn. It is not an essential component of adequate total health care."* Good penile hygiene accomplishes as much. If the ventral surface of the glans is not covered by preputial tissue, *hypospadias* is present. Hypospadias is characterized by an anomalous position of the urethral meatus on the ventral portion of the glans penis, rather than at its center. It may also be situated on the ventral surface of the penile shaft anywhere along its length.

In term infants the *testes* are in the *scrotum*. In premature infants the testes are in the inguinal canal, or they may not be palpable. The scrotum varies in size in relation to maturity. In premature infants it is small and close to the perineum. In term babies the scrotum is large, hanging loosely at a greater distance from the perineum. The term infant's scrotum is rugated (wrinkled) over its entire surface, back to its perineal attachment. The scrotum of the premature infant is less extensively rugated, becoming smoother toward the perineal attachment. Scrotal rugation is one of the external signs used for the assessment of gestational age (see Chapter 5). A *hydrocele* is frequently observed in the scrotum, particularly in term infants. It is a unilateral (sometimes bilateral) accumulation of fluid that surrounds the testis. When a hydrocele is unilateral, the affected side of the scrotum is larger,

appearing tightly cystic. Transillumination of a hydrocele reveals a striking translucency. In an inguinal hernia the scrotal contents are comprised of intestine or fluid (or both). It is thus opaque to transillumination, or considerably less translucent than the hydrocele. A hydrocele usually disappears spontaneously in a few days or weeks.

Female genitalia

In term babies the *labia minora* are sometimes more prominent than the *labia majora;* in premature infants this is almost the rule. The *clitoris* varies in size. It may be so large as to confound determination of the baby's sex. The diagnosis of adrenogenital syndrome, an endocrine disorder that involves excessive secretions of androgenic and other hormones from the adrenal gland, may then be made. In the affected neonate, life-threatening electrolyte disturbances and dehydration may occur rapidly within a few days after birth.

The *hymenal tag* is a normal redundant segment of the hymen that pro-

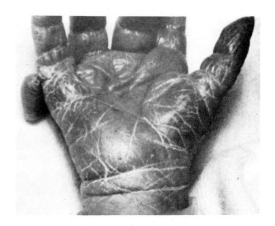

Fig. 6-19. Digitus postminimus (see text). Hypotrophic finger hangs by a thin pedicle from lateral aspect of fifth finger.

trudes from the floor of the vagina and disappears in several weeks. During the first week of life, a milk-white mucoid discharge, which is sometimes blood tinged, may be evident in the vagina. This is a physiologic manifestation of maternal hormonal influences that disappears within 2 weeks.

Extremities

The extremities should be examined for malformations and trauma. Malformations frequently involve the fingers. *Polydactyly* is an excessive number of digits on the hands or feet. In its most common form it consists of a rudimentary digit (digitus postminimus) attached to the lateral aspect of the little finger by a thin pedicle (Fig. 6-19). It is treated by firmly tying a silk suture around the pedicle, close to the surface of the normal fin-

ger. Gangrene of the anomalous digit ensues in a few days, and it falls away. Less commonly an extra, fully formed digit is present. *Syndactyly* is the fusion of two digits into one structure (Fig. 6-20), and it most commonly involves the toes.

Fractures have been discussed in Chapter 2. The clavicle, humerus, and femur are respectively involved in descending order of frequency. Fractures should be suspected in any baby who fails to move one extremity as extensively as the others. Malposition and a visible

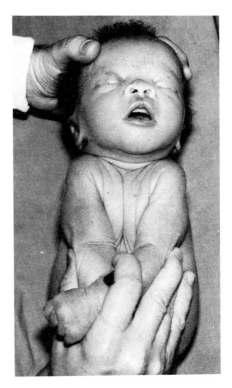

Fig. 6-21. Cleidocranial dysostosis (congenital absence of clavicles). If clavicles were not examined as a routine part of examination, this major syndrome would not have been identified in the neonate, when it should be. Shoulders are drawn anteriorly, and when compressed, they meet in midline.

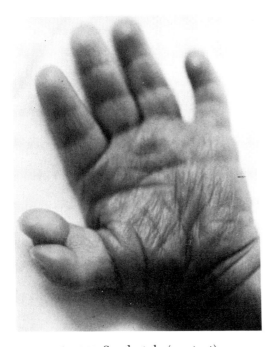

Fig. 6-20. Syndactyly (see text).

local deformity at the fracture site are often helpful signs.

Clavicles must be palpated to ascertain their presence as well as to detect fractures. Absence of the clavicles, either total or segmental, is characteristic of *cleidocranial dysostosis* (Fig. 6-21), an inherited disorder of bone formation in the skull, the clavicles, and occasionally the pubic bone. Absence of the clavicles permits innocuous anterior displacement of the shoulders so that they almost meet in the midline (Fig. 6-21).

Congenital ring constrictions (annular or amniotic bands) are poorly understood malformations that occur infrequently. They affect the extremities, which are thought to become entangled in a local early rupture of the amniotic membrane. Subsequent growth occurs in the presence of constricting amniotic bands. In the extreme, amputation occurs, either of an extremity somewhere along its length or of one or more digits. Milder expressions of this disorder are seen as banded depressions of the skin that are much like a tight rubber band around the extremity (Fig. 6-22). The most common sites of involvement in order of frequency are the fingers, toes, ankle, leg, forearm, and arm. Amniotic bands and the amputations with which they are sometimes associated may involve more than one extremity but are usually unilateral.

Neurologic evaluation

Abnormal neurologic signs may be transient or persistent. They may disappear by the time the infant is discharged from the nursery, or they may be present throughout the nursery stay. Predictions of later brain dysfunction cannot be made with consistent accuracy on the basis of neurologic abnormalities during the newborn period.

Observations should be made with as little disturbance to the baby as possible. Reflexes that require the greatest degree of disturbance should be elicited toward the end of the examination. Thus *spontaneous movements* should be studied first. Infants who are generally depressed will move very little or not at all. They are hypotonic as well. Intrauterine asphyxia, or hypoxia at any time, is the most common cause of this neuromuscular abnormality. Drugs administered to the mother are also frequent causes of depression. These drugs include analgesics (Demerol), hypnotics (barbiturates, magnesium sulfate, alcohol), and local anesthetics (lidocaine). Central nervous

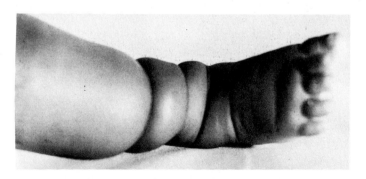

Fig. 6-22. Congenital amniotic bands above the ankle.

system infections, bacterial or nonbacterial, and metabolic disturbances (hypoglycemia, hypothyroidism) also cause depression. Trauma to the central nervous system, most often in the form of cerebral contusion or subdural hematoma, is an additional cause of diminished or absent spontaneous activity.

Spontaneous hyperirritability and exaggerated responses to ordinary tactile or acoustic stimuli are abnormal. These responses may range from severe agitation or jitteriness to frank convulsions. They may thus be manifested as localized twitches, gross rhythmic repetitive jerks of one or more muscle groups (myoclonus), or generalized clonic convulsions. There is little to be gained in attempting to localize central nervous system lesions based on these localized convulsive phenomena, since in the neonate there is generally no such correlation. There is also little use in attempting to differentiate between a severely agitated state characterized by ceaseless movement and a frank convulsion. Usually they are of equal significance. These irritative phenomena are most common during recovery from asphyxia, after a period of depression. They also occur in babies of narcotic-addicted mothers (heroin or morphine withdrawal) and among infants of mothers who are habituated to barbiturates (phenobarbital withdrawal). Hypocalcemia, hypomagnesemia, and hypoglycemia may cause irritative phenomena. Neonatal hyperthroidism and pyridoxine dependency are rare causes. Maternal administration of local anesthetics such as lidocaine may produce depression at first, but this is followed by convulsions. Intracranial hemorrhage and, occasionally, central nervous system infection may also produce irritative responses early in their courses.

Asymmetry in movement of the extremities indicates weakness, paralysis, or bone fracture. In brachial plexus palsy, for example, the affected upper extremity is hypoactive or immobile. Failure to move the lower extremities suggests a spinal cord injury. Asymmetry of movement or tone is always abnormal.

Muscle tone is extremely important in the neurologic evaluation of neonates. The normal infant maintains some degree of flexion in all the extremities, and extension by the examiner of any one of them is followed by at least a partial return to the previous position of flexion. Flexion posture is less pronounced in premature infants. Infants who experience intrauterine hypoxia are hypotonic; they may not be flexed at rest. Furthermore, straightening of the extremities is not followed by return to flexion. Poor head control, described later, is additional evidence of abnormally diminished muscle tone.

The elicitation of certain reflex responses is essential for assessment of the infant's neurologic status. The *grasp reflex* is normally strong in term infants. It is elicited by placing a finger across the palm at the base of the fingers. In response, the examiner's finger may be grasped so firmly that, using both hands, the infant can often be raised off the surface of the crib. This response is considerably more feeble in premature babies or in depressed infants. It is asymmetric in some cases of brachial plexus palsy (Klumpke type), being absent or weak on the affected side.

The *rooting reflex* is activated by lightly stroking the angle of the lips. The baby turns his head to the stroked side. Recently fed infants and those who are lethargic or depressed merely purse the lips or do not respond at all. Vigorous infants turn the head briskly and instantly, pursuing the finger as long as contact with the lips is maintained.

The *suck* is evaluated by inserting a sterile nipple into the mouth. In normal infants, particularly those who are hungry, the response is immediate, coordinated, and forceful. Recently fed infants, premature babies, and those who are depressed respond with varying degrees of feebleness.

The *knee jerk* is normally brisk. It is weak in depressed infants, exaggerated to the point of clonus (repetitive jerks) in irritated ones, and asymmetric in babies who have spinal cord lesions, fractures of the femur, or bone and joint infection of the examined extremity.

Ankle clonus is elicited by placing two fingers against the anterior sole of the foot and abruptly, with a short, brisk movement, dorsiflexing it. The response will

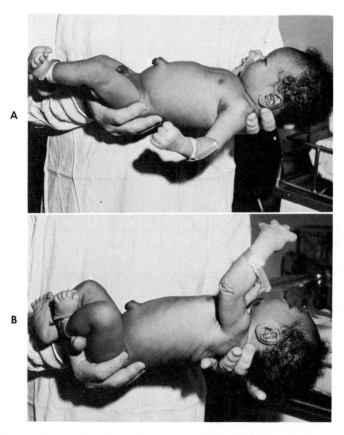

Fig. 6-23. Moro reflex. **A,** The baby is supported beneath the sacrum and upper back, including the occiput. The head is level with the body. **B,** The head is allowed to fall backward. In response, the upper extremities are abruptly thrust upward and outward while the knees and hips are rapidly flexed. Compare changes in position of the head and upper and lower extremities. Compare also this normal response to that in brachial plexus palsy (Fig. 2-15).

usually consist of several repetitive jerks (beats) of the foot or none at all. If more than eight to ten beats occur, the baby is probably in an irritated state.

Head control in the normal neonate is more effective than is generally realized. With the infant supine the examiner takes the wrists and lifts him slowly to a sitting position. The normal term infant reinforces the maneuver by contracting the shoulder and arm muscles, followed by flexion of the neck. As the sitting position is reached, the infant controls his head by action of neck muscles and thus prevents it from falling forward onto the chest. In many babies the head falls forward but is soon righted to the erect position. Hypotonic infants, such as those with Down's syndrome or those who are hypoxic, have little or no head control, and they do not respond to traction by activating the muscles of the arms and shoulders. The neck is extremely lax, and the head bobbles in any direction dictated by the combined effects of body position and gravity. There is no attempt to assume an erect posture once the head has fallen to either side or onto the chest.

The *Moro reflex* is demonstrable in all normal neonates (Fig. 6-23). It is often erroneously elicited by slapping the bassinet or jerking it. Some examiners abruptly pull a blanket from under the baby. Others lift him slightly off the crib surface by the wrists and allow him to fall back. The most consistent responses are obtained by holding the baby in a supine position with both hands, one palm beneath the sacrum and buttocks and the other beneath the occiput and upper back. By suddenly slipping the hand down from the occiput onto the back, the head is allowed to fall through an angle of approximately 30 degrees, thus activating the Moro reflex. The normal response is characterized by straightening of the arms and elbows away from the body and by extension of the wrists and fingers. This is followed by return of the upper extremities onto the chest in a position of passive flexion. A cry often accompanies the baby's startled response. Reflex movement of the hips and knees occurs quickly and is of short duration. If an extremity does not respond fully, a localized neurologic defect or fracture is suspect. Suboptimal vigor of the overall response occurs in depressed infants, whereas in premature infants the response is disorganized and incomplete to varying degrees.

Transillumination of the skull is a useful procedure if neurologic disorder is suspected. It is performed with a strong light source from a flashlight fitted with a rubber collar that fits snugly to the skull. In a dark room devoid of light leaks, the examiner must first become dark-adapted. As a rule, dark adaptation is present when the light, placed into the examiner's palm, is transmitted through the hand so that shadows of the distal metacarpal bones are clearly visible as light penetrates the soft tissue between them. The flashlight is then applied to the scalp tightly, and while the snug fit is maintained to avoid light leak, it is moved over the surface of the head. We use a two-battery flashlight. With it, a flare of light greater than 1.5 to 2 cm beyond the rim of the rubber fitting is considered abnormal. The entire cranium lights up like a red electric bulb in babies who have congenital absence of the cerebral hemispheres (hydranencephaly). In this instance the cranial vault is filled with fluid instead of brain tissue. These infants may behave normally during the newborn period. Severe hydrocephalus produces the same phenomenon. Abnormal light flare is seen locally over subdural hematomas or porencephalic cysts (local absence of cerebral tissue).

A number of conditions cause abnormal light transmission that is not indicative of a brain disorder. Most understandable and common is edema of the scalp, which may occur in infiltration of intravenous fluids being given into a scalp vein or in caput succedaneum. The water-logged scalp transmits more light over a greater area. In the region of the anterior fontanelle, abnormal light transmission is also misleading. The flare of light increases and may extend beyond 2 cm because of the absence of bone. Infants who weighed less than 1250 grams at birth, have grown rapidly, and are approximately 1 month of age may often manifest generalized abnormal light transmission. This does not indicate developing hydrocephalus nor cerebral malformation. It is apparently the result of normal enlargement of the subarachnoid space, which seems to occur during this period of rapid growth. Serial measurements of *both head and chest circumferences* will reveal that the apparent rapid growth of the head is actually a component of growth of the entire body. Misinterpretation of this normally increased transillumination, combined with failure to assess head enlargement as a normal component of overall body growth, has resulted in numerous needless pneumoencephalograms, ventriculograms, and other extensive neurologic inquiries.

Final impression of the infant's neu-rologic status must be formed with great caution. The neurologic examination is not in itself inadequate, but the nature of the neonate's neurologic disorders makes it difficult to localize the disorder or, in marginal situations, to be certain there is any disorder at all. Certainly one cannot take the sum of abnormal findings and arrive at a conclusion in a manner more appropriate for a bookkeeper than a clinician. The incidence of false-positive and false-negative signs is high. Furthermore, repeated observations are absolutely indispensable because abnormal signs are often transient, disappearing in a matter of hours. Extremes are seldom a puzzle; the gross abnormalities and the unequivocal normal state cause little difficulty for the clinician. The in-between phenomena are notoriously troublesome in the total physical examination generally, and in the neurologic evaluation particularly.

REFERENCES

Behrman, R. E.: The fetus and the neonatal infant. In Vaughan, V. C., McKay, R. J., and Behrman, R. E., editors: Nelson's textbook of pediatrics, Philadelphia, 1979, W. B. Saunders Co.

Korones, S. B.: The newborn: perinatal pediatrics. In Hughes, J. G., editor: Synopsis of pediatrics, ed. 5, St. Louis, 1980, The C. V. Mosby Co.

Lucey, J. F.: Examination of the newborn. In Reed, D. E., Ryan, K. J., and Benirschke, K., editors: Principles and management of human reproduction, Philadelphia, 1972, W. B. Saunders Co.

Paine, R. S.: Neurologic examination of infants and children, Pediatr. Clin. North Am. **7**:471, 1960.

Phibbs, R. H.: Evaluation of the newborn. In Rudolph, A. M., editor: Pediatrics, New York, 1977, Appleton-Century-Crofts.

CHAPTER 7

Basic principles and clinical significance of acid-base, fluid, and electrolyte disturbances

ACID-BASE BALANCE

In newborn babies almost all serious illnesses eventually involve an acid-base imbalance that in itself may be more hazardous to the baby's survival than the primary disease process. The infant often can be sustained by partial or complete correction of the acid-base disturbance while the primary pathophysiology runs its course. In hyaline membrane disease, for example, there is no effective therapy for eradication of the basic pulmonary pathology (atelectasis), but with spontaneous appearance of adequate quantities of a phospholipid substance known as surfactant, the atelectasis tends to resolve spontaneously in a few days (p. 198). In the meantime, if no attempt is made to correct biochemical abnormalities that arise from the primary pulmonary disorder, death is inexorable in severely affected infants. Diarrhea is another case in point. Whether or not antibiotics are ultimately effective in eliminating the etiologic agent (and most often they are not), fluid therapy must be instituted early to rectify the life-threatening acidosis and dehydration that develop so rapidly. Although the diarrhea usually subsides in several days, acid-base balance and optimal hydration must be maintained during its course if the baby is to survive.

An understanding of acid-base disturbances is essential if the nurse is to correlate laboratory data with the clinical course of the disease process and thus assess an infant's progress accurately. Appreciation of the rationale of appropriate therapy is indispensable if the nurse is to participate intelligently in its administration. The discussion that follows will summarize pertinent acid-base factors that are operative in the production of life-threatening illness. Emphasis on terminology is appropriate because understanding of terms and mastery of concepts are inseparable.

pH, acids, and bases

pH. At any given moment acid-base status is determined by the concentration of hydrogen ion (H^+) present in body fluids as a result of the production, neutralization, and elimination of various acids. The higher the concentration of hydrogen ion, the more acid the fluid, and conversely the lower the concentration of hydrogen ion, the more alkaline the fluid. The acidity of a fluid, whether blood, plasma, or urine, is expressed as its *pH*. The mathematic derivation of pH is such that a rise or fall indicates a change of hydrogen ion concentration in the opposite direction. The pH of a solution is therefore inversely proportional to the concentration of hydrogen ion within it. A pH of 4.0 is more acid than a pH of 5.0, but not simply one fifth more acid as is superficially apparent from the difference between the two values. Rather, there is a tenfold difference between the two figures because, being negative and logarithmic, each figure represents a multiple of minus 10, or the number of places to the right of a decimal point. Thus a pH of 4.0 represents 0.0001 gram of hydrogen ion per liter of solution. This representation is ten times greater than a pH of 5.0, which indicates 0.00001 gram of hydrogen ion per liter. Other translations of pH values are listed here to emphasize the large differences in acidity that are indicated by various pH units:

pH 1.0 indicates 0.1 gram of hydrogen ion per liter

pH 2.0 indicates 0.01 gram of hydrogen ion per liter

pH 3.0 indicates 0.001 gram of hydrogen ion per liter

pH 4.0 indicates 0.0001 gram of hydrogen ion per liter

A solution with a pH of 1.0 thus contains a hydrogen ion concentration 100 times greater than a solution with a pH of 3.0, or 1000 times greater than at pH 4.0. The reader should again note that the greater the pH value, the less the concentration of hydrogen ion. The accepted normal values for the pH of arterial blood in newborn infants at 24 hours of age is 7.35 to 7.44. The range of pH values compatible with life is 6.8 to 7.8. Most clinically important deviations occur between 7.00 and 7.25. These values represent enormous increases in hydrogen ion concentrations compared with the seemingly small differences between the numbers themselves. Compared with 7.35, a pH of 7.20 represents an increase of 40% in hydrogen ion concentration; pH of 7.10 represents an increase of approximately 80%, and at pH 7.00 the blood is over twice normal acidity (actually an increase of 124%).

Acids. Acids are substances capable of surrendering hydrogen ion (H^+) when in solution. The strength of their acidity depends on the extent to which the hydrogen ion is dissociated from its molecule when in solution, and this varies from one acid to another. Hydrochloric acid (HCl) is powerful because it is dissociated almost completely when in solution, thereby surrendering greater amounts of hydrogen ion than most other acids. The resultant high concentration of hydrogen ion in solution renders a lower pH than other, less-soluble acids in similar concentration. Carbonic acid (H_2CO_3), for example, does not dissociate as readily as hydrochloric acid; it surrenders fewer hydrogen ions in solution and is therefore a considerably weaker acid.

Bases. Bases are alkaline molecules capable of accepting hydrogen ions. When an acid is added to a base in solution, the dissociated hydrogen ion becomes bound to the base, with the resultant formation of a weaker acid. The base thus acts as a buffer by diminishing the potential acidity of a solution. Buffering is indispensable to the continuous maintenance of acid-base balance. In the neonate it is often overwhelmed by pathophysiologic events such as asphyxia, pulmonary dysfunction, or diarrhea. Therapeutic measures to enhance the buffering capacity of blood are therefore applied without delay.

Physiologic maintenance of acid-base equilibrium

Normal metabolism entails a relentless production of acids, principally carbonic acid, which must be neutralized and ultimately eliminated from the body. These acids are categorized as volatile and non-volatile (or fixed) acids. Carbonic acid (H_2CO_3) is volatile because it is constantly converted to carbon dioxide (CO_2) in the blood and eliminated in the gaseous state through the lungs. The nonvolatile, or fixed, acids are principally lactic, sulfuric, and phosphoric acids. They are buffered in blood and excreted through the kidneys. The three principal mechanisms by which acid products of normal metabolism are neutralized or eliminated are buffering activity in blood, elimination of carbon dioxide (volatile acid) through the lungs, and excretion of fixed acid through the kidneys. The respiratory apparatus directly controls blood levels of carbonic acid; the kidneys directly regulate the concentrations of bicarbonate buffer and hydrogen ion in the blood.

Buffers and buffer pairs. A buffer is a substance that, by its presence in a solution, is capable of minimizing changes in pH caused by the addition of acids or bases. Thus when a strong acid or base is added to a solution that contains a buffer, a weaker acid or base is formed and the change in pH is thus minimized. Buffers exist in pairs that are normally in sufficiently high concentration to stabilize changes in pH. These pairs are comprised of a weak acid and its salt. The principal buffer pairs in blood are sodium bicarbonate/carbonic acid ($NaHCO_3$/H_2CO_3) and sodium proteinate/acid protein. The protein buffer system resides predominantly in hemoglobin. The first member of each pair is a salt; the second member is a weak acid. The hydrogen ion concentration in blood, and therefore the pH, is determined by a *ratio of the constituents that comprise each buffer pair*; the proportion of bicarbonate to carbonic acid (normally 20:1) is the most important determinant. The ratio may be altered by a decrease in bicarbonate or an increase in carbonic acid, thus elevating hydrogen ion concentration and lowering pH.

Buffering of nonvolatile acids. Normally the changes in pH of body fluids caused by the addition of lactic and other nonvolatile acids are minimized and held within physiologic limits principally by the buffering activity of the bicarbonate/carbonic acid system. In this reaction lactic acid is buffered by sodium bicarbonate and converted to sodium lactate plus carbonic acid. Sodium lactate is excreted through the kidneys, and carbonic acid is excreted in the gaseous state (CO_2) through the lungs. These events are represented in the following formulas:

(1) HL (lactic acid) + $NaHCO_3 \rightarrow$
$$Na\ lactate + H_2CO_3$$

(2) $H_2CO_3 \rightarrow H_2O + CO_2$

Other nonvolatile acids also combine with sodium bicarbonate to form salts and carbonic acid.

Buffering of volatile acid (H_2CO_3). Carbonic acid is produced in greater quantity than any other acid during the course of normal tissue metabolism. It is buffered in the erythrocyte by hemoglobin. From tissue fluid it crosses capillary walls to enter the plasma and thence into erythrocytes. By a series of reactions within erythocytes it is converted to bicarbonate, which is released into plasma as sodium bicarbonate. Thus the carbon dioxide that originates in tissues is largely carried in plasma as sodium bicarbonate. The acid change in pH that would have occurred is held within normal limits by the production of bicarbonate in the red blood cells.

Stabilizing influence of the respiratory ap- **paratus.** The concentration of carbonic acid in plasma is determined by the amount of carbon dioxide that is present (P_{CO_2}), which in turn is largely dependent on the capacity of the respiratory apparatus to ventilate normally. In the fetus this process depends on normal placental function. The quantity of carbon dioxide excreted through the lungs increases with the depth and the rate of respiration. The depth and rate of respiration are subject to neural control of the respiratory center in the medulla of the brain, which is exquisitely sensitive to changes in blood pH. The respiratory center directs an increase in rate to eliminate more carbon dioxide when blood pH declines; it directs a decrease in rate to conserve carbon dioxide when the pH is elevated. If the ratio of bicarbonate to carbonic acid falls below normal as a result of an elevated carbonic acid concentration, pH declines. The respiratory rate is then accelerated in response to stimulation of the medullary respiratory center. An increased amount of carbon dioxide is blown off, the ratio of bicarbonate to carbonic acid is restored toward normal, and the pH of blood now rises. On the other hand, if blood pH rises abnormally, as it may when excessive doses of intravenous sodium bicarbonate are administered, the ventilatory rate is slowed. Carbon dioxide is retained, and the level of carbonic acid rises. Although the absolute quantities of carbonic acid and bicarbonate are now increased, their ratio is closer to normal and the pH declines. Ultimately excess bicarbonate is excreted by the kidneys, whereas temporarily retained carbon dioxide is eventually eliminated through the lungs.

Stabilizing influence of the kidneys. Whereas the respiratory apparatus directly regulates the concentration of volatile acid, the kidneys control the blood content of nonvolatile acid. This is primarily accomplished by the excretion of hydrogen ion plus the simultaneous conservation of bicarbonate. In contrast to the rapidly activiated compensatory efforts of the lungs, the kidneys respond more slowly, but they tend to carry compensatory mechanisms closer to completion.

Classification of acid-base disturbances

Disturbances in acid-base equilibrium may culminate in a diminished pH (acidosis) or an increased pH (alkalosis). Changes in either of these directions are caused by primary disorders of ventilation (respiratory acidosis and alkalosis) or primary disorders of general metabolism, renal function, or both (metabolic or nonrespiratory acidosis and alkalosis). The distinctions and variations of these disturbances are defined here, having been distilled from a broad literature. When appropriate, the biochemical deviation is described in association with the pathophysiologic event that gives rise to it. Over the years biochemists and physiologists who are concerned with the problems of acid-base balance have been at odds regarding proper definitions of various disturbances. There is frequent mention, in a voluminous literature, of the advantages and pitfalls of a "physiologic language" or a "laboratory language." For us the definitions presented here have facilitated the teaching and clinical applications of the concepts they describe. Table 7-1 summarizes the attributes of the various types of acid-base disturbance and their degrees of compensation.

Uncompensated disturbance. The uncompensated abnormalities defined here are characterized in each instance by the presence of an abnormal pH. The same

Table 7-1. Attributes of acid-base disturbances according to type and degree of compensation

Disturbance	Blood pH	Blood P_{CO_2} (mm Hg)	Blood HCO_3^- (mEq/L)
Normal	7.35 to 7.44	30 to 35	20 to 24
Metabolic acidosis			
Uncompensated	Lowest	Normal	Low
Partially compensated	Low	Low	Low
Fully compensated	Normal	Lowest	Low
Metabolic alkalosis			
Uncompensated	Highest	Normal	High
Partially compensated	High	High	High
Fully compensated	Normal	Highest	High
Respiratory acidosis			
Uncompensated	Lowest	High	Normal
Partially compensated	Low	High	High
Fully compensated	Normal	High	Highest
Respiratory alkalosis			
Uncompensated	Highest	Low	Normal
Partially compensated	High	Low	Low
Fully compensated	Normal	Low	Lowest

underlying abnormalities also exist in compensated forms. They are described later in this chapter.

Acidosis is a condition that causes an inordinate accumulation of acid (nonvolatile or volatile) or loss of base. The net result is an increase in hydrogen ion concentration and thus a diminution of blood pH to levels below normal.

Alkalosis is a condition that causes an excessive accumulation of base or a loss of acid (nonvolatile or volatile). The net result is a decrease in hydrogen ion concentration and thus an increase in blood pH to levels that are above normal.

Metabolic (nonrespiratory) acidosis occurs with an increase in the concentration of nonvolatile acids as a result of (1) deranged metabolism in which there is overproduction of acids, (2) disrupted renal function with impaired excretion of nonvolatile acids, and (3) excessive loss of base through the gastrointestinal tract (diarrhea) and rarely through the kidneys (renal tubular acidosis).

Metabolic (nonrespiratory) alkalosis is characterized by an increased concentration of base (bicarbonate). In the neonate it is most frequently caused by inappropriately large therapeutic doses of sodium bicarbonate. Repeated vomiting due to pyloric stenosis is occasionally encountered, causing metabolic alkalosis because a significant quantity of hydrochloric acid is lost in vomited gastric secretions. Rarely metabolic alkalosis results from an excessive renal loss of hydrogen ion or from renal retention of bicarbonate.

Respiratory acidosis follows decreased pulmonary gas exchange with resultant retention of carbon dioxide (increased P_{CO_2}). Perinatal asphyxia and hyaline membrane disease are the most common neonatal clinical entities in which respiratory acidosis occurs.

Respiratory alkalosis, caused by respiratory dysfunction, is characterized by an abnormally low P_{CO_2} resulting from excessive elimination of carbon dioxide during hyperventilation. It is most frequently encountered in therapy with mechanical ventilators that are incorrectly set to deliver respiratory rates and tidal volumes in excess of physiologic needs.

Compensated disturbances. Although definitions in the preceding paragraphs are based on an abnormal pH, acid-base disturbance can also be operative in the presence of a normal or nearly normal pH, provided certain compensatory mechanisms are effective. A description of the data in Table 7-1 is presented in the paragraphs that follow.

Compensation is a physiologic process that occurs in response to an antecedent (primary) derangement of acid-base balance. It tends to restore the ratio of buffer pairs toward normal. If compensation is complete, a normal ratio is reestablished and the pH is normal even though concentrations of the individual members of a buffer pair are abnormal. However, the original source of acid-base disturbance may still exist. The importance of recognizing these compensated disorders cannot be overestimated, since their corrective effects are often only temporary. The underlying disturbance, masked by these compensatory responses, requires cautious therapy.

Compensated metabolic (nonrespiratory) acidosis is characterized chiefly by hyperventilation for the reduction of P_{CO_2} to levels below normal. Hyperventilation is the compensatory process activated by accumulation of nonvolatile acid that consumes available base (bicarbonate). The excretion of volatile acid (CO_2) through the lungs must be increased to lower carbonic acid concentration to match the lowered level of bicarbonate and thus to restore the sodium bicarbonate/carbonic acid ratio in that buffer pair. In this compensated state the pH is normal or almost normal, but both the P_{CO_2} and the serum bicarbonate concentrations are low.

Compensated metabolic (nonrespiratory) alkalosis involves hypoventilation that is activated for the purpose of diminishing the elimination of carbon dioxide. Since the primary disturbance is accumulation of bicarbonate, retention of volatile acid (CO_2) tends to restore the ratio between sodium bicarbonate and carbonic acid. In this compensated state the pH is virtually normal, but the P_{CO_2} and serum bicarbonate concentrations are elevated.

Compensated respiratory acidosis involves retention of bicarbonate as a result of adjustment in renal function. Since the primary disturbance is accumulation of carbon dioxide, and thus an increase in carbonic acid, the rise in bicarbonate tends to restore the bicarbonate/carbonic acid ratio toward normal. In a fully compensated state the pH is normal, but P_{CO_2} and serum bicarbonate are increased. Whereas the renal mechanism seeks to restore pH by conserving bicarbonate, the respiratory apparatus attempts to eliminate the accumulated carbon dioxide. The clinically evident result of this activity is tachypnea.

Compensated respiratory alkalosis also involves adjustment of renal function. The primary disturbance is caused by hyperventilation with excessive elimination of carbon dioxide and resultant decline of P_{CO_2}. The kidney thus acts to increase excretion of bicarbonate to restore the bicarbonate/carbonic acid ratio to normal. In the fully compensated state pH is normal, but P_{CO_2} and serum bicarbonate are individually diminished although in normal ratio.

Mixed disturbances of acid-base balance. Some clinical disorders simultaneously give rise to disturbances of the respiratory and metabolic components of acid-base balance. These are called mixed disturbances, and they are characterized by a concurrence of respiratory and metabolic acidosis or alkalosis. In neonates the most commonly encountered variety is mixed acidosis associated with severe perinatal asphyxia and hyaline membrane disease. In mixed respiratory and metabolic acidosis, the combination of retained carbon dioxide and diminished bicarbonate causes a considerable decrease in pH.

Laboratory procedures for measuring acid-base status

The advent of microtechniques for the direct measurement of blood gases and pH has been a boon to the management of sick neonates. Rational therapy to rectify acid-base disorders is currently based on these procedures. Serial determinations are indispensable during the entire course of an illness because blood gas content and pH may change rapidly and repeatedly. Infants on mechanical respirators, for instance, must be monitored repeatedly and at frequent intervals for blood gas and acid-base status.

The collection of samples should be accomplished with precision and with a minimum quantity of blood. The blood P_{CO_2}, P_{O_2}, and pH can be measured from as little as 0.1 ml. Indwelling umbilical artery catheters are commonly utilized as a source of arterial blood samples. If this route is unavailable, capillary blood obtained by heel prick may be used for P_{CO_2} and pH determinations. Capillary blood P_{O_2} is not accurate. This method of collection requires warming of the heel with a moist pack for a minimum of 5 minutes to dilate capillaries and arterioles. The sample thus obtained is arterialized capillary blood.

An inordinate delay in performing determinations after collection of samples usually causes inaccurate results if the blood is kept at room temperature. The pH drops and the P_{CO_2} rises because continued glycolysis in the red blood cells produces lactic acid in the sample. The average pH error in normal blood that is analyzed 20 minutes after collection is only minus 0.01 unit. Errors are minimal and clinically insignificant if the blood is stored in ice. Determinations can then be made up to 2 hours later with only a slight fall in pH (less than 0.015 unit). Exposure to room air is another pitfall to be avoided. In these circumstances the P_{CO_2} falls considerably because it escapes to lower carbon dioxide tensions in the atmosphere, and this causes the pH to rise. When blood is exposed to the atmosphere, P_{O_2} is also altered, since it tends to equilibrate with the oxygen tension of room air, which is approximately 140 mm Hg.

Heparin is the only acceptable anticoagulant for collection of blood samples. Other anticoagulants, such as citrate, oxalate, and EDTA, have significant effects on blood pH. Tubes utilized for capillary samples are commercially prepared with proper amounts of heparin to prevent clotting.

Capillary blood samples are useless for P_{O_2} determinations because they do not correlate with arterial blood levels. Oxygen tension must be monitored from blood taken directly from an artery. This is especially important for premature infants who are given supplemental oxygen; hyperoxia may cause retrolental fibroplasia (p. 219). Arterial samples are obtainable from an umbilical artery catheter or from punctures of the radial, bra-

chial, or temporal arteries. Determinations of pH and P_{CO_2} in capillary blood are valid, however, because they are well correlated with arterial values if the sample is properly collected. However, difficulty arises when the extremities are poorly perfused for any reason. Venous stasis is evident in distressed infants whose extremities are cyanotic. Stasis of capillary blood lowers pH and augments P_{CO_2}; both of these values may thus differ considerably from those of arterial blood, therefore precluding reliable reference to such data for therapy.

Most neonatal special care units utilize blood gas and pH measurements for the characterization of acid-base status. Ideally personnel and laboratory should be close at hand so that results are available within minutes after they are ordered. The parameters pertinent to acid-base evaluation are as follows:

pH is a measure of hydrogen ion concentration. It expresses the end result of buffer activity and *in itself does not indicate whether an abnormality originates in respiratory or nonrespiratory dysfunction.* Normal values range from pH 7.35 to 7.44.

P_{CO_2} expresses the partial pressure of carbon dioxide dissolved in plasma. *Deviations from normal are indicative of disorders in the respiratory apparatus.* Normal neonatal values range from 30 to 37 mm Hg.

Plasma bicarbonate measures total bicarbonate concentration. Normal values are between 20 and 25 mEq/L.

Base excess (B.E.) or deficit is a value that is calculated rather than directly measured by the laboratory (see later). It is expressed as a positive or negative value. The negative value is sometimes referred to as a base deficit. Base excess indicates, in milliequivalents per liter, the quantity of blood buffer base remaining after hydrogen ion is buffered. It thus expresses the combined buffering capacity of plasma bicarbonate and hemoglobin. Normal neonatal values range from +4 to −4 mEq/L.

Alignment nomogram. Base excess is calculated from the alignment nomogram reproduced in Fig. 7-1. The computation of base excess is possible when hemoglobin concentration and any two of the following parameters are known: blood pH, P_{CO_2}

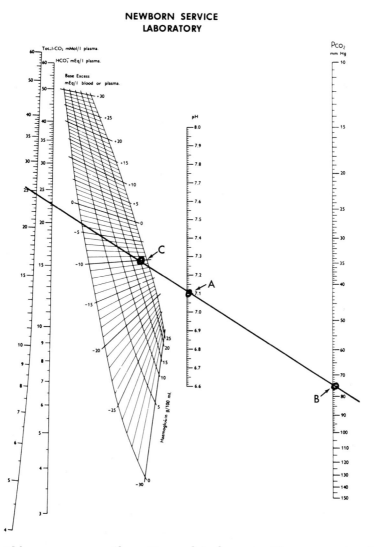

Fig. 7-1. Acid-base nomogram (from Siggaard-Andersen) with an example of plotted data from a sick infant. (See text for explanation.) (Modified from Winters, R. W., Engel, K., and Dell, R. B.: Acid-base physiology in medicine, a self-instruction program, Cleveland, 1967, The London Co.)

plasma bicarbonate, or total carbon dioxide content of plasma. The variables most commonly utilized in newborn laboratories are pH and P_{CO_2}.

Assume that an infant in rather severe respiratory distress is admitted to your facility. Blood samples are collected soon after admission, and the following information is forwarded to you:

pH = 7.10 (normal = 7.35 to 7.44)

P_{CO_2} = 75 mm Hg (normal = 30 to 37 mm Hg)

Hemoglobin = 20 grams/100 ml

The values for pH and P_{CO_2} are plotted on their appropriate scales at points *A* and *B*, as shown on the nomogram. A line is drawn through points *A* and *B* across all four scales. The base excess is read at minus 10 mEq/L at point *C*, where the drawn line intersects a grid line representing hemoglobin concentration of 20 grams/100 ml. The plasma bicarbonate concentration can now also be read at 23 mEq/L. If only the pH and bicarbonate are know (as well as the hemoglobin concentration), base excess and P_{CO_2} can be derived by drawing a line through points corresponding to the known values.

Basis of therapy. Intravenous sodium bicarbonate is occasionally utilized to correct a negative base excess (base deficit). Sodium bicarbonate is available in ampules of a 7.5% solution containing 0.88 mEq/ml. For ease of calculation it is satisfactory in clinical situations to consider the concentration as 1.0 mEq/ml. The dose of sodium bicarbonate is computed from the following formula:

mEq of $NaHCO_3$ to be given =
Base deficit × 0.3 × Body weight in kilograms

The factor 0.3 represents the approximate portion of body weight composed of extracellular fluid. If the infant whose base deficit was 10 mEq/L weighs 2500 grams, calculation of the dose of sodium bicarbonate is as follows:

$$\begin{aligned} \text{mEq of } NaHCO_3 &= 10\,\text{mEq} \times 0.3 \times 2.5\,\text{kg} \\ &= 10 \times 0.75 \\ &= 7.5 \end{aligned}$$

Thus 7.5 ml of the 7.5% solution of sodium bicarbonate will be required. It must always be diluted because the extremely alkaline pH may damage blood vessels near the site of infusion. The required dose should be mixed with at least an equal quantity of water for injection or with 10% glucose water. Generally one fourth to one half of the calculated dose is injected (after dilution) over a period of 2 to 5 minutes, and the remainder is added to intravenous fluid already dripping. In some centers the entire dose is infused, particularly if the infant is profoundly ill. See p. 77 for further discussion.

Summation

Principles of acid-base relationships apply to the management of all neonates admitted to the intensive care nursery. Mechanisms by which these normal relationships are disrupted and restored are operative in every sick baby. Acid-base imbalance is a by-product of the entire spectrum of primary neonatal disorders. It occurs in response to cold stress, during respiratory embarrassment, in gastrointestinal disturbances, as a result of all types of infectious disease, in disorders of the central nervous system, during postoperative periods, and even during the normal birth process. Preoccupation with the obvious symptomatology of these primary disorders often diverts attention from the subtle and perhaps more sinister effects produced by acid-base imbalance. These effects can be identified with certainty only by recourse to laboratory data. It is thus imperative for the neonatal nurse to comprehend the significance of these data.

FLUIDS AND ELECTROLYTES
Changes in quantity and distribution of body water during maturation

As gestational and postnatal ages increase, body water content decreases. Total body water (TBW) diminishes from 67% of body weight in postneonatal infants to 60% in older children and adults. In the neonate, however, water is 78% of body weight for a term infant, 80% at 32 weeks of gestation, and 95% in a 13- to 14-week fetus. The premature infant has more total body water than the term infant. Postnatal management requires consideration of these and other significant differences.

The distribution of water between the extracellular and intracellular compartments also changes with age. The percent of extracellular fluid (ECF) is greatest in the young. Thus, ECF comprises 20% of body weight in adults and children, 25% in postneonatal infants, 45% in term infants, and 60% in the 5-month fetus. The increased total body water in term and premature infants is largely extracellular.

As the ECF compartment contracts with age, intracellular fluid (ICF) expands from 20% of total weight in a 5-month fetus, to 30% at term, and 40% in adulthood. Total body water, and ECF within it, decreases with age. Conversely, the younger the premature infant, the greater the proportion of ECF. An abrupt change in fluid content occurs regularly in the 3 to 5 days following birth, whether the infant is premature or term. The most premature of infants (very low birth weight) normally lose up to 15% of their body weight, and virtually all of it is ECF. Prevention of this normal fluid loss by intravenous replacement is ill-advised.

Body composition; chemical anatomy

Water and solids. As the fetus grows, solid material increases while water content decreases. The 300-gram fetus has a body content of 7% to 8% protein; the term infant has 12.5%. Fat is virtually absent in a fetus of less than 1500 grams because it is only deposited toward the end of normal gestation and at an accelerated rate. In term infants, fat comprises 16% of total body weight.

Distribution of water and solutes: the compartments (ECF and ICF). As traditionally conceived, TBW is divided into extracellular and intracellular compartments (Fig. 7-2). ECF refers to water outside

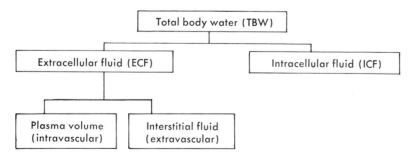

Fig. 7-2. Distribution of body water among principal compartments. (See text.)

the cells; ICF is water within them. As unrealistic as it may be, it is nevertheless useful to think of a different solution in each of two compartments (ECF and ICF), one separated from the other by a continuous semipermeable membrane. The membrane allows free bidirectional movement of water between the compartments. It is semipermeable (rather than freely permeable) because it limits diffusion of electrically charged particles (ions) and blocks passage of large particles that are dissolved in water. Ionic passage does occur normally in certain conditions that require an expenditure of energy by the membrane, such as the sodium pump mechanism, or by the action of hormones, neuromuscular activity, and changes in membrane porosity. Transfer of ions also occurs in disorders that alter the integrity of the membrane to allow abnormal passage of water, particles, or both. Disruption of function is associated with asphyxia, shock, congestive heart failure, severe infections, acid-base imbalance, and dehydration.

Extracellular water and solutes (ECF). Extracellular fluid is distributed between two "spaces": extravascular (interstitial) space and intravascular space. Interstitial fluid surrounds the cells of the body. It comprises approximately two thirds of the total extracellular fluid volume. Plasma volume comprises one third of extracellular fluid volume. The principal difference between plasma and interstitial fluid is their protein content. Plasma contains a considerable amount of protein; interstitial fluid has virtually none. Plasma proteins are normally present in amounts between 5 and 6 grams/dl; 94% to 95% of the plasma is water. The electrolytes are almost entirely dissolved in the water fraction. Capillary membranes are normally impermeable to protein;

electrolytes traverse them freely. The plasma fluid within capillaries, and the interstitial fluid outside them, contain virtually identical concentrations of all the electrolytes that are characteristic of extracellular fluid. The water within red blood cells, while literally "intracellular," is nevertheless considered part of the extracellular compartment, mainly because the red cells are unlike other cells elsewhere. The extracellular fluid is therefore a continuous compartment of water and solutes, even though one portion of it is outside the vascular space and the other is within it.

The *solutes* of ECF are substances dissolved in its water. Electrolytes, being electrically charged, are dissolved in water as *ions*. The molecules of other substances, such as glucose and urea, are also dissolved in water, but they are not electrically charged and are thus considered *nonionic particles. Cations* are ions that have a *positive electrical charge; anions* have a *negative charge.* Normal electrolyte balance requires the total positive charge to equal the total negative charge; the sum of the cations must equal that of anions. This is to say that the total milliequivalent content of each of the two types of ion is equal. The term *milliequivalent* is a quantitative expression of positively or negatively charged particles. This is traditionally expressed as milliequivalents in a liter of fluid (mEq/L). The total of all cations in plasma (and thus also in interstitial fluid) is 155 mEq/L. The total of anions is identical. Sodium (Na^+) is the principal cation of extracellular fluid. Its normal concentration is 142 mEq/L. The other cations are potassium (K^+) at 5 mEq/L, calcium (Ca^{++}) at 5 mEq/L (also often expressed as 10 mg%), and magnesium (Mg^{++}) at 3 mEq/L. The major anion of ECF is chloride

(Cl⁻); the normal concentration of chlorides in plasma is 105 mEq/L. The remaining anions are bicarbonate (HCO_3^-) at 25 mEq/L, sulfate ($SO_4^=$) and phosphate ($PO_4^=$), which together comprise 9 mEq/L, and proteins (Prot⁻) at 16 mEq/L. When in solution, glucose and urea do not dissociate into ionic particles; their quantity is therefore not expressed as mEq/L, but rather as mg/dl.

Intracellular water and solutes (ICF). Although the intracellular space contains fluid that varies in composition from one type of tissue to another, that compartment can validly be considered as a single one that is comprised of "millions of little bags of water, all doing the same thing at the same moment."* In contrast to the *capillary* membrane in the ECF space, the *cellular* membrane in the ICF space does not admit free passage of cations and allows very little to anions. When these particles normally traverse cell membranes, they do so by action of transport systems that involve an energy expenditure by the membrane. The energy is derived from chemical reactions within the membrane. As a result of the limited permeability of cell membranes, the ionic separation of ICF and ECF is such that their percent composition differs greatly. Yet, when transfer of ions from one compartment to the other is essential for normal metabolism, the membrane's transport systems accommodate it. The integrity and interdependence of ICF and ECF are thereby preserved.

ICF is more inaccessible to study than ECF; thus, less is known about its precise composition. Within an individual cell, fluid of varying constituency is contained in substructures, such as the nucleus and mitochondria. It is nevertheless well established that the major cation of ICF is potassium (K⁺); in ECF the major cation is sodium (Na⁺). The concentration of ICF potassium is approximately thirty times greater than ECF potassium. Potassium is essentially an intracellular cation. The other intracellular cations are magnesium (Mg⁺⁺) and sodium (Na⁺). Although all these cations are also present in the ECF, their concentrations differ considerably between the two compartments. The intracellular concentration of magnesium (Mg⁺⁺) is ten to fifteen times greater than the extracellular concentration. Magnesium is therefore considered primarily an intracellular ion. The concentration of sodium (Na⁺) in the ICF is only about one fifteenth that of the ECF, and sodium is thus primarily an ECF cation. The concentrations of intracellular anions also differ from that of the extracellular ones. Chloride (Cl⁻) is almost nonexistent in the ICF, 2 mEq/L in the cells compared with 105 mEq/L outside them. The reverse relationship exists for phosphate

Table 7-2. Ionic concentrations in ECF and ICF

Ions	ECF (mEq/L)	ICF (mEq/L)°
Cations		
Sodium (Na⁺)	142	10
Potassium (K⁺)	5	150
Calcium (Ca⁺⁺)	5	None
Magnesium (Mg⁺⁺)	3	40
Anions		
Chloride (Cl⁻)	105	2
Bicarbonate (HCO_3^-)	25	12
Phosphate ($PO_4^=$) and Sulfate ($SO_4^=$)	9	126
Protein (prot⁻)	16	60

*Concentrations of ICF ions are assumed.

*From Weil, W. B., and Bailie, M. D.: Fluid and electrolyte metabolism in infants and children, New York, 1977, Grune & Stratton, Inc., p. 20.

($PO_4^=$) and sulfate ($SO_4^=$) because together they comprise 126 mEq/L in the ICF and only 9 mEq/L in the ECF. There are 12 mEq/L of intracellular bicarbonate (HCO_3^-) as contrasted with 15 mEq/L of the extracellular anion. ICF protein is 60 mEq/L; ECF protein is only 16 mEq/L. These distinct differences are maintained by the semipermeable cell membranes. The reader has probably already noticed that identical ions are contained in both major fluid compartments; it is their concentrations that vary so considerably. Table 7-2 lists the ionic concentrations of ICF and ECF.

Osmolality and the exchange of water between compartments. A solution exerts osmotic pressure in relation to the number of dissolved particles (solute) within it. The greater the number of particles in a unit of water, the higher the osmotic pressure. These particles may be ionic (Na^+, Cl^-, K^+, and so forth) or nonionic (glucose, urea). Osmotic pressure is not related to the size or weight of particles or to their electrical charge; it is directly determined by the number of dissolved particles in a unit of water—the concentration of particles in the solution. Magnesium chloride ($MgCl_2$) dissociates into one magnesium ion and two chloride ions. In solution, the three ionic particles of the $MgCl_2$ molecule exert a greater osmotic pressure in the same volume of water than sodium chloride (NaCl), which dissociates into only two ionic particles, one sodium and one chloride ion. Glucose and urea do not dissociate into ions. Theirs are nonionic molecular particles. *Together, the ionic and nonionic particles in solution account for the total osmotic activity of the solute.* The term *milliosmole (mOsm)*, expresses the unit of osmotic pressure exerted by the solute. *Osmolality* refers to the quantity of milliosmoles per *kilogram* of water

(mOsm/kg). *Osmolarity* refers to the number of milliosmoles per *liter* of water (mOsm/L). The values of osmolality and osmolarity approximate each other so closely that both terms can be used interchangeably.

Osmotic pressure of one solution is exerted on that of another when both are separated by a semipermeable membrane. If a difference in osmolality exists, the result is a *net flow* of water into the more concentrated solution until the concentration of particles (milliosmoles) in both solutions is equal. An exchange of water thus occurs between intravascular fluid (plasma) and interstitial fluid and then between interstitial fluid and intracellular fluid. The transfer of water across a membrane between two solutions is actually a continuous bidirectional one. However a greater volume of water flows into a more concentrated solution, as less is simultaneously transferred in the opposite direction, into the more dilute solution. Thus the *net flow* of water is said to be in the direction of the solution of higher osmolality, and ultimately its osmolality decreases—it becomes more dilute. Constant bidirectional exchange of water occurs across all cell membranes. The difference in osmolality between the two compartments is thus minimized or eliminated, not by exchange of electrolytes across the cell membrane, but by transfer of water in response to discrepant particulate concentrations (osmolality). If sodium (as in $NaHCO_3$, for instance) is infused into the vascular space, it eventually permeates capillary walls (membranes) into the interstitial fluid, but it is very slow to cross the cell membrane from the interstitial space. In the meantime, the resultant heightened osmolality of interstitial fluid produces a transfer of water from within the cells to the extracellular compartment (intersti-

tial fluid) in an attempt to equalize osmotic pressure. The result is a loss of water from cells. When large quantities of
sodium are infused over a short period,
the increased intravascular osmolality
causes movement of fluid from the interstitial space into blood vessels with a resultant increase in intravascular volume.
When this occurs in the fragile capillaries
of the premature infant's brain, rupture of
capillary walls causes intracranial hemorrhage. This is the basis for caution in
the administration of NaHCO$_3$ for metabolic acidosis (p. 77).

Physiologic mechanisms for the maintenance of fluid and electrolyte balance

Fluid input and loss. The sole sources of
input for the normal term neonate are
breast milk or formula. The sick neonate,
until he recuperates, receives fluids and
electrolytes only by the intravascular
route. Consideration of the type and
quantity of fluid that is given must be
based on a knowledge of how it is lost.
Fluid is lost from the body through three
methods; evaporative loss from skin and
lungs, direct loss from the kidneys, and
direct loss from the gastrointestinal tract.
Evaporative and renal losses are of pri-

mary importance in the neonate. Stool
losses, while they occur consistently, are
not clinically significant in the sick baby
unless diarrhea or loose stools (see Phototherapy, p. 183) are present. Table 7-3
lists average water losses by the various
routes discussed.

**Insensible water loss (IWL) and the effects
of environmental factors.** Evaporative loss
occurs visibly in the form of sweat and in-
visibly in the form of insensible water
loss (IWL) from the skin and respiratory
tract. Sweating is negligible or absent in
babies less than 36 weeks of gestation
(p. 90). IWL comprises 35% to 45% of
total water losses. The smaller the baby,
the greater the IWL. Approximately 30%
of IWL is from the respiratory tract. The
quantity thus lost can be influenced significantly by increasing the humidity of
inspired air. If very high levels of humidity are provided, respiratory losses may
be reduced by as much as 55%. Cutaneous IWL varies considerably because
it is influenced by factors that are operative in the baby and in the environment.
The most fundamental of the intrinsic
factors is gestational age. The less mature
the baby, the greater the evaporative
losses in any given environmental circumstances. This occurs for several reasons. The immature baby's surface area
per kilogram of body weight is significantly larger than that of the mature infant; the skin is thinner and more copiously vascularized, and body water
content is higher. The immature infant,
especially if birth weight is less than
1500 grams, is therefore particularly vulnerable to changes in the environment.
The environmental factors that may increase or decrease IWL are:

1. High ambient temperature (increase)
2. High ambient humidity (decrease)
3. Radiant warmers (increase)

Table 7-3. Mean water loss (ml/kg/day)

	750-1000 grams	1001-1250 grams	1251-1500 grams
First 2 weeks			
IWL	62	52	35
Urine	72	72	72
Stool	7	7	7
Second 2 weeks			
IWL	48	35	30
Urine	80	80	80
Stool	10	10	10

4. Plastic shield (radiant warmer) (decrease)
5. Plastic shield (incubator) (decrease)
6. Plastic "bubble blanket" (decrease)
7. Phototherapy (increase)

High ambient temperature, when above the level required for maintenance of normal body temperature, increases water loss through the skin. Needlessly high environmental temperatures increase the metabolic rate, which is associated with enhanced water loss through the skin. Losses from the respiratory tract are also augmented because the infant's respiratory rate increases in such circumstances.

High ambient humidity diminishes evaporative losses. Heightened humidity principally affects respiratory water loss, which has been shown experimentally to diminish by 55%. Considerably less effect is exerted on cutaneous losses, which in the same experiments, were diminished by only 18%.

Radiant warmers enhance IWL significantly, and this has been a major objection to their protracted use. Studies of this phenomenon have consistently demonstrated greater insensible losses under the warmers than in incubators. These losses vary depending on the type of warmer utilized, size and gestational age of the infant, and probably the postnatal age as well. Under radiant warmers, IWL increases by one half to three times the amount expected in an incubator. Such losses are notably increased in babies whose gestational ages are 30 to 32 weeks or less and whose birth weights are below 1500 grams, but especially below 1250 grams. They also vary with the type of warmer. In one study, the KDC warmer was associated with a mean insensible loss of 84 ml/kg/24 hours in small premature infants. Under the Air Shields and Ohio warmers, small babies lost approximately 60 ml/kg/24 hours by IWL. These quantities may not be specifically applicable to every infant managed on a radiant warmer because they are mean values. Variations in gestational age and size exert a significant influence on these average figures for IWL. Nevertheless, the trend is clear and the data are important; the role of radiant warmers must be considered when monitoring the water balance of sick infants. *A baby who is managed in an incubator will require less fluid than one who is on a warmer, if other factors do not differ significantly.*

Heat shields on radiant warmers, if they are the proper type, can reduce IWL imposed by radiant energy. In one study, the use of a cylindric Plexiglas shield (identical to the one shown in Fig. 4-7 on p. 98) was associated with a 25% diminution of evaporative losses. However, the authors did not recommend routine use of these shields because for hypothermic infants the radiant energy of the warmer was less effective in maintaining core temperature. We have measured the quantity of radiant energy delivered to infants beneath this Plexiglas shield, and we have found that radiant energy does not pass through the Plexiglas. Body temperature may thus be supported only by the increased heat that is generated within the Plexiglas wall, not the radiant energy delivered to the baby. In contrast, the heat shield shown in Fig. 4-8 on p. 99 utilized a Saran Wrap covering. It did not reduce the measured quantity of radiance delivered to the body surface. Our data also indicate that evaporative losses are reduced by approximately 50% when these particular shields are used (p. 100). When heat shields are used in incubators, heat loss and IWL are reduced (p. 100). These data were derived from a study in which use of the Plexiglas heat shield was associated with a mean decline in IWL of 25%. The infants in that study weighed 695 to 1770 grams at birth. Averages from infants whose birth weights vary so widely are often misleading when specific application to an individual infant is required. Although the average decline in IWL for all birth weights was approximately 25%, IWL decreased by as much as 45% among infants who were 1250 grams or less. *Plexiglas shields are effective in incubators; their routine use on radiant warmers is ill-advised.*

Plastic "bubble blankets" were used in one study to minimize water loss on premature infants who were managed in incubators. The plastic blanket, used for commercial packing of fragile merchandise such as china and crystal, is light and transparent. It produced a 70% reduction in IWL. Water loss was 65 ml/kg/24 hours without the blanket, 16.2 ml/kg/24 hours with it. Similar studies on radiant warmers have not been reported.

Phototherapy exerts a substantial influence on evaporative water loss. Under phototherapy, increased amounts of water are lost through the skin, from the respiratory tract because respiratory rate is increased, and from the gastrointestinal tract because frequent loose stools contain abnormally large quantities of water. Among term infants who receive phototherapy while in an incubator, one can expect a 40% increase in the IWL, and a 160% increase in water loss from stool. These data were derived from term infants, who being otherwise well could compensate for their losses by increasing their oral intake of formula. It is plausible to assume that increased losses incurred on small, seriously ill infants are even more significant, and if neglected, more hazardous. Phototherapy is often used for infants who are under radiant warmers. The addition of phototherapy to babies under 1500 grams who are already on radiant warmers increases IWL by almost 50%. It thus follows that if an infant is transferred from an incubator to a radiant warmer, fluid intake must be increased in anticipation of increased IWL; if phototherapy is also initiated, fluid intake must be increased still more.

Renal water loss. Although renal loss accounts for 50% to 60% of total water loss, it varies considerably depending on the volume of water available and the amount of solute that must be excreted (solute load). The kidney regulates the *amount* of urinary solute in response to the requirements of electrolyte and acid-base balance. It also regulates the *concentration* of solute in response to requirements of water balance. Although it varies widely within physiologic limits, solute excretion is continuously obligatory. Solute is derived from intake of protein and electrolyte and from metabolic processes. It is largely comprised of urea, sodium, chloride, and potassium. The intake of fat and carbohydrate need not be considered in this context because they do not impose a solute load on the kidney. These substances are metabolized to CO_2 and water. When urine concentration is maximal, the kidney allocates minimal quantities of water to excrete its solute load, thereby conserving water when it is needed.

The capacity of the kidney to concentrate and dilute is most accurately reflected as *milliosmoles per liter (mOsm/L)* of urine. Specific gravity is also used for the same purpose, and though it is not quite as accurate, there is an acceptable correlation between it and osmolar values.

At term, the neonate can maximally concentrate urine to approximately 600 mOsm/L (sp. gr. = 1.020), compared with the adult's and older child's capacity of 1400 mOsm/L (sp. gr. = 1.040). Maximal dilutional capacity of both term and premature infants is approximately 50 mOsm/L (sp. gr. = 1.001). Concentrating capacity is diminished at lower gestational ages. If inappropriately large amounts of water are lost by IWL, less water is available to the kidney for excretion of solute. At maximal urine concentrations, urine osmolalities are high. When the amount of available water is insufficient for a solute load, solutes are retained. Serum sodium becomes elevated (over 150 mEq/L), and a corresponding abnormal rise in serum osmolality occurs (over 300 mOsm/L). The baby now has hyperosmolar dehydration because a large IWL was not considered in the calculation of water requirements.

If water intake is suboptimal, the kidneys excrete less urine to preserve water balance, yet a fixed amount of solute must be excreted if normal electrolyte and acid-base balance is to be maintained. Renal concentration compensates for the unavailability of water by utilizing less water for solute excretion. The neonate can concentrate only half as well as the older child; the premature infant concentrates even less. It follows that there is less tolerance to insufficient water input, or to uncompensated excessive water loss such as IWL.

Role of hormones in the maintenace of fluid and electrolyte equilibrium. *Antidiuretic hormone* (ADH) and *aldosterone* play prominent roles in water and electrolyte homeostasis.

ADH produces an antidiuretic effect — it diminishes the volume of water excreted by the kidneys, in the extreme producing severe oliguria, water retention, and overhydration. On the other hand, the absence of ADH increases renal water loss, producing severe polyuria and life-threatening dehydration in the extreme. ADH increases the permeability of renal tubular epithelium to water. Water thus moves from within the renal tubules to the interstitial tissue, and it is retained rather than excreted. In the absence of ADH, renal tubular epithelium is virtually impermeable to water so that an abnormally large volume is excreted. Between the extremes of antidiuresis (severe water retention) and diuresis (abnormally large water loss), varying blood levels of ADH exert appropriate control in response to a fluctuating physiologic need for water retention and excretion. The release of ADH from the posterior pituitary gland may increase or decrease in response to stimuli from osmoreceptors in the hypothalamus, which themselves respond to changes in plasma osmolality. Thus, renal water retention occurs if plasma osmolality is high, and diuresis occurs when plasma osmolality is low. A typical sequence of events may be described as follows. When ECF (and thus plasma) is inappropriately concentrated, the hypothalamic osmoreceptors stimulate ADH release. The increased circulating ADH arrives at the renal tubular epithelium to increase its permeability to water. A greater amount of urinary water is now reabsorbed from the tubules, urine volume decreases, and urine osmolality increases. The water thus retained is incorporated into the ECF, and the previously elevated plasma osmolality is reduced. Now reduced plasma osmolality stimulates osmoreceptors to diminish release of ADH, and less water is reabsorbed from the tubules. Urine becomes more dilute, urinary flow is increased, and renal water loss is enhanced. *Renal water excretion varies inversely with the level of circulating ADH.*

The rate of ADH secretion is also influenced by intravascular volume. Receptors that are sensitive to changes in blood pressure (baroreceptors) are situated in the aorta, the carotid arteries, and wall of the atrium. If blood pressure rises, these structures become distended, and the baroreceptors are stretched. In that state they convey impulses to the hypothalamus to diminish the release of ADH. Renal water excretion increases as indicated by a lower urine osmolality. In neonates, hypotension is a more frequent occurrence. The decrease in blood pressure stimulates baroreceptors to signal an increased release of ADH. Renal tubules become more permeable, and water is transferred to renal interstitium. Urinary water loss diminishes, and urine osmolality increases. Retention of water represents an attempt to maintain blood pressure by increasing intravascular fluid volume.

In summary, ADH exerts its powerful influence on the volume of water that is lost from the kidneys by promoting or inhibiting the reabsorption of water from renal tubules. ADH is released in response to a need for retention or excretion of water to compensate for abnormal osmolality of extracellular fluid, and for abnormal intravascular volume.

Aldosterone is a mineralocorticosteroid that is secreted by the adrenal cortex. It promotes the reabsorption of sodium across renal tubular epithelium. This mechanism, well known in older children and adults, has been identified in low birth weight infants. An excessive intake of sodium causes a decline in blood aldosterone levels. This produces an increase of urinary sodium excretion by inhibiting reabsorption from the tubules.

Stool loss. The volume of water lost from the gastrointestinal tract is insignificant unless a large number of loose or watery stools are excreted, as in babies with diarrhea. When phototherapy is applied, the water content and volume of stools increase. This does not often cause clinical difficulty.

Disorders of fluid and electrolyte balance

Dehydration. Physiologic equilibrium requires a normal volume of body water, a normal content of solute therein, and a normal distribution of both between the intracellular and extracellular compartments. Dehydration almost always entails a reduced volume of body water in the ICF as well as the ECF. In severe dehydration, blood volume is ultimately reduced because plasma water is so depleted. Dehydration is produced when (1) fluid input is diminished and water loss does not decrease; (2) fluid loss increases and is not matched by an increased input; and (3) increased loss is combined with decreased input. In most instances, dehydration in the neonate occurs when more water is lost than is administered.

Three types of dehydration are clearly identifiable. *Isotonic dehydration* is the result of excessive loss in which water and solute are of the same proportion as in normal body fluids. Serum sodium concentration and osmolality are thus normal because proportional loss of solute and water does not change the concentration of electrolytes in the remaining body fluids. *Hypertonic dehydration* occurs when the volume of lost water is proportionately greater than the quantity of lost solute. Body fluids are thus deprived of greater amounts of water than solute. The result is an abnormal elevation of serum sodium concentration and osmolality. The body fluids that remain are thus hypertonic. *Hypotonic dehydration* is the result of excessive losses that contain more solute than water when compared with normal concentrations in body fluids. The relatively greater loss of solute diminishes serum sodium concentration and serum osmolality. The residual body fluids are hypotonic.

The most frequent cause of dehydration is failure to administer the proper amounts of fluid and electrolytes for physiologic equilibrium, particularly in very small premature infants. Hypotonic dehydration is rare; isotonic dehydration occurs more frequently. Hypertonic dehydration is the most frequent consequence of inadequate fluid administration. In this respect, IWL is probably the most important consideration. Its variations, as influenced by gestational age, size, and use of radiant warmers and phototherapy, are often unappreciated. If IWL is not approximated by adequate fluid input, dangerous *hypertonic dehydration* occurs because water, not solute, is lost through the skin. Some degree of compensation for the excessive serum sodium concentration can be expected from an increased excretion of sodium by the kidneys. Decreased renal excretion of water partially compensates for the IWL, but all this renal activity cannot prevent serious water depletion in the face of a protracted inadequacy in fluid administration.

Some *congenital malformations of the kidney* (renal dysplasia and severe hydronephrosis) are characterized by an inability to concentrate urine effectively. The resultant water loss proportionately exceeds the loss of solute, and hypertonic dehydration becomes apparent. *Diarrhea* is not a frequent occurrence in the neonatal intensive care unit, except during outbreaks of infection. Dehydration develops rapidly, particularly in the smallest babies. It is generally isotonic, although hypertonic dehydration is not unusual. The use of *theophylline* for apnea of prematurity has become pervasive. Theophylline causes diuresis, often with a disproportionately large loss of sodium. Either hypotonic or isotonic dehydration may result, depending on the volume of water that accompanies the loss of sodium. Hypertonic dehydration follows *fever* or *high ambient temperature*.

Overhydration. Overhydration refers to an excess of total body water that may be produced by a large input of fluid, a severe diminution in water loss, or a combination of both. Overhydration is usually hypotonic, sometimes isotonic. Hypertonic overhydration is rare, usually occurring postoperatively in presence of oliguria and injudicious fluid and solute administration.

The clinical signs of overhydration depend on the amount of interstitial fluid that has accumulated (subcutaneous edema) and the extent to which intravascular volume is increased (pulmonary edema, cardiac failure). Edema is the cardinal sign of interstitial fluid accumulation. It usually pits with relatively little pressure, but pitting edema is not present in early overhydration. Furthermore, the neonate is usually supine and unless the examiner attempts to demonstrate pitting at the flanks and back, its presence will be missed because fluid aggregates in dependent areas. Edema of subcutaneous tissue is itself benign, even though it can be unsightly and it may contribute to pressure ulcers. If however, plasma volume is expanded, the ultimate result is pulmonary edema and cardiac failure. Overhydration is also characterized by an inordinate weight gain. Whether or not edema is in evidence, inappropriate weight gain indicates overhydration. The most common clinical situations in which overhydration occurs are (1) administration of inappropriately large volumes of fluid and (2) the syndrome of inappropriate ADH (SIADH).

Administration of inappropriately large quantities of fluid is usually the result of an uninformed estimate of the neonate's fluid needs. Ongoing monitoring of fluid balance is indispensable if overhydration is to be avoided. Acute overhydration from intravascular fluids rapidly leads to pulmonary edema, particularly in smaller premature infants. In them, the lungs have been likened to a "sump" in which interstitial fluid accumulates rapidly, even in the absence of cardiac failure. When overhydration develops gradually, it is more likely to produce obvious edema. Pulmonary edema then appears later if the administration of excessive fluid is not curtailed.

The *syndrome of inappropriate ADH (SIADH)* refers to oversecretion of the antidiuretic hormone. It occurs most often in term infants, although it affects premature infants more frequently than is generally realized. SIADH has been reported at a gestional age as low as 27 weeks. Whether in premature or term infants, virtually all reported instances of SIADH have occurred in association with brain injury due to asphyxia, intracranial hemorrhage, and meningitis. Generally, the onset of SIADH in premature infants has been observed at 5 days to 2 weeks of age. In term infants, SIADH occurs most often after perinatal asphyxia. Typically, Apgar scores are low and resuscitation is required in the delivery room. Meconium aspiration is frequently identifiable in these asphyxiated infants. Most of them first convulse at 6 to 12 hours of age. Cerebral edema is indicated by a tight bulging fontanelle and separated sutures.

It is in such infants that oversecretion of ADH often occurs. The mechanism by which ADH is copiously released in asphyxiated infants is not understood.

Heightened levels of ADH produce massive reabsorption of water from the renal tubules, considerably exceeding the normal process of compensation for serum hyperosmolality that was described earlier in this chapter. These elevated levels of ADH are initiated in the presence of normal blood volume and serum osmolality. Severe water retention, plus continued renal excretion of small quantities of sodium, results in severe hyponatremia. Serum sodium may be as low as 110 mEq/L. A unique aspect of SIADH is the high urine osmolality and diminished urine output that occurs and persists even though serum osmolality is low. Abnormally high ADH levels cause massive tubular reabsorption of water; urine osmolalities are thus considerably higher than those of the serum. In contrast to SIADH, overhydration resulting from excessive fluid administration is associated with low (or normal) serum osmolality and low urine osmolality as well. In both instances of overhydration, serum sodium concentration is low because water is retained, not because excessive sodium is lost. This is called *dilutional hyponatremia.* The criteria for the diagnosis of SIADH are hyponatremia and serum hyposmolality, urine hyperosmolality, and normal adrenal and renal function.

SIADH is primarily an inability to excrete water through the kidneys because of massive tubular reabsorption. Fluid input must be severely restricted between 30 and 50 ml/kg/24 hours. The addition of sodium to administered fluids in an attempt to correct hyponatremia is contraindicated. Some authors advocate that daily maintenance requirement of sodium be given (2 to 3 mEq/kg); others do not add sodium to fluid infusions.

Ongoing assessment of fluid and electrolyte status

The ongoing assessment of fluid and electrolyte status requires several laboratory determinations. Protracted intravascular fluid administration should not be attempted unless such data are available to *personnel who understand their significance.*

The most immediate concern of ongoing assessment is the detection of renal compensatory activity that is called into play by a surfeit or a paucity of infused fluid. At that point imbalance has not yet occurred, and the correction of existing therapy will avoid it. *The earliest recognizable response to inappropriate fluid therapy is the concentration or dilution of urine.* The kidneys concentrate urine to preserve water when input is insufficient to match loss. Conversely, the kidneys dilute urine so that water excretion is increased when input exceeds loss. *This compensatory renal activity is reflected in the urine osmolality or specific gravity, well in advance of abnormalities in serum.* Assuming normal renal function, a urine osmolality between 100 and 300 mOsm (sp. gr. = 1.008 to 1.012) indicates optimal water balance. Furthermore, within these limits, osmolality is associated with a normal urine volume. Osmolalities between 300 and 400 mOsm suggest that somewhat less than an optimal volume of fluid is being given. Hypertonic urine that is over 400 mOsm indicates a need to increase fluid input until osmolality is 100 to 300 mOsm. If urine osmolality is below 100 mOsm, the quantity of fluid input should be de-

creased. Specific gravity is a more commonly utilized procedure for the determination of urine concentration because it is simple and rapid and does not require laboratory personnel. We prefer urine osmolality because it can be better correlated with serum osmolality when assessing the development of serious fluid imbalance. Whether expressed as osmolality or specific gravity, periodic determination of urine concentration is the most valuable screening procedure for careful monitoring.

Monitoring for dehydration. Insufficient fluid input is indicated early by concentrated urine (greater than 300 to 400 mOsm). If an inadequate amount of fluid input is allowed to continue, water in the intravascular space diminishes and the increased plasma osmolality is compensated for by movement of water from the interstitial space into the blood vessels. Blood volume and plasma osmolality are thereby temporarily maintained within normal limits (270 to 300 mOsm). Next, body weight decreases to the extent of net water loss, even before the plasma becomes hyperosmolar. Significant weight loss is the first indication of *uncompensated* imbalance. As dehydration progresses, the osmolality of plasma and interstitial fluid rises and serum sodium concentration also becomes abnormally high (over 150 mEq/L). An osmolar discrepancy has now developed between the ECF and ICF, producing movement of fluid from the intracellular space into the interstitial and intravascular spaces. These compensatory activities ultimately become ineffective; plasma volume due to net water loss eventually becomes so diminished as to produce an increased hematocrit and plasma protein level due to hemoconcentration. Diminished blood volume causes shock. Even before shock

Table 7-4. Water imbalance: sequence of events and abnormal values

Dehydration (input<loss)	Overhydration (input>loss)
↓ Urine volume (<1 ml/kg/hr) ↑ Urine osmolality (>400 mOsm) ↑ Urine sp. gr. (>1.012) ↓	↑ Urine volume (>3 ml/kg/hr) ↓ Urine osmolality(<100 mOsm) ↓ Urine sp. gr. (<1.008) ↓
Weight loss (5% to 15%/24 hours) ↓	Weight gain (5% to 15%/24 hours) ↓
↑ Serum sodium (>150 mEq/L) ↑ Serum osmolality(>300 mOsm) ↓	↓ Serum sodium (<130 mEq/L) ↓ Serum osmolality (<270 mOsm) ↓
Dry skin, mucous membrane ↓ Skin turgor ↓	Subcutaneous edema Pulmonary edema ↓
↑ Hematocrit (≥ 10%) ↑ Serum protein (>6 gm/dl) ↓ Blood volume (variable) ↓	↓ Hematocrit (≥10%) ↓ Serum protein (<4 gm/dl) ↑ Blood volume (variable) ↓
Shock	Cardiac failure

develops, the skin becomes dry to touch; its turgor is diminished. Mucous membranes lose the sheen that is normally imparted by moisture; they appear dull and dry. The anterior fontanelle is depressed, presumably because the volume of cerebrospinal fluid is diminished. All these abnormal physical signs become apparent late in the process of dehydration. *This entire sequence of events began with the appearance of hyperosmolar urine (over 400 mOsm) when renal compensation was still effective. Dehydration could have been prevented early by increasing the volume of infused fluid.*

Systematic monitoring should also include total fluid input, urine output, urine and serum osmolalities, serum electrolytes, blood urea nitrogen, body weight determination at least every 12 hours, total serum protein and hematocrit, and postoperative fluid losses from sites of surgical repair.

Monitoring for overhydration. Fluid input in excess of loss is indicated early by di-

lute urine (less than 100 mOsm). In these circumstances, plasma fluid increases transiently until excess water diffuses into the interstitial space. At some point, fluid volume in both spaces is increased and osmolality of ECF is reduced relative to that of ICF. There ensues a movement of water from the interstitial space into the intracellular space. *Uncompensated* imbalance is first manifested by an inordinate gain in body weight. Serum osmolality is low (less than 270 mOsm), and serum sodium concentration is correspondingly diminished to less than 130 mEq/L. Subcutaneous edema appears if the process of overhydration is gradual; pulmonary edema appears first if the process is rapid. In the extreme, fluid overload leads to congestive heart failure. *This sequence of events began with the appearance of dilute urine (less than 100 mOsm), when compensation could have been effected by diminishing water input.* Table 7-4 lists the sequence of these events and, when applicable, the approximate values that indicate their abnormal nature.

Systematic monitoring must also include total fluid intake and urinary output, blood urea nitrogen, serum electrolytes, total protein, hematocrit, and a recording of weight at least every 12 hours.

Maintenance requirements of fluids and electrolytes

Fluids. Maintenance fluid is administered to replenish the total water loss that occurs from skin, lungs, and kidneys. Water losses are directly related to expended energy as measured in calories. The usual figure given for total water loss in the neonate is 100 ml/100 cal expended. However, in babies who are between 1 and 4 kg, energy expenditure is closely related to body weight. Fluid requirements are therefore accurately expressed as ml/kg of body weight.

Since several factors are known to profoundly influence the loss of water, it is impossible to recommend specific fluid volumes that are applicable in all circumstances. Fluid requirements differ according to the microenvironment provided for infant management such as incubators, radiant warmers, or open bassinets. Requirements vary with weight, gestational and postnatal age, type of illness, humidity during respiratory support, and use of phototherapy or heat shields. They even differ from one commercial brand of radiant warmer to another. Therefore, in providing maintenance fluid, one estimates the standard amount required, alters that quantity according to the presence of influencing factors, and then makes further alterations in response to the available monitoring data.

Intravascular fluid is generally admin-

Table 7-5. Maintenance volumes of intravascular fluid by birth weight for the first 2 weeks of life

Birth weight (grams)	ml/kg/24 hours
750-1000	130-160
1001-1250	120-150
1251-1500	110-140
1501-2500	100-130
2501 and over	70-100

istered within a volume range that is selected according to birth weight and microenvironment. In any given nursery, successful experience generally dictates the quantity of fluids that are customarily administered. Table 7-5 lists intravascular fluid volumes according to birth weight during the first 2 weeks of life. There is little change in these ranges during the ensuing 2 weeks.

Fluid intake should be decreased by 25% of stated quantities during the first 2 days of life. Increases in fluid volume may be required when ambient temperature is higher than usual, with use of radiant warmers and phototherapy, and in the presence of fever, hyperactivity, increased work of respiration (respiratory distress), and fluid drainage from postoperative wounds. The extent to which these conditions impose an increased fluid requirement can only be estimated with the aid of ongoing monitoring data.

Fluid maintenance requirements may diminish if a heat shield is utilized in an incubator or on a radiant warmer, when a plastic "bubble blanket" is applied to the baby, and when the humidity of inspired air is high. Fluid restriction is necessary in the presence of renal failure from any cause, inappropriate ADH syndrome, congestive heart failure, and patent ductus arteriosus with a significant left-to-right shunt.

Electrolytes. Daily requirements of sodium and potassium are each 2 mEq/kg and for chloride, 2 to 4 mEq/kg. Infants who are less than 1500 grams often require 3 to 4 mEq/kg of sodium daily, often much more because of large renal sodium losses.

REFERENCES

Behrman, R. E.: The use of acid-base measurements in the clinical evaluation and treatment of the sick neonate, J. Pediatr. 74:632, 1969.

Bell, E. F., and Oh, W.: Fluid and electrolyte balance in very low birth weight infants, Clin. Perinatol. 6:139, 1979.

Bell, E. F., Neidich, G. A., Cashore, W. J., and Oh, W.: Combined effect of radiant warmer and phototherapy on insensible water loss in low birth weight infants, J. Pediatr. 94:810, 1979.

Driscoll, J. M., and Heird, W. C.: Maintenance fluid therapy during the neonatal period. In Winters, R. W., editor: The body fluids in pediatrics, Boston, 1973, Little, Brown & Co.

Fanaroff, A. A., Wald, M., Gruber, H. S., and Klaus, M. H.: Insensible water loss in low birth weight infants, Pediatrics 50:236, 1972.

Kildeberg, P.: Clinical acid-base physiology; studies in neonates, infants and young children, Baltimore, 1968, The Williams & Wilkins Co.

Marks, K. H., Friedman, Z., and Maisels, M. J.: A simple device for reducing insensible water loss in low-birth-weight infants, Pediatrics 60:223, 1977.

Mendoza, S. A.: Syndrome of inappropriate antidiuretic hormone secretion (SIADH), Pediatr. Clin. North Am. 23:681, 1976.

Moylan, F. M. B., et al.: Inappropriate antidiuretic hormone secretion in premature infants with cerebral injury, Am. J. Dis. Child. 132:399, 1978.

Oh, W.: Disorders of fluid and electrolytes in newborn infants. Pediatr. Clin. North. 23:601, 1976.

Oh, W., and Karecki, H.: Phototherapy and insensible water loss in the newborn infant, Am. J. Dis. Child. 124:230, 1972.

Report of Ad-hoc Committee on Acid-Base Terminology: Current concepts of acid-base measurements, Ann. N.Y. Acad. Sci. 133:251, 1966.

Weil, W. B., and Bailie, M.D.: Fluid and electrolyte metabolism in infants and children, New York, 1977, Grune & Stratton, Inc.

Weinberg, J. A., Weitzman, R. E., Zakauddin, S., and Leake, R. D.: Inappropriate secretion of antidiuretic hormone in a premature infant, J. Pediatr. 90:111, 1977.

White, A., Handler, P., and Smith, E.: Principles of biochemistry, New York, 1968, McGraw-Hill Book Co.

Williams, P. R., and Oh, W.: Effects of radiant warmer on insensible water loss in newborn infants, Am. J. Dis. Child. 128:511, 1974.

Winters, R. W.: Terminology of acid-base disorders, Ann. N. Y. Acad. Sci. 133:211, 1965.

Winters, R. W., Engel, K., and Dell, R. B.: Acid-base physiology in medicine, a self-instruction program, Cleveland, 1967, The London Co.

Wu, P. Y. K., and Hodgman, J. E.: Insensible water loss in preterm infants: changes with postnatal development and non-ionizing radiant energy, Pediatrics 54:704, 1974.

Yeh, T. F., et al.: Reduction of insensible water loss in premature infants under the radiant warmer, J. Pediatr. 94:651, 1979.

Disorders of the lungs

Although reports on the incidence of pulmonary disorders may vary from one source to another, there is universal agreement that these diseases are the most frequent causes of neonatal morbidity and mortality. Broadly categorized, they are due to perinatal misadventures that impair adaptation to extrauterine life, to prenatal and postnatal infections, to congenital anomalies, and to extrapulmonary disorders such as cardiac failure, which secondarily give rise to respiratory dysfunction. This chapter describes the adaptive mechanisms responsible for adjustment to extrauterine respiration and the major clinical entities that are associated with respiratory distress.

FETAL CARDIOPULMONARY APPARATUS
Pulmonary circulation

The fetal circulation is described in Chapter 1. However, allusion to its pulmonary component is pertinent to the present discussion, particularly in reference to the changes that accompany the first breath (see later). The fetal lung is perfused by only 5% to 7% of cardiac output as a result of the high vascular resistance created by constricted pulmonary arterioles and collapsed alveolar capillaries. Most of the blood emanating from the right ventricle is thus shunted from the main pulmonary artery into the ductus arteriosus, bypassing the lungs. In the mature circulation, all blood from the right ventricle enters the pulmonary circulation directly. Blood supply to the fetal lung is further minimized by diversion of a major portion of inferior vena caval blood into the left atrium by way of the foramen ovale, thus constituting another pulmonary bypass. Establishment of normal extrauterine respiration requires that these fetal pathways be converted to the mature pattern very soon after birth. Further discussion of these changes may be found on p. 202.

Development of the fetal lungs

At 24 days the *primitive lung bud* appears as a localized pouch from the ventral surface of the *embryonic gut* (endoderm). This segment of gut will ultimately develop into the esophagus; the lung bud will be the trachea (Figs. 8-1 and 8-2). Persistence of a connection between the two structures is the basis for one of several possible types of tracheoesophageal fistulas (p. 258). At 26 to 28 days the lung bud divides into two structures that will become the two major bronchi. Subsequent growth progresses into surrounding mesenchyme (mesoderm), which becomes incorporated into pulmonary structures as differentiation proceeds; branching of each terminal structure continues as it grows laterally and downward into the pleural space, carrying with it the surrounding mesenchyme. The right and left branches of the original single bud thus give rise to successive generations of bronchi, bronchioles of diminishing size, alveolar ducts, and alveoli. The mesenchyme that surrounds these developing airway structures ultimately differentiates into blood vessels, muscle, connective tissue, cartilaginous plates in the bronchi, and the connective tissue that supports and separates alveolar and other structures in the lung.

By 6 weeks the *segmental bronchi* are formed, and at 12 weeks the *major lobes* are delineated. *Respiratory bronchioles* are differentiated at approximately 16 weeks; from them, at about 24 weeks, alveolar sacs are formed. At birth, they are considerably smaller and more shallow than at 1 and 2 months of age. Meanwhile, capillaries have been differentiating from the surrounding mesenchyme since the twentieth week. At 25 to 26 weeks, if live-born, an infant may breathe air successfully if appropriate postnatal support is instituted and if prenatal complications do not preclude survival. At this stage an increased number of capillaries is in direct contact with air spaces that may be functional postnatally. A number of terminal units for air-exchange are nevertheless not yet morphologically equipped for extrauterine life. Fewer capillary walls are in contact with potential air spaces, and the remaining mesenchyme (connective tissue) is so abundant that lung compliance will be severely restricted after birth. At 27 to 28 weeks

larger numbers of capillaries are in contact with the walls of *alveolar sacs* (alveolar membranes), which themselves have increased in number. The alveolar sacs now comprise most of the cross sectional area of the lung, whereas previously, bronchioles were the most prominent structures. Connective tissue spaces between terminal units are still relatively extensive, however. Lung compliance is low as a result, and in addition, these wide connective tissue spaces may account for the ease with which fluid accumulates within them postnatally. In infants born at this early stage of gestation, the interstitial connective tissue may retain fluid in sponge-like fashion. Furthermore, the relatively large interstitial

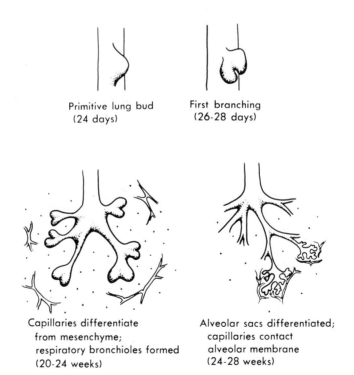

Primitive lung bud
(24 days)

First branching
(26-28 days)

Capillaries differentiate
from mesenchyme;
respiratory bronchioles formed
(20-24 weeks)

Alveolar sacs differentiated;
capillaries contact
alveolar membrane
(24-28 weeks)

Fig. 8-1. Development of primitive lung bud and subsequent branching into surrounding mesenchyme. (Modified from Avery, M. E., and Fletcher, B. D.: The lung and its disorders in the newborn infant, Philadelphia, 1974, W. B. Saunders Co.)

space in such infants may well account for interstitial emphysema (p. 248) unassociated with an ensuing pneumothorax, which is seen so often in more mature neonates. The wider interstitium also impedes exchange of gases between air sacs and capillaries. At 28 to 29 weeks further differentiation occurs at the distal ends of airways. Terminal saccules are lined with mature type II cells from which surfactant is released. From 30 to 33 weeks new alveolar units appear rapidly. Interstitial tissue is still relatively extensive; alveolar walls are thicker than in the mature infant. At 34 to 36 weeks mature alveolar structures are in evidence. Most pulmonary growth is attributable to new alveoli. Postnatal ventilation at this gestational age is more af-

fected by perinatal misadventure than by immaturity of structure or function. If unstressed, the neonate at this gestational age can survive by his independent capacity to ventilate and produce surfactant for alveolar stability.

Congenital malformations can be better understood with some knowledge of pulmonary development. Agenesis of the lung and tracheal stenosis are the result of maldevelopment in the earliest differentiation of the primitive lung bud. Tracheoesophageal fistulas of various types probably originate during the earlier branching of the lung bud. Defective deposition of bronchial cartilage from embryonic mesenchyme results in the syndrome of deficient cartilaginous rings. The bronchi collapse during inspiration

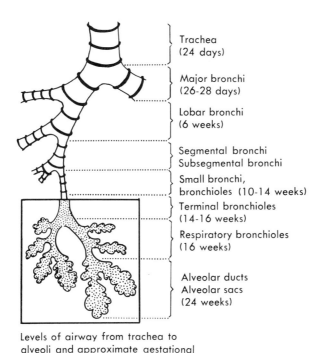

Trachea
(24 days)

Major bronchi
(26-28 days)

Lobar bronchi
(6 weeks)

Segmental bronchi
Subsegmental bronchi

Small bronchi,
bronchioles (10-14 weeks)

Terminal bronchioles
(14-16 weeks)

Respiratory bronchioles
(16 weeks)

Alveolar ducts
Alveolar sacs
(24 weeks)

Levels of airway from trachea to alveoli and approximate gestational week of formation

Fig. 8-2. Branching pattern of respiratory tract. The mature structures are indicated, with approximate gestational age of formation.

for lack of supporting tissue. Congenital lung cysts probably result from detachment of respiratory bronchioles, alveolar ducts, and sacs from the proximal airways with which they should normally be continuous. They may enlarge because trapped fluid, secreted by cells in respiratory bronchioles and alveoli, accumulates continuously.

The fetal lungs are metabolically active structures, even though they have no real function until the advent of extrauterine respiration. The blood vessels are narrow, and the alveoli are filled with fluid. Lung fluid differs in origin and composition from amniotic fluid. Lung fluid is derived from cells in the respiratory tract. It is less viscous, and it contains a lower protein concentration than amniotic fluid. Lung liquid must be evacuated soon after birth during the establishment of normal respiration. Its diminished viscosity presumably facilitates postnatal evacuation.

Postnatal lung growth is a vigorous, active process. The chest diameter increases rapidly in early infancy, mostly because of increased number of alveoli and respiratory bronchioles. The term baby is born with 24 million alveoli. At 3 months there are 77 million, and in the adult, 200 to 600 million. The alveolar sacs are considerably more shallow in the neonate, being 50 μm in diameter, compared with 100 to 200 μm in older children and 200 to 300 μm in the adult. The surface area available for gas exchange in the adult is about twenty times greater than in the neonate, which is close to the average increase of adult over neonatal body weight.

Intrauterine fetal breathing movements

It has only been in recent years that human fetal breathing movements have been identified unequivocally as such. A considerable amount of investigation in lambs preceded work on the human fetus. As in the lamb, human intrauterine breathing movements are episodic, being present in a normal pregnancy 70% of the time. They have been recorded as early as 13 weeks of gestation. The rate varies from 30 to 70 respirations per minute. The movements are identifiable by ultrasound techniques, but occasionally the mother can perceive them as localized movements of her abdomen, particularly near term. Since research on the subject has just begun, knowledge is limited. The incidence of breathing episodes is diminished in some high-risk pregnancies, such as those in which diabetes, hypertension, or toxemia is present. Apparently a fall in breathing incidence, accompanied by gasps, is a sinister sign that seems to be associated with subsequent death of small-for-dates babies. Fetal asphyxia apparently precipitates episodes of irregular gasping movements. Fetal breathing is a new parameter for monitoring, and it may become valuable in the detection of fetal distress. Whether there is validity in the speculation that without previous practice the respiratory muscles would be weak at birth, remains to be seen.

FIRST BREATH

Insight into the changes involved in the baby's first breath provides a sound basis for the understanding of pulmonary disturbances of the neonatal period, particularly hyaline membrane disease. During intrauterine life, exchange of oxygen and carbon dioxide occurs across the placental membrane from one liquid medium to another. After birth this exchange occurs across the alveolar membrane between a gaseous medium (air in the alveolus) and a liquid one (blood in alveolar capillaries). Among the many changes the infant undergoes at birth, the most abrupt and crucial ones are concerned with adaptation of respiratory function to a gaseous environment. Several requirements must be satisfied before the lungs can assume and maintain these functions:

1. *Respiratory movements must be initiated.*

2. *Entry of air must overcome opposing forces if the lungs are to expand.*

3. *Some air must remain in the alveoli at the end of expiration so that the lungs do not collapse (establishment of functional residual capacity).*

4. *Pulmonary blood flow must be increased, and cardiac output must be redistributed.*

Although these events transpire simultaneously, they lend themselves well to sequential description.

Initiation of respiratory movements

The precise roles of the various stimuli that bombard the infant to initiate his respiratory movements after birth have not been clarified. Their separate effects are difficult to delineate. The identification of intrauterine respiratory movements has given rise to the idea that extrauterine breathing is a continuation of fetal respiratory movements. The neonate may therefore be well practiced by virtue of his fetal experience. If this experience explains the ease with which regular respirations are established after birth, additional explanation is required for the greatly enhanced vigor with which the first extrauterine breaths are executed.

Asphyxia is a significant stimulator of the first breath. Low arterial P_{O_2}, low pH, and high P_{CO_2} are each known to stimulate respiratory movement under certain conditions. They initiate impulses from the carotid and aortic chemoreceptors that are transmitted to the respiratory control center in the medulla. These asphyxial changes are present to some extent at birth in most normal newborn infants, and they are considered potent stimulators of the first breath. Before the onset of respiration, oxygen saturation of umbilical venous blood (from the placenta to the fetus) varies from 9% to 96%, whereas in umbilical artery blood (returning to the placenta), it ranges from 0% to 67%; yet many of these transiently hypoxemic infants are vigorous. In a substantial number of them, oxygen saturations are below 10%. Some have no measurable oxygen at all, and yet most of them breathe spontaneously within seconds after delivery. The average P_{CO_2} at birth is elevated to 58 mm Hg, and the mean pH is depressed to 7.28. These asphyxial chemical changes also activate chemoreceptor nerve endings in the carotid arteries and the aortic arch. These short periods of asphyxia are presumably components of the normal birth process. They are characterized by absence of metabolic acidosis (normal buffer base), although respiratory acidosis (high P_{CO_2} and diminished pH) is present. The first breath may well be a deep inspiratory gasp, stimulated by hypoxia of the central nervous system, that is not unlike the gasps that follow fetal asphyxia. On the other hand, protracted asphyxial episodes are obviously not normal. They are characterized biochemically by metabolic acidosis (diminished buffer base) in addition to respiratory acidosis (hypercapnia) and hypoxemia. Short asphyxial episodes are thought to be powerful stimuli to the first breath; prolonged asphyxial episodes depress it.

Another important stimulus to the onset of respiratory movement is the abrupt drop that occurs in the infant's ambient temperature on arrival in room air. The baby leaves a fluid intrauterine environment of 98.6° F (37° C) and is thrust into a dry ambient temperature of 70° to 75° F (21° to 24° C) in an air-conditioned delivery room. This sudden change in environmental temperature stimulates nerve endings in the skin, with subsequent transmission of impulses to the medullary respiratory control center. This is probably an intense stimulus, and the response is instantaneous. The rapid onset of breathing requires an instantaneous response. At birth, the impact of a cold temperature on the skin (Chapter 4) is probably a further stimulus to breathing. Lambs fail to breathe when delivered into a normal saline bath that is at normal body temperature. The same phenomenon has been noted in human infants. During the first few minutes after delivery, core temperature falls at a rate of approximately 0.2° F (0.1° C) per minute, whereas the decline in skin temperature is three times as great. These temperature changes are apparently within physiologic limits. Purposeful excessive cooling of depressed infants is contraindicated. It causes profound depression due to an abnormal fall in body temperature, which produces the penalties of severe cold stress, including hypoxia (p. 90).

The tactile stimulation provided during ordinary handling of infants at birth is probably of only minor significance in the initiation of respiratory movement. Although the traditional slaps to the heels or buttocks may have some influence in stimulating respiratory movement in normal babies, the time so expended on depressed infants is better utilized for more effective resuscitative measures.

The net result of the initial extrauterine activity of respiratory muscles is the creation of lower pressure within the lungs than in the atmosphere. This negative intrathoracic pressure "invites entry" of air into the lungs. The negative pressure created by expansion of the thorax is largely accomplished by descent of the diaphragm, by contraction of its muscle fibers. The contribution of intercostal muscles to thoracic expansion is relatively minor. The air that is "sucked in" as a result of the normal activity of the diaphragm must now reach the alveoli by overcoming forces that obstruct its free flow.

Entry of air into the lungs and expansion of alveoli

The forces most important in opposing the entry of air into the lungs are exerted by surface tension in the alveoli and by the viscosity of lung fluid in the entire respiratory tract. Surface tension forces are minimized by *surfactant* in the alveoli. Lung fluid is evacuated into lymphatic vessels and blood capillaries if the lungs expand normally. Initial negative intrathoracic pressures may reach 60 to 80 cm H_2O. The volume of inspired air has been measured as high as 80 cc. At end expiration much of it remains in the lungs as residual air.

Surface tension and surfactant. Surface tension forces are produced by an imbalance in the attraction of one molecule for an adjacent one. Consider a cup of liquid. Below the surface its molecules are attracted to and repelled from each other with equal force from all directions because they are completely surrounded by other molecules. However, the situation is different in the surface layer of molecules because the molecular forces of attraction cannot be equal from all directions. The air above the surface layer exerts little upward pull, and the balance of forces thus favors downward and horizontal directions. The force exerted by this imbalance in intermolecular attraction at the uppermost level of molecules is called surface tension. It produces a constant tendency for contraction of a surface area. Now apply this concept of surface area contraction to the spherical inner surface of alveolar walls. In the absence of a counteracting influence (surfactant) and in the presence of an interface with air, surface tension tends to contract alveolar surfaces, thus promoting alveolar collapse.

Alveoli of the lung are similar to a conglomerate of bubbles. Alveolar walls are largely liquid; they envelope air within them. Since an air-liquid interface is present (much like that just described for the uppermost molecular layer of water in a cup), surface-active forces are operative. Intermolecular attraction contracts the surface area of the liquid wall of the bubble (alveolus). Furthermore, in accordance with a law of physics (LaPlace), the smaller the bubble, the stronger the forces of surface tension. Therefore the smaller the bubble, the greater its tendency to collapse as a result of unopposed surface forces. Ultimately the bubble (alveolus) collapses completely (atelectasis).

Pulmonary surfactant is a mixture of approximately ten compounds. It is described as a unique lipoprotein that is predominantly comprised of lecithins, and to a lesser extent, of cholesterol, neutral lipids, or other phospholipids. Quantitatively, the major component of surfactant is phosphotidylcholine (PC). It is also the compound that is most active in lowering surface tension forces. Another important component of surfactant is

phospotidylglycerol (PG). The PG fraction of surfactant is far smaller than that of PC, but interest in PG stems from the close correlation of lung maturity with its first appearance. It may be that PG is the compound of most critical functional significance in maturation of the lung.

Surfactant is synthesized by type II alveolar cells (pneumonocytes). It is stored for a relatively long period prior to its discharge from these cells on the alveolar membrane, where it forms a continuous film on the surface. At this site, it functions to diminish the collapsing (atelectatic) effect of surface tension forces on the alveoli.

In the normal lung, surface tension is minimized or eliminated by surfactant, a complex substance principally composed of lipoprotein that is elaborated by type II cells in the alveolar wall. It appears in the fetal lung at approximately 22 to 24 weeks of gestation. Without surfactant, unopposed surface tension forces increase directly with shrinkage of alveoli during expiration, ultimately resulting in alveolar collapse (atelectasis). However, in the presence of surfactant the effects of surface tension forces are eliminated or minimized. As alveoli shrink in the presence of surfactant during normal breathing, surface tension forces diminish rather than increase in magnitude because the surfactant layer, by becoming compressed, is made thicker; in this state surfactant counteracts surface forces most effectively. Conversely, the surfactant layer is thinned as alveoli expand during normal inspiration, and in this attenuated state the lining layer is less effective in diminishing surface tension. The influence of surfactant is therefore least at peak inspiration, when alveolar expansion is greatest. At this point, recoil of the expanded lung is relatively unopposed, and the deflation required for expiration is facilitated. The alveolar lining layer (surfactant) functions principally to maintain alveolar stability (residual expansion at end-expiration) once air has entered the alveolus.

Lung fluid.   Since 1948 it has been realized that the lungs secrete fluid that ultimately is added to amniotic fluid. A number of animal experiments in which fetal tracheas were ligated in utero have confirmed this original suggestion. In these circumstances, lungs at term were found to be overdistended with retained fluid and considerably heavier than lungs that were not ligated at the trachea. Even at an earlier date (1941), accumulation of pulmonary fluid was noted in a human fetus whose anomalous lung was not connected to the trachea. Fetal lung fluid presents a major opposing force to entry of air during the first breath. As the chest emerges from the birth canal, 30 to 40 ml of fluid are squeezed from the lung through the nose and mouth. With complete delivery of the chest, brisk recoil of the rib cage occurs, at which time 7 to 42 cc of air are "sucked" into the upper airway to replace the expressed fluid. The expulsion of lung fluid is often observable during delivery when the head is first exteriorized, while the chest is compressed in the birth canal by pressures up to 95 cm H_2O. Approximately one third of the total quantity of lung fluid may be "squeezed out" during vaginal delivery. Some term infants are apparently capable of absorbing all of the lung fluid without oral drainage because breathing begins immediately after cesarean delivery. On the other hand, transient tachypnea of the newborn (RD II) (see later) is more frequent in term infants born by cesarean section. This disorder is thought to be caused by delayed absorption of lung

fluid. Most lung fluid is evacuated across alveolar membranes through the lymphatic vessels and blood capillaries. The rate of fluid evacuation by each of these routes has not been clearly defined, but data from rabbits and lambs indicate increased lymph flow during the first breath and for several hours thereafter. Protein content (300 mg/100 ml) of lung fluid approximates amniotic fluid, and it has been suggested that this protein concentration would require evacuation by way of the lymphatics during the first breaths. Disappearance of lung fluid is far more rapid in rabbits delivered vaginally (several hours) than by cesarean section (several days). The mechanical effect of vaginal delivery is apparently an important factor in fluid evacuation. Absorption by lung capillaries and removal through lymphatics are also significant. Presumably these observations hold true for the human fetus.

Several mechanisms seem to be active in promoting the removal of lung fluid during the first few breaths. First, the continuous secretion of this fluid comes to a halt at birth. The secreting cells are inactivated by some unknown mechanism. It is clear from conclusive experiments in animals, however, that lung fluid does not accumulate postnatally. Second, the pressure relationship between the airway (alveoli) and interstitial tissue is altered when descent of the diaphragm generates negative pressures up to 80 or 100 cm H_2O. Pressure in the interstitial tissue is therefore considerably lower than in the alveoli, and fluid is forced to flow from alveoli to interstitial space along this pressure gradient. Third, expansion of the lungs has been shown to stretch alveolar walls with resultant enlargement of their pores. In the neonate these pores are six to ten times larger after lung expansion than they were before such expansion in the fetus. Now, the increased permeability of alveolar membranes and the previously described changes in pressure gradients combine to promote displacement of fluid to the interstitial tissue and then to the lymphatics and capillaries. The fourth active mechanism for removal of lung fluid involves the decrease in pulmonary vascular pressure and the increase in pulmonary blood flow that are inherent in the first breath and in adaptation to extrauterine life (see later). With these vascular changes, fluid that was displaced into the interstitium is subsequently "pulled into" blood vessels and lymphatics for ultimate evacuation.

Aeration of the lungs and evacuation of long fluid are inseparable requirements of normal postnatal breathing. Removal of liquid occurs in two stages: displacement from alveolar spaces to interstitial tissue and from there into lymph and capillary blood vessels. In the normal term infant, displacement to interstitial tissue is rapid, often instantaneous. Complete removal into lymph and blood vessels may take up to 5 or 6 hours.

Establishment of functional residual capacity (FRC)

If normal respiration is to follow the first breath, some air must remain in the alveoli at the end of expiration to maintain them in a partially expanded state. The volume of this retained air is the lung's *functional residual capacity*. The ability to retain the air is called *alveolar stability*.

In normal term human lungs, the first expansion may require an opening pressure as high as 60 to 80 cm H_2O. At the end of expiration the pressure is again zero, but if all is well, the lungs retain

about 40% of their fully expanded volume, since some air remains in the alveoli; functional residual capacity is thus established. It reaches its neonatal maximum by the end of 3 hours. From this partially expanded state the second inspiration is accomplished with minimal effort because now small pressure changes can produce relatively extensive inflation. During the second inspiration a high opening pressure is not necessary, since the lungs are already partially expanded at rest. The lung thus is approximately 40% inflated at zero intrathoracic pressure. Failure to retain air, together

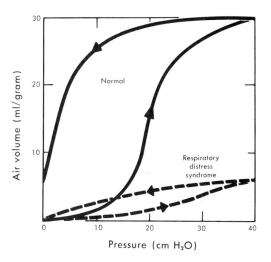

Fig. 8-3. Pressure-volume curves for normal lungs (solid lines) and surfactant-deficient lungs (broken lines). Normal lung expands maximally at 40 cm H_2O. Note that descending limb does not return to 0 level, indicating partial expansion at end-expiration (alveolar stability). The hyaline membrane disease curve peaks at a low expansion for 40 cm H_2O because lung compliance is poor. The curve returns to 0, indicating alveolar collapse at end-expiration (no alveolar stability). (From Klaus, M. In Barnett, H., editor: Pediatrics, ed. 15, New York, 1972, Appleton-Century-Crofts, Publishing Division of Prentice-Hall, Inc.)

with the resultant collapse of alveoli, is precluded by the presence of surfactant. Expansion of the immature lung is quite different, presumably because surfactant activity is diminished. At the end of expiration, at zero pressure, the alveoli collapse in response to unopposed surface tension forces (absence of surfactant). The difference between normal and abnormal expansion is graphically depicted in Fig. 8-3. Thus, with failure to establish functional residual capacity, each succeeding inflation requires the same amount of opening pressure as the first breath. The work of respiration is considerably increased, and continuity of alveolar gas exchange is not established. This phenomenon is of fundamental significance in the pathogenesis of hyaline membrane disease.

Increased pulmonary blood flow and redistribution of cardiac output

Cardiovascular adaptation to extrauterine life proceeds simultaneously with pulmonary adaptation. Five attributes of the fetal circulation must be altered if the mature cardiovascular pattern is to evolve. These fetal characteristics fall into two broad categories:

1. *Pulmonary-systemic pressure relationships*
   High pulmonary artery pressure due to increased pulmonary vascular resistance
   Low aortic systemic pressure (placental circuit)
2. *Sites of venous admixture (right-to-left) shunts)*
   Foramen ovale
   Ductus arteriosus
   Ductus venosus

Pulmonary-systemic pressure relationships
Fetal aortic blood pressure lower than pulmonary artery pressure. The placenta

receives 40% to 50% of the fetal cardiac output. The fetal placental vessels are apparently not supplied with nerve endings; they are generally relaxed. Therefore they offer little resistance to the flow of blood. The placenta therefore constitutes a low-resistance circuit. The blood that perfuses it comes from the fetal aorta and returns to the fetal inferior vena cava, thus making it a prominent low-resistance component of the *systemic circulation*. Clamping of the cord eliminates the placental vascular bed, thus reducing considerably the total intravascular space in the systemic circuit; in consequence, at birth the aortic blood pressure is raised. Simultaneously, return flow to the inferior vena cava is reduced by severance of the placenta, and a small drop in pressure occurs in the venous side of the circulation.

Pulmonary artery pressure higher than aortic pressure. This is the result of extremely high pulmonary vascular resistance to blood flow in the fetus. Resistance to blood flow through the lungs is so high as to permit only 5% to 7% of cardiac output to perfuse them, in contrast to the low-resistance placental circuit, which accommodates 40% to 50% of cardiac output. If the lungs expand sufficiently, vasodilatation produces a precipitous fall in pulmonary vascular resistance within the first few minutes after birth. Resistance has been calculated to fall by 80% from fetal levels. A more gradual reduction in resistance transpires over the next 6 to 8 weeks. With the abrupt diminution of resistance comes an equally abrupt increase in pulmonary blood flow. Within minutes after the establishment of adequate ventilation, pulmonary perfusion has increased approximately fivefold. Relaxation of the pulmonary arterioles is principally in the precapillary segments. An overwhelming stimulus to this vasodilatation is the increase in blood P_{O_2} that follows the first few breaths. Of secondary significance is the dilatation of capillaries that results from elimination of their compression by alveolar fluid as air enters the alveoli.

High fetal pulmonary arteriolar resistance is not solely a function of constriction. The relative thickness of the muscle layer of these arterioles is considerably greater than it will be later in postnatal life. Thus the gradual diminution of vascular resistance that occurs over the first 6 to 8 weeks is related to thinning out of the muscle layer, rather than to ongoing relaxation of existing muscle. In summary, initial lung expansion and adequate oxygenation diminish blood pressure in the pulmonary circuit by forcefully stimulating pulmonary arteriolar relaxation. At the same time, blood pressure in the systemic circuit increases because of greater resistance brought about by severance of the placenta. With this reversal of relative blood pressures in the pulmonary and systemic circuits, the stage is now set for elimination of the fetal sites at which venous admixture occurs (right-to-left shunt).

Fetal sites of venous admixture (right-to-left shunts)

Closure of the foramen ovale. The foramen ovale is an aperture in the interatrial septum. It is covered by a thin flap of tissue that can open like a swinging door in only one direction—into the left atrium. Since, in the fetus, pressure in the right atrium is higher than that in the left (because pulmonary circuit pressure is high), the flap remains open, permitting most of the well-oxygenated blood from the inferior vena cava to flow from the right atrium into the left atrium. The position of the flap is thus a function of the pressure relationship between both atria. If pressure in the right atrium is *higher* than that in the left, the flap is open and blood flows from the right to left atrium. This is normal for the fetus. When pressure in the right atrium is *lower* than that of the left, the flap closes. This is normal for the neonate. Lung expansion during the first breath causes an abrupt decline in pulmonary vascular resistance and a marked increase in pulmonary blood flow. The amount of blood that flows into the left atrium is therefore increased (pulmonary venous return), causing the left atrial pressure to rise slightly. Right atrial pressure falls because of lowered pulmonary vascular resistance. The pressure relationship between the atria is now reversed. When the left atrial pressure increases over that of the right, the swinging flap of tissue abuts against the margins of the foramen ovale. The foramen is now *functionally* closed, and one site of right-to-left shunting is eliminated. The tissue flap does not become immovably adherent to the atrial septum for several months. It is held in the closed position by the higher left atrial pressure. If right atrial pressure again becomes higher than that on the left (the baby is suddenly asphyxiated), the foramen will reopen.

Closure of the ductus arteriosus. The fetal ductus arteriosus is a large vessel, almost equal in diameter to the pulmonary artery. When it constricts, its substantial muscle layer has the capacity of obliterating the lumen. Constriction of the ductus arteriosus occurs in response to the increased blood P_{O_2} that occurs during the first few breaths. Vasoconstrictive response of the ductus to oxygen is in contrast to the vasodilating response of pulmonary arterioles. If the lungs do not expand normally, failure of P_{O_2} to rise causes sustained ductus patency. Normally, functional closure (constriction) is complete by 15 hours after birth in term infants. Anatomic closure (fibrosis) is usually complete by 3 weeks of age. In premature infants the ductus remains patent for much longer, and variable, periods because the capacity to constrict in response to augmented oxygen tension is not yet developed. The reasons for this lack of response have only recently begun to unfold. The ductus remains patent throughout fetal life because of compounds within its tissue that are known as *prostaglandins*. These substances exist in a number of molecular variations. They are synthesized within virtually every tissue in the body. Their functions vary according to the organ (tissue) in which they are synthesized and according to their molecular structure. In the ductus, prostaglandin E_1 and E_2 exert a vasodilatory effect. Prostaglandins remain in the ductal tissue of premature infants after birth, and it is believed that their presence inhibits the constrictive effect of oxygen after postnatal breathing. The physiologic mechanism by which the vasodilatory effect of prostaglandin E_1 and E_2 is ultimately inhibited has not yet been clarified. The prostaglandins are formed within cells by an enzyme complex known as *prostaglandin synthetase*. The activity of this enzyme can be inhibited pharmacologically by *prostaglandin synthetase inhibitors*. Inhibition impedes formation of prostaglandins, and when this occurs in a patent ductus arteriosus, the vessel proceeds to constrict. Indomethacin is a potent prostaglandin synthetase inhibitor that has been shown clinically to bring about constriction of the ductus in premature infants. Conversely, in animal experiments, infusion of prostaglandin E_1 or E_2 reversed the

constrictive effects of indomethacin. In these experiments, the prostaglandins maintained ductal patency. Discussion of the clinical significance and treatment of patent ductus arteriosus is presented later in this chapter.

Prior to completion of anatomic closure in term or premature babies, the ductus may reopen in response to lowered blood oxygen tension. The older the infant, the less likely is the ductus to reopen. With ductal closure, another fetal right-to-left shunt is eliminated.

Closure of the ductus venosus. The ductus venosus is a channel that, in the fetus, connects the portal (hepatic and intestinal) venous circulation with the inferior vena cava. In the fetus, umbilical vein blood passes through the liver, into the ductus venosus, to the inferior vena cava, and thence to the heart. The mechanism of closure of the ductus venosus is unknown. After birth, very little blood flows through it. Anatomical closure (fibrosis) is completed in 3 to 7 days.

In summary, changing pressure relationships are responsible for elimination of the fetal sites of right-to-left shunting. With adequate lung expansion, an increase in pulmonary blood flow occurs. This is brought about by the diminished vascular resistance that results from dilatation of pulmonary vessels. Almost all subsequent changes in circulation are a consequence of decreased pulmonary vascular resistance associated with normal lung expansion. Increased blood flow through the lungs leads to a larger flow into the left atrium, thereby raising left atrial pressure above that in the right atrium. When this occurs, the foramen ovale closes, thus eliminating the fetal right-to-left shunt at this site. The ductus arteriosus begins gradual closure by constriction of its wall as a result of a rising arterial P_{O_2}. Earlier, diminished ductus blood flow is a function of changes in pressure relationships between the pulmonary and the systemic circulations. As pulmonary blood pressure declines with lung expansion, pressures in the pulmonary and systemic circuits are almost equalized. There is thus gradual elimination of the pressure gradient that directed fetal blood from the pulmonary artery through the ductus into the aorta. Constriction of the ductus in response to increased oxygenation when prostaglandin synthesis is inhibited physiologically, plus the change in pressure relationships between the pulmonary and systemic circulations, therefore combine to obliterate another fetal site of right-to-left shunting.

What causes the pulmonary vascular bed to dilate and thus receive a greater flow of blood? Perhaps the most powerful influence is an increase in arterial P_{O_2}. Conversely, hypoxia constricts pulmonary vasculature. Most of this activity occurs in the precapillary arterioles. With the establishment of extrauterine respiration, the increase of arterial P_{O_2} exerts very different effects on pulmonary arterioles and the ductus arteriosus. The former relax as P_{O_2} rises; the latter constricts. The alveolar capillaries dilate as the lung expands and alveolar fluid is replaced by air during the first few breaths.

HYALINE MEMBRANE DISEASE (RESPIRATORY DISTRESS SYNDROME, RDS I)

Hyaline membrane disease (HMD) is also known as idiopathic respiratory distress syndrome (IRDS), or simply as respiratory distress syndrome (RDS). It is an acute disorder that is symptomatic at birth or soon thereafter. Primarily char-

acterized by respiratory distress, it occurs almost exclusively in premature infants. Its natural course is 3 to 5 days in duration. In the United States it is estimated that 12,000 infants die of hyaline membrane disease annually.

Incidence and prognosis

Hyaline membrane disease occurs in 1% to 2% of total live births in all races and in all socioeconomic groups. Reports of incidence are quite variable, but a common trend has been noted in all parts of the world. It is almost exclusively a disease of premature infants, rarely occurring in babies born at term. Furthermore, the incidence varies from one birthweight group to another. It is most common among infants who weigh between 1000 and 1500 grams, next most frequent in those between 1500 and 2000 grams, and it is least common between 2000 and 2500 grams. In general, 10% to 20% of all premature infants are affected. In the 1000- to 1500-gram group, the one of highest incidence, hyaline membrane disease has been reported to affect as many as 57% of babies. Severe respiratory distress is even more frequent in babies below 1000 grams. In them the clinical picture differs from classic hyaline membrane disease. This disorder occurs in 65% of infants in this lowest birth weight category.

Case fatality rates are too variable to quote precisely, but as one might expect, the lower the birth weight, the less likely is survival. Although recent advances in therapy have diminished the percentage of mortality impressively, it remains high nevertheless.

Pathophysiology

Comprehension of the pathophysiology of hyaline membrane disease requires familiarity with the events of the first breath. In essence, hyaline membrane disease is a partial persistence of, or reversion to, the fetal cardiopulmonary state. Whatever other factors may influence the course of events, the central difficulty seems to be a deficiency in surfactant activity. Hyaline membrane disease is fundamentally a developmental disorder. The maturation of surfactant synthesis has been amply demonstrated by extensive studies. They have thus far confirmed the validity of L/S ratio measurements, which indicate that, with a few exceptions, the lungs are capable of normal extrauterine function at approximately 35 gestational weeks. The central

significance of a developmental concept seems plausible because the disease preponderantly affects premature infants; term infants are rarely affected. A well-defined sequence of biochemical events must transpire in utero before maturation of the lungs is established. If birth occurs prior to completion of this sequence, the neonate with premature lungs is incapable of normally coping with a gaseous environment.

The principal factors that are operative in the evolution of hyaline membrane disease are depicted in Fig. 8-4. The narrative that follows will refer to the numbered squares in the diagram. The *persistent fetal state (1)* implies *surfactant deficiency* and increased *pulmonary vascular resistance* as well. The latter would ordinarily disappear in the presence of normal lung expansion, but this disappearance is precluded in the premature lung because of surfactant deficiency. In most instances there is probably enough functional surfactant present at birth to accommodate reasonably effective breathing. Thus, at birth, and for a short time thereafter, some infants breathe with little or moderate difficulty. Soon respiration becomes more labored as surfactant is dissipated. Consequently, normal functional residual capacity (alveolar stability) is not possible. Alveoli that are inflated during inspiration are again collapsed at end expiration. Each breath is like the first; collapsed alveoli require reinflation. The work of respiration is thus relatively tremendous; an effort similar to that expended for the first breath must be mounted for each one that follows. As the infant becomes more feeble, he fails to open more alveoli. *Atelectasis (2)*, already present at birth to some extent, now becomes more widespread. Pulmonary hypoperfusion from vaso-

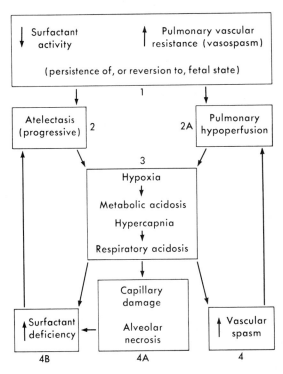

Fig. 8-4. Principal intrapulmonary factors in pathogenesis of hyaline membrane disease. (See text.)

spasm has been present from the beginning (2A). These two factors (2, 2A) produce *hypoxia* and *hypercapnia (3)*. As hypoxia becomes prolonged, anaerobic glycolysis is activated for the production of glucose from glycogen. The by-product of this process is an increased quantity of lactic acid, which causes *metabolic acidosis (3)*. Furthermore, carbon dioxide cannot be blown off due to atelectasis and the paucity of blood that delivers it to the lungs. The resultant retention of CO_2 (hypercapnia) causes *respiratory acidosis (3)*; blood pH is therefore diminished considerably.

Hypoxia and acidosis accentuate preexisting *vascular spasm (4)*, which in turn increases *pulmonary hypoperfusion (2A)*. Hypoxia and acidosis also inflict *capillary damage* and *alveolar necrosis (4A)*, both of which aggravate *surfactant deficiency (4B)* by impairing its production. As a consequence, *progressive atelectasis (2)* is unabated.

Failure of lung expansion and persistence of high vascular resistance result in increased blood pressure in the pulmonary circuit. Venous admixture (right-to-left shunt) through the foramen ovale, as it existed in utero, is maintained after birth. If pressure in the pulmonary circuit is sufficiently high in relation to aortic pressure, a right-to-left shunt (pulmonary artery to aorta) is also present at the ductus arteriosus. The effect of these extrapulmonary shunts is to divert blood from the lungs and thus add to their hypoperfusion. To a variable extent, the fetal cardiopulmonary circulation persists in each patient.

This entire sequence of events can be ascribed to failure of lung expansion and inability to establish alveolar stability as a result of a primary surfactant deficiency. Surfactant deficiency is enhanced by in-

trauterine asphyxia. Asphyxia causes pulmonary vasoconstriction in utero. The resultant ischemia impairs surfactant production.

The incidence of intrauterine asphyxia in premature infants is indeed higher than in term babies, but the majority of infants who have hyaline membrane disease give no evidence of antecedent stress. Acute asphyxia probably accentuates the maturational inadequacy.

Lung compliance is diminished in hyaline membrane disease. Compliance is a function of the elasticity of lung tissue. It expresses the capacity of the lung to increase in volume in response to a given amount of applied pressure during inspiration. The lungs in hyaline membrane disease require far more pressure than normal lungs for equal amounts of expansion. Pressures of 35 cm H_2O, which usually expand normal lungs, cause little inflation of lungs with hyaline membrane disease. The abnormal lung tissue is thus said to be "stiffer," or less distensible. Compliance is expressed in milliliters (volume change) per centimeter of water (pressure change), or ml/cm H_2O. Compliance of normal newborn lungs is 4 to 6 ml/cm H_2O; in hyaline membrane disease it is one fourth to one fifth as much. The stiffness of affected lungs, and thus their limited distensibility, contributes significantly to the work of breathing in these sick babies. It also permits therapy with positive end-expiratory pressure (discussed later).

The role of the hyaline membranes in disruption of pulmonary function has not been delineated. In years past they were believed to arise solely from aspiration of vernix and other particulate matter in amniotic fluid. It has become evident, however, that they are principally the product of cellular necrosis in the alveoli and terminal respiratory bronchioles. Hyaline membranes do not in themselves cause atelectasis. They probably contribute to diminution of compliance.

Predisposing factors

Prematurity is virtually a constant predisposing factor; complications of pregnancy and labor play an additional major role. Maternal bleeding and other causes of fetal asphyxia are associated with the disease but not in the majority of babies. Maternal diabetes is an important predisposing factor in itself; it also predisposes to the disease because of the high incidence of prematurity among infants of diabetic mothers (p. 306). The role of cesarean section is still debated. The causes of fetal distress that urgently necessitate cesarean section seem to be the decisive factors. Most studies indicate that elective cesarean (performed in the absence of detectable fetal difficulty) are not associated with an increased incidence of the disease. On the other hand, there is impressive evidence for a contributory role by cesarean section itself.

Morphologic pathology

At autopsy the lungs are purple red, resembling the consistency of liver. They contain little or no air in contrast to normal lungs, which are salmon pink and spongy by virtue of their air content. The microscopic appearance is characterized by widespread atelectasis and hyaline membranes. These membranes are present only in previously aerated portions of the lung, and with usual staining techniques in microscopic sections they may vary in color from pale pink to red (eosinophilic). Generally they have a homogeneous, waxen appearance. They line the surfaces of alveoli and terminal respiratory bronchioles. Epithelial cells are necrotic or absent in areas occupied by membranes and in collapsed alveoli.

Clinical manifestations

Infants with hyaline membrane disease were previously believed to be free of abnormalities for the first few hours of life, but as more careful observations were made, it became obvious that the majority of affected babies had some sort of respiratory difficulty at birth or within 2 hours thereafter. If there is truly no respiratory distress within 3 hours after delivery, the diagnosis of hyaline membrane disease is not tenable. In the past, errors were due to infrequent observation, failure to appreciate the more subtle signs of respiratory difficulty, and failure to perform Apgar scoring at birth.

Increased respiratory rate (over 60 respirations per minute) is the most common sign of abnormal ventilation. Occasionally an expiratory grunt or sigh is the only perceptible sign. The expiratory grunt is a fascinating phenomenon. It is an effort to obstruct exhalation of air temporarily and thus, by increasing "back pressure," to maintain some degree of alveolar expansion to increase functional residual capacity. The epiglottis is held so that the glottis is closed. Pressure mounts within the respiratory tract as the outflow of air is obstructed. When the epiglottis is abruptly released, the sudden rush of air over the vocal cords produces a grunt. Infants who grunt can raise their arterial P_{O_2} by 10 to 20 mm Hg. Since the exhalation of air must be obstructed by closure of the glottis, passage of an endotracheal tube eliminates the grunt. However, this should not be interpreted as a contraindication to intubation of severely affected infants who require such therapy.

Retraction of the chest wall during inspiration is a classic sign of respiratory distress or, more specifically, diminished lung compliance. Retractions indicate a failure to fill the lungs with air during efforts exerted by respiratory muscles, especially the diaphragm. They thus indicate inadequate distention of the lungs during inspiration. Retractions are not always a sign of intrinsic lung disease, although this is their most frequent cause. They may also result from obstruction of airflow in the nose, larynx, trachea, or major bronchi. In hyaline membrane disease, airflow is diminished by incomplete expansion of the lungs, which is due to diminished compliance. The lungs are stiffer than normal, and they fail to inflate fully as the diaphragm descends to enlarge the thorax. Negative pressure persists in the pleural space between the chest wall and the unexpanded lungs, and since the lungs do not expand to fill this space, the flexible chest wall is pulled inward. The net result is retraction of the chest wall.

In addition to *tachypnea, grunting,* and *retractions, flaring of the external nares* is also a frequent sign of respiratory distress. Auscultation of the chest reveals generalized *diminution of breath sounds* and, occasionally, *crepitant rales. Apneic episodes* occur in severely affected babies. They are an ominous sign, particularly when observed during the first 24 hours of life. *Cyanosis* in room air is the rule.

Cardiac signs are not ordinarily prominent. The heart rate is usually quite variable, but it becomes fixed as the disease increases in severity. Bradycardia (less than 100 beats/min) occurs when hypoxemia is severe. Cardiac failure is rare.

Pallor is the result of peripheral vaso-constriction, rather than anemia. *Edema,* which is common in normal premature babies, is more frequent and severe in those with hyaline membrane disease. *Pitting edema* of the hands and feet appears within the first 24 hours and resolves by the end of the fifth day.

Decreased body temperature is frequently observed. In mildly or moderately involved infants it is correctable in an optimal thermal environment, but in severely affected infants it often defies remedial measures. Ambient incubator temperatures of 95° F (35° C) or more may be required to raise the body temperature.

Specific central nervous system signs are few. The muscles are universally *flaccid,* and the infant is *hypoactive* or *motionless.* Severely ill infants assume a frog-leg position, with the mouth open and the head fallen to one side.

Retractions continue for approximately 3 to 5 days and then diminish. Tachypnea often persists for several days afterward. Improvement is signaled by diminution of retractions, increased muscle tone and spontaneous activity, and frequent voiding accompanied by resolution of edema. Death is unlikely after 72 hours except for infants with complications such as intracranial hemorrhage, pneumonia, or pulmonary hemorrhage.

Laboratory data

Except for the recently described foam stability test on gastric aspirate, there are no specific laboratory tests for the diagnosis of hyaline membrane disease. The characteristic biochemical abnormalities (hypoxemia, hypercapnia, and acidosis) are identical to those of perinatal asphyxia and postnatal respiratory failure from any cause. In severely ill infants in room air the arterial P_{O_2} is below 40 mm Hg (normal lower limit: 50 mm Hg), the arterial P_{CO_2} is over 65 mm Hg (normal upper limit: 45 mm Hg), and the pH is below 7.15 (normal: 7.35 to 7.45).

Hypoxemia. Inadequate ventilation plus poor perfusion of tissues combine to cause low arterial oxygen tensions. Restoration of normal levels is the primary aim of therapy. Hypoxemia induces metabolic acidosis because lactic acid production increases. It also causes pulmonary arteriolar constriction with intrapulmonary right-to-left shunting because alveoli are bypassed. Other deleterious effects of hypoxemia include damage to capillary endothelium all over the body, impaired metabolic response to cold stress, and ultimately a low systemic blood pressure from diminished cardiac output.

Hypercapnia. Accumulation of carbon dioxide in the blood is due to inadequate ventilation caused by atelectasis and hypoperfusion. A rising arterial P_{CO_2} signifies deterioration of pulmonary function. In the extreme, arterial P_{CO_2} may exceed 100 mm Hg.

Acidosis. Mixed respiratory and metabolic acidosis is the rule in hyaline membrane disease. Early in the course of the disease respiratory acidosis may predominate, but soon a metabolic component also appears. The arterial pH may approach 6.8 terminally. The deleterious effects of acidosis include pulmonary vasoconstriction, irregular heartbeat, depression of myocardial function, dilatation of cerebral vessels that imposes a hazard of cerebral hemorrhage, further impairment of surfactant activity, and detachment of bilirubin from albumin to cause kernicterus at unexpectedly low serum bilirubin concentrations (p. 294).

Other blood chemical values. Serum elec-trolyte values may remain relatively unaltered, except for potassium, which increases as a result of hypoxic cellular injury in untreated or unsuccessfully treated babies. Lactic acid levels rise in conjunction with hypoxemia. Serum bilirubin levels are generally higher in babies with hyaline membrane disease; this is apparently related to depressed liver function (p. 291).

Foam stability test (shake test) on gastric aspirate. The foam stability test was first described for amniotic fluid (p. 15), for which it is generally used as a screening procedure preliminary to L/S ratio determination. The presence of surfactant causes the formation of stable bubbles (foam) in a test tube of amniotic fluid that is shaken for 15 seconds after the addition of 95% ethanol. If surfactant is absent, bubbles are not formed. The test is negative.

The same procedure on gastric aspirate taken from the baby within an hour after birth is useful in distinguishing hyaline membrane disease from other causes of respiratory distress. One-half milliliter gastric aspirate is mixed with an equal quantity of normal saline. The resultant 1 ml mixture is added to 1 ml of 95% ethanol and shaken briskly for 15 seconds. The test tube is left standing in room air, and the result is read after 15 minutes. The test tube must be viewed from above against a black background in good light. The test is positive if a complete ring of bubbles is present in the meniscus. A positive shake test indicates that surfactant is present and that, with rare exception, hyaline membrane disease will not ensue. A negative test is indicated by complete absence of bubbles. It predicts almost certainly that hyaline membrane disease will follow. An intermediate result is comprised of bubble patterns that form a ring around one third of the circumference of the meniscus or less. Most of these babies will have hyaline membrane disease. Properly executed, this procedure could aid substantially in determining the need for transfer of an infant to a regional center.

Radiologic findings

The typical x-ray appearance of the lungs is well correlated with the morphologic pathology of the disease. Almost every author who writes about it describes a reticulogranular pattern that is diffuse over both lung fields, occasionally involving one lung more than the other. The general impression one receives on viewing such a film is that the lungs appear clouded or similar to ground glass. White density is particularly prominent and homogeneous at the hilar areas. Close inspection peripheral to the hilar

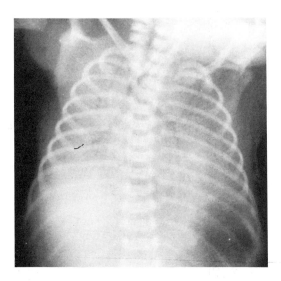

Fig. 8-5. Radiologic appearance of severe hyaline membrane disease. The lungs are dense. The cardiac shadow is barely discernible in left chest. Prominent black streaks emanating from both hilar areas are air bronchograms.

regions reveals tiny, closely spaced, comma-like densities that sometimes suggest a heavy snowfall at night. Each of these small densities is an atelectatic area of lung. At the hilar regions, and for some distance peripherally, dark streaks represent air-filled bronchi, which are easily discerned against the white background provided by the collapsed lung. These dark streaks are called air bronchograms. Hilar densities, a diffuse reticulogranular pattern, and air bronchograms are thus the cardinal radiologic features of hyaline membrane disease (Fig. 8-5).

Treatment

There is to date no definitive treatment for hyaline membrane disease. The therapeutic approaches of confirmed benefit are supportive in nature. This discussion is limited to the most successful ones. They are directly concerned with providing effective ventilation, correcting acid-base imbalance, providing optimal environmental temperature, and maintaining normal hematocrit and blood pressure.

Oxygen therapy. Nothing is more critical to tissue metabolism than an adequate supply of oxygen. The most important aspect of total therapy for hyaline membrane disease is the provision of oxygen. *Once the need for such therapy is apparent for any disorder, its adequacy must be ascertained and its hazards averted by continuous monitoring of arterial oxygen tensions.* In this section, before discussion of practical considerations, it seems fitting to discuss the physiologic principles that underlie rational oxygen therapy, its benefits, and its hazards.

Physiology of oxygen transport: the basis for rational oxygen therapy. The erythrocyte is the vehicle for transport of oxygen. Its basic function is to take up oxygen from the lungs and deliver it to the tissues, carrying sufficient quantities to effect rapid diffusion from capillaries to tissue cells. The performance of this function depends on a number of factors that include an adequate fraction of inspired oxygen ($F_{I_{O_2}}$), normal pulmonary function, blood volume, cardiac output, perfusion, and distribution of blood to tissues. Other aspects are intrinsic to blood. They involve arterial pH and temperature, hemoglobin concentration, and the affinity of hemoglobin for oxygen. Several definitions must be considered before continuing this discussion.

Partial pressure of oxygen, or oxygen tension (P_{O_2}). Management of oxygen therapy is based on monitored levels of arterial oxygen tensions (Pa_{O_2}), expressed in millimeters of mercury (mm Hg). The partial pressure of a gas is the measured force it exerts in its tendency to escape from a liquid to a gaseous medium or from one compartment to another, much like the pressure exerted by escaping bubbles in champagne. It is called "partial" when the gas in question is only one of several in a common liquid (or chamber) that exert pressure simultaneously. In arterial (or venous) blood, with the subject breathing room air, partial pressures are measurable for oxygen, carbon dioxide, nitrogen, and water vapor. Total pressure of these gases—that is, their aggregate driving force to escape—is approximately 750 mm Hg. The pressure exerted by oxygen itself, or partial pressure (arterial P_{O_2}), is about 90 mm Hg. The tension attributable to carbon dioxide, the arterial P_{CO_2}, is usually 40 mm Hg. The remaining partial pressures are exerted by nitrogen. The P_{O_2} is thus the driving force of oxygen, which will move it from one compartment to another— from alveoli to pulmonary capillaries if P_{O_2} is higher in alveoli than in capillaries,

and from capillaries to tissues if partial pressure in the capillaries is higher than in tissue fluid. The same principle is operative for movement of oxygen from tissue fluid to individual cells. Movement of CO_2 in the opposite direction, from tissues to blood and thence to alveoli, is governed by a similar pattern of pressure differences. Movement of gas from a higher to a lower partial pressure is movement governed by a *pressure gradient*. If normal arterial blood (P_{O_2}, 90 mm Hg) is exposed to room air (P_{O_2}, 160 mm Hg), oxygen will enter the blood until equilibrium is established, that is, until both have a P_{O_2} of 160 mm Hg. On the other hand, with arterial P_{CO_2} of 40 mm Hg and atmospheric P_{CO_2} of 0 (there is virtually no CO_2 in air), carbon dioxide will ultimately disappear from blood, having moved into room air. The pressure gradient for oxygen movement was from room air to blood; arterial P_{O_2} rose. For carbon dioxide it was in the opposite direction; arterial P_{CO_2} declined. This is precisely what occurs when blood collected for blood gas determination is inadvertently exposed to room air. Blood gas determinations in these circumstances are invalid.

Oxygen content. The oxygen content of whole blood is the total amount of the gas in 100 ml of whole blood. Normal oxygen content is 20.6 ml (vol %). This includes 20 ml bound to hemoglobin and 0.6 ml (approximately 3% of the total) dissolved in plasma.

Oxygen capacity. Oxygen *capacity* must be distinguished from oxygen *content*. Oxygen-carrying capacity is the maximal amount of the gas that hemoglobin can theoretically hold. Oxygen content is the actual amount held. Most oxygen in blood is bound to hemoglobin. Each gram of hemoglobin has the capacity to bind 1.34 ml of oxygen. If the hemoglobin concentration of whole blood is 15 grams/100 ml, the calculated capacity at this concentration is 15 × 1.34, or 20.1 ml of oxygen/100 ml of blood.

Oxygen saturation. Referring only to hemoglobin, oxygen saturation is given as a percentage value that is calculated by dividing the amount of oxygen bound to hemoglobin by the maximal amount that can be bound (oxygen capacity). Normal oxygen saturation is 96% to 98%. Oxygen saturation is governed by the P_{O_2} and by the affinity of hemoglobin for oxygen.

Affinity of hemoglobin for oxygen. Fetal hemoglobin differs from adult hemoglobin. Among its unique attributes is the ability to bind more oxygen at any given P_{O_2}. Therefore, at any given P_{O_2}, oxygen saturation of fetal hemoglobin is higher than the adult's. Fetal hemoglobin thus has a greater affinity for oxygen than adult hemoglobin. The fetal red blood cell therefore takes up more oxygen in the lungs, but this phenomenon is of little overall significance. Of greater potential importance is the fact that increased affinity also causes less oxygen to be released to the tissues. Conversely, when oxygen affinity is reduced, as in the adult, more oxygen is unloaded to the tissues at any given Pa_{O_2}. Hemoglobin releases bound oxygen in response to a lower tissue oxygen tension (P_{O_2}). In the neonate, the tension must fall farther before fetal hemoglobin releases oxygen, since it is held more avidly than in the adult.

The molecular configuration of fetal hemoglobin differs from that of the adult. This difference, plus the quantity of organic phosphates in the red blood cells, determines the affinity of hemoglobin for oxygen. The principal organic phosphate in the erythrocyte is 2,3-diphos-

phoglycerate (2,3-DPG). A diminished interaction between fetal hemoglobin and DPG in the neonatal erythrocyte results in greater affinity for oxygen. Greater interaction between adult hemoglobin and DPG results in less oxygen affinity. If the neonate is transfused with fresh adult blood, more oxygen is released to tissues.

The oxygen-hemoglobin dissociation curve. Normally there is a predictable correlation between oxygen saturation and P_{O_2}. Plotted on a graph in which the percentage of saturation is arranged vertically, and P_{O_2} horizontally, a typical S-shaped curve results when the plotted points are joined. Dissociation curves for fetal and adult hemoglobins are shown in Fig. 8-6. The saturation of fetal hemoglobin (vertical scale) is higher than the adult's at all P_{O_2} levels because there is a greater affinity for oxygen. Stated differently, the same percentage of saturation occurs at a lower P_{O_2} in fetal hemoglobin than in the adult's. This can be clearly discerned by reference to the two shaded vertical bars that indicate zones in which cyanosis is visible, corresponding to fetal and adult values for oxygen saturation of hemoglobin. Cyanosis is apparent when blood is between 75% and 85% saturated with oxygen. These saturations occur at P_{O_2} levels of 32 to 41 mm Hg in the neonate and 42 to 52 mm Hg in the adult. Fig. 8-6 demonstrates why the newborn is considerably less oxygenated than the adult when cyanosis first becomes discernible. The fetal dissociation curve is said to be shifted to the left of the adult's.

The position of the curve (shifted right or left) actually indicates the affinity of hemoglobin for oxygen. When the affinity is decreased, as in the adult, more oxygen is released to tissues at any given oxygen tension. Saturation at any oxygen

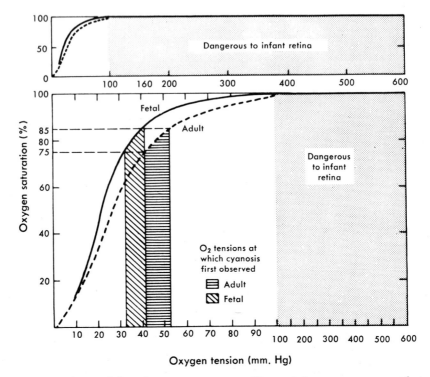

Fig. 8-6. Oxygen-hemoglobin dissociation curves. Cyanosis becomes apparent between 75% and 85% saturation, correlating to lower oxygen tension in neonates than that in adults. Scale at top shows the curves in relation to toxic levels. (From Klaus, M., and Meyer, B. P.: Pediatr. Clin. North Am. **13**:731, 1966.)

tension is therefore less than in the neonate. Saturation at any given P_{O_2} decreases as affinity diminishes. The oxygen-hemoglobin dissociation curve is thus shifted to the right. If affinity is increased, as in the neonate, less oxygen is unloaded to tissues at any given Pa_{O_2}. Saturation at any Pa_{O_2} is therefore greater than in the adult. The curve is now said to be shifted to the left.

Two factors intrinsic to blood exert a major influence on affinity of hemoglobin for oxygen. Affinity diminishes as blood pH decreases and as temperature increases; the curve shifts to the right. Affinity increases as blood pH rises and temperature falls; the curve shifts to the left. The increased affinity caused by lower temperatures explains a common phenomenon. In bitter cold weather, earlobes are bright red because the blood within them is chilled. Affinity for oxygen increases; saturation at any given Pa_{O_2} is thus also increased, and the curve is shifted to the left, as in the neonate. The P_{O_2} of earlobe blood may be relatively low, but the increased saturation renders it bright red because hemoglobin retains more oxygen, releasing less to tissues as a result of its greater affinity for oxygen.

Practical aspects of oxygen administration

Dose and blood level; monitoring $F_{I_{O_2}}$ and blood gases. Oxygen is like any drug; it must be administered in proper dosage.

Unlike many drugs, however, the dose required for optimal and harmless effect varies widely from one infant to another and from time to time in the same infant. Appropriate doses of oxygen can be maintained only by monitoring its ambient concentrations and measuring the ultimate effect of such concentrations on the infant's arterial oxygen tension. The ultimate measure of optimal therapy is the arterial P_{O_2}. Carbon dioxide tension and pH are always determined on the same blood sample. A detailed record of these serial determinations must be kept, particularly in reference to the percentage of inhaled oxygen that is provided. The ambient concentration should always be measured when a blood sample is collected.

By any method of administration, from the simple oxygen hood to the complex mechanical ventilator, oxygen is a medication that requires proper dosage $F_{I_{O_2}}$ and repeated blood level determinations (arterial P_{O_2}). Pa_{O_2} over 100 mm Hg is currently considered hyperoxemic; under 50 mm Hg it is hypoxemic. For sick babies who require supplemental oxygen, there is no Pa_{O_2} that can be predictably correlated with any particular $F_{I_{O_2}}$. In most neonatal intensive care units, current practice maintains Pa_{O_2} between 50 and 70 mm Hg; some regulate at 60 to 80 mm Hg. These levels are achievable at widely varying inspired oxygen concentrations. An infant who is profoundly ill from hyaline membrane disease may require an $F_{I_{O_2}}$ of 1.00 (100% oxygen) to maintain a Pa_{O_2} of 50 mm Hg. During recovery 5 days later, the same $F_{I_{O_2}}$ may produce toxic Pa_{O_2} of over 200 mm Hg. Similar radical changes in $F_{I_{O_2}}$ requirements can occur within an hour or less.

The dose of oxygen is always expressed as its fraction of inspired air ($F_{I_{O_2}}$). The day has long since passed when oxygen can properly be ordered in liters per minute. This designation merely expresses flow rate of the gas, not its concentration in inspired air. Orders for oxygen administration given as liters per minute betray a sad lack of information about adequate therapy.

The dose of oxygen must be monitored continuously. Use of any of several varieties of oxygen analyzers is mandatory for this purpose. At present we prefer an analyzer that is placed in line so that the air mixture is monitored continuously. The $F_{I_{O_2}}$ should be determined every hour. We provide prescribed oxygen concentrations through a blender that regulates simultaneous inflow of air and oxygen by adjusting an indicator to the desired level.

The arterial blood level of oxygen should be determined at least every 4 hours for sick babies, often at much shorter intervals (15 minutes) for the most acutely ill infants, and at least every 6 hours for babies who are not acutely ill. These scheduled assessments are particularly necessary for premature infants.

Sites of blood sampling. For blood gas determinations, we use arterial blood samples exclusively. They are drawn from an umbilical artery catheter, or from the radial, brachial, or temporal arteries by needle puncture. In our laboratory approximately 25% of over 45,000 annual blood gas/pH determinations are drawn by puncture of those peripheral arteries. Determinations are made around the clock every day of the week.

Although the great majority of neonatal units use arterial blood for these assessments, a few facilities consider capillary blood samples to be adequate. Blood is collected by heel prick from a foot that has been warmed for 5 to 10 minutes.

Others prick the lateral aspect of a finger, over one of the digital arteries. Capillary blood values of 35 to 55 mm Hg are said to correspond to arterial tensions of 40 to 65 mm Hg. If capillary P_{O_2} is above 60 mm Hg, the arterial level may exceed 150 mm Hg. Most centers do not rely on capillary samples for monitoring P_{O_2}.

Collection of arterial samples through an umbilical artery catheter is widely practiced. Most centers insert the catheter tip to a level between the third and fourth lumbar vertebrae, which is just above the aortic bifurcation and below the origins of the renal arteries. In sick infants who have a right-to-left shunt through the ductus arteriosus, blood taken from the descending aorta is a mixture of oxygenated blood from the left ventricle and deoxygenated blood from the right ventricle that has passed through the ductal shunt. It is a postductal specimen because it came from the descending aorta below (distal to) the ductus opening. If the ductal shunt is substantial, postductal arterial P_{O_2} is at least 15% lower than preductal blood. Arterial blood collected from the right arm and from the temporal artery is preductal. The right subclavian artery (to the right arm) and the carotid arteries (to the head) branch from the proximal portion of the aortic arch. Aortic blood from the left ventricle passes these branches before it reaches the distal end of the arch where the ductus arteriosus connects to the aorta. It is thus unmixed with ductal blood. If a right-to-left shunt is present, ductus arteriosus blood empties into the aorta. This blood is from the right ventricle. It is deoxygenated (venous) blood that has not perfused the lungs. Its presence in postductal aortic blood may lower the P_{O_2} substantially. Arterial P_{O_2} levels in samples from the right radial and brachial arteries, and from either of the temporal arteries, are not mixed with postductal blood. These P_{O_2} levels are thus the same as in blood that perfuses the brain and the eyes. In severe hyaline membrane disease, with a right-to-left ductal shunt, the preductal P_{O_2} is considerably higher than the postductal one. Similarly, if an infant is hypotensive, the relatively higher pressure in the pulmonary circuit produces a significant shunt across the ductus. Postductal P_{O_2} in blood from the umbilical artery is therefore substantially lower than in blood from the right radial artery and, in many instances, does not reflect oxygen tension of blood that perfuses the eyes. The Pa_{O_2} in samples from the left radial artery may be similar either to the right radial artery or to postductal aortic samples, since the left subclavian artery (to the left arm) may originate from the aorta at the level of the ductus, slightly above it or slightly below. In the vast majority of infants, Pa_{O_2} in the left arm is similar to that in postductal blood taken from an umbilical artery catheter.

Monitoring with transcutaneous oxygen tension measurement (tcP_{O_2}). The necessity for frequent arterial blood gas samples ultimately requires repeated arterial punctures, usually taxing the ingenuity of staff and the well-being of babies. Futhermore, the resultant values are applicable to conditions that existed at the moment of sampling. We obviously have no idea what the oxygen tension is when blood is not taken. Neonatologists have long felt the need for a *noninvasive* technique by which blood gases can be monitored *continuously*. Several attempts to provide such devices have been concerned with P_{O_2} electrodes implanted at the tip of an indwelling umbilical artery catheter. Their limitations have restricted widespread use.

A device has been developed to measure oxygen tension by securing an electrode to the skin. The transcutaneous oxygen sensor can produce P_{O_2} values from the warmed skin (tcP_{O_2}) that are generally well correlated with arterial P_{O_2}. Continuous readout of oxygen tensions is possible. In addition, the device indicates the state of skin perfusion.

In healthy neonates a marked variation in tcP_{O_2}, mostly influenced by respiratory rate, is noted. An apneic episode causes a drop in tcP_{O_2} in seconds, and if apnea is sustained, the rate of fall is constant at 30 mm Hg/min. Crying infants have a marked drop in tcP_{O_2} usually between 20 and 50 mm Hg. When crying ceases, the tcP_{O_2} curve rises to normal. The difficulty in obtaining valid Pa_{O_2} in crying infants by traditional methods of arterial blood sampling is well known.

Warmth and humidity of oxygen. Oxygen must be warm and humid, regardless of the mechanism that is used to deliver it. This requires equipment that permits regulation of heat in a water reservoir through which oxygen flows before entering the respiratory tract. The infant pays dearly when cold, dry oxygen is thoughtlessly administered.

In an oxygen hood, ambient temperatures about the head and body should be similar. This cannot be accomplished unless oxygen is warmed. Prolonged oxygen therapy by mask is contraindicated, not only because F_{IO_2} cannot be regulated, but also because cold stress is inflicted on the face. Even if the oxygen is warm, the velocity of flow from the mask results in increased heat loss by convection (Chapter 4). The need for warmth and humidity is often overlooked when oxygen is administered by means of hood or mask. Most caregivers are not familiar with the exquisite thermal sensitivity of nerve endings in the skin of the face and forehead, believing that requirements for

thermal environment are met by warming the rest of the body. *If face and forehead are chilled, the infant reacts as though totally cold stressed even when the rest of the body is kept warm.*

In the application of continuous positive airway pressure (CPAP) by either the nasal or endotracheal route, warmth and humidity are indispensable because oxygen is introduced directly over mucosal surfaces. Dry gas increases evaporative fluid loss from the extensive mucosal surfaces, thus augmenting evaporative heat loss. Additionally, mucosal integrity is threatened by the sustained drying effect of unhumidified oxygen. Secretory material, usually copious in small infants, becomes inspissated when humidity is lacking. Resultant obstruction of the respiratory passages, particularly the smaller ones, causes atelectasis.

Hypoxia: detection, prevention, and penalties. Generally, a Pa_{O_2} less than 50 mm Hg is considered hypoxemic. A number of infants may tolerate somewhat lower levels for some time, but it is unsafe to regularly maintain arterial tensions at these lower levels. The acute effects of hypoxemia must be understood; they are often difficult to identify with certainty from clinical manifestations. The clinical recognition of hypoxemia on the basis of *cyanosis* is far from a simple matter. Several factors influence the recognition of cyanosis, including color and thickness of skin, number of capillaries, hemoglobin level, and serum bilirubin. Add to these variables the type and intensity of light, as well as the differences in perception among observers, and one can readily appreciate the complexity of this clinical situation. In the neonate, acrocyanosis (including circumoral involvement) that is present 24 to 48 hours after birth is of no significance insofar as arterial oxygen tensions are concerned. Cyanosis is not uniformly discernible on all areas of the body, even when oxygen saturations in blood are as low as 70%. Cyanosis of the lips (and perhaps the tongue) is most reliably correlated with hypoxic Pa_{O_2} levels; yet one in ten infants whose lips are not cyanotic may actually be hypoxic. Conversely, 28% of infants whose lips are blue are not hypoxic. They have no need for supplemental oxygen, and they will be needlessly exposed to the risk of pulmonary toxicity and retrolental fibroplasia if it is given. Hands, nailbeds, and circumoral areas are even less reliable. They frequently appear to be cyanotic in spite of normal oxygen saturations. The trunk and ears yield a high percentage of false-negative observations; they often appear pink in babies who are actually hypoxemic. *The clinical diagnosis of hypoxia is therefore unreliable. Cyanosis may be absent in hypoxic babies, and it may be present in those who are well oxygenated. Its presence over different parts of the body is variable, and there is little consistency among observers in the ability to recognize it.*

At this point in the discussion, it would be advisable to review the oxygen-hemoglobin dissociation curves (Fig. 8-6). Cyanosis is not visible until saturations fall between 75% and 85%. At these saturations the neonate's Pa_{O_2} is between 32 and 42 mm Hg. Cyanosis in the older child and adult is identifiable at higher Pa_{O_2} levels. The clinical message of the dissociation curve is clear. The pink baby in respiratory distress may be hypoxemic; when cyanosis finally appears, catastrophe may be at hand. The Pa_{O_2} may already be as low as 32 mm Hg. *The ill effects of hypoxemia had transpired while the baby was pink.* The acute responses to hypoxia began as the Pa_{O_2} fell below 50 mm Hg.

Diminished tissue oxygenation causes *metabolic acidosis* due to overproduction of lactic acid during anaerobic glycolysis. Peripheral vasoconstriction due to acidosis and hypoxemia may cause pallor and a transient rise in blood pressure.

Anaerobic glycolysis also depletes glycogen stores rapidly because more glycogen is required for glucose production. *Hypoglycemia* is therefore another penalty of hypoxia.

The most immediate response to a drop in oxygen tension is *constriction of pulmonary arterioles*, which is greatly accentuated if metabolic acidosis is also present. Hypoxemia worsens because ventilation is impaired by the resultant pulmonary hypoperfusion. Furthermore, surfactant production may diminish as a consequence of alveolar ischemia. One can now see that the fetal cardiopulmonary state is returning: pulmonary artery blood pressure rises, and a shunt is reestablished from the right to the atrium through the foramen ovale. In the extreme, as in sudden asphyxia from aspiration of a feeding, a right-to-left shunt also appears across the ductus arteriosus.

The thermogenic response to cold stress is reduced or eliminated at Pa_{O_2} levels of 30 to 40 mm Hg. Thus *hypothermia* may develop while the baby is pink. Babies who are marginally hypoxic may become extremely restless. They cry continuously, and their aimless body movements are ceaseless.

The babies who are most often at risk without blood gas determinations are premature, dyspneic, but pink for several hours after birth, though their hyaline membrane disease is progressive. Alveoli collapse continually. They may receive unmeasured oxygen. They remain hypoxic, but there is no clinical indication of hypoxia. Pulmonary vasoconstriction progresses relentlessly. In this pink baby the meager supply of surfactant that was present at birth is dissipated quickly, and more alveoli collapse as time passes. At 8, 12, or perhaps 18 hours they are suddenly apneic, cyanotic, and hypotensive. Therapy should have been instituted while they were pink.

Brain damage due to hypoxia may be evident either while the baby is still in the nursery or not until several months later. There is no Pa_{O_2} level that can be regularly correlated with central nervous system damage. Acute and protracted episodes of hypoxia are known to injure brain tissue, but the duration of episodes, the extent to which arterial oxygen tension must decline, and the influence of other variables, such as acidosis and hypoglycemia, have not been defined precisely. There is agreement, however, that these factors produce signs of central nervous system dysfunction immediately after the hypoxic episode or chronically thereafter.

Reducing the $F_{I_{O_2}}$. In the presence of generalized cyanosis, it is advisable to abruptly increase the concentration of inspired oxygen. This is generally understood and widely practiced. However, it is not as generally appreciated that a reduced need for oxygen requires gradual diminution of ambient concentrations. Except for circumstances in which therapy is maintained for less than a few hours, an abrupt change to considerably lower concentrations is contraindicated. "Turning off the oxygen" after administering it in high dosage for some time is a dangerous practice. The longer the duration of therapy, the greater the hazard of abrupt discontinuation; sudden cyanosis and respiratory collapse may follow. This serious reaction is a result of sudden pulmonary vasoconstriction. Called "flip-flop," it is a retrogression that is sometimes more severe than the original dis-

order. It may persist for several hours or days, or it may be fulminant, leading to death. Usually a decrease of 5 or 10 percentage points every 3 to 4 hours is well tolerated, but variations should be expected. Infants who have received oxygen for over a week because of intrinsic lung disease may not adjust to such a regimen. They may require decrements as small as 3% to 5% every few hours, or even every 24 hours. On the other hand, infants with relatively normal lungs who have received oxygen for less than a few hours and have recovered from perinatal asphyxia may require—and will tolerate—a rapid decrease to avert hyperoxia.

Hyperoxia: oxygen toxicity. The detection of oxygen overdosage is as sensitive as the identification of oxygen deprivation. Here the concern is with the etiologic relationship between retrolental fibroplasia and high arterial oxygen tensions. The absolute upper limit of safety and the length of time oxygen therapy is tolerated have not been documented. At present the consensus is that an arterial P_{O_2} in excess of 100 mm Hg increases the likelihood of eye injury and is of no value in the treatment of hypoxemia. There are no clinical signs to indicate when this limit has been surpassed. *During oxygen therapy the infant's future vision is therefore dependent on a careful monitoring regimen that includes frequent measurement of $F_{I_{O_2}}$ and arterial oxygen tensions.* To date, the principal toxic effects of oxygen in the neonate have been noted in the eyes and in the lungs.

Retrolental fibroplasia (RLF, retinopathy of prematurity) is a disease of the eyes related to hyperoxemia in premature infants. After its first description in 1942, and in the decade that followed, an intensive worldwide search for its cause took place. Approximately three dozen etiologic possibilities were investigated. The ophthalmologic and pediatric literatures were inundated with hopeful hypotheses and all sorts of apparent documentations, but not until 1951 was valid evidence presented for the destructive effects of oxygen. It emanated from Australia, and confirmation from England and the United States soon followed. Thus in the short course of 10 years, a disease was unearthed, its cause was defined, and a regimen for its prevention was established. Retrolental fibroplasia occurs primarily in premature infants; the shorter the gestational age, the greater the vulnerability. In these infants, therapeutic hyperoxygenation causes changes in the retinal vasculature that may ultimately destroy the normal architecture of the eye and result in total blindness. There is no doubt that the disease is caused by inordinately high levels of oxygen in retinal capillaries of premature infants. It also has been documented in term infants who received oxygen therapy and in premature infants who did not, but these instances are exceptional. Realization of the role of oxygen overdosage was soon followed by rigid restriction of therapeutic oxygen to ambient concentrations below 40%, and as a result the disease virtually disappeared. However, in 1958 attention was called to an increased mortality rate in infants with hyaline membrane disease, and this increased rate was shown to be a function of the restrictive policies that came to govern oxygen administration. At just that time, the "do not disturb" attitude toward sick neonates had begun to yield to more aggressive approaches, and in this context the administration of oxygen was liberalized. It also became apparent that the relationship of arterial P_{O_2} to ambient oxygen concentrations was not fixed, but that it

was influenced by the infant's pulmonary function. A concentration of 40% was shown to be inadequate for many severely distressed babies. Today, mortality from hyaline membrane disease has indeed diminished, but at the cost of a resurgence of retrolental fibroplasia.

The disease begins during oxygen therapy. Oxygen does not diffuse through the cornea or sclera. RLF is therefore not directly related to a high F_{IO_2}, as in bronchopulmonary dysplasia (see later), but rather it is a function of high Pa_{O_2} levels. Retinal arterial constriction appears, and it persists during the therapeutic period as long as hyperoxemia is present. Within 1 or 2 months after treatment is terminated, the vessles dilate and proliferate; retinal edema then appears. At any time up to this stage, the process may come to a halt, with no resultant visual disturbance, or perhaps only a slight to moderate one. If extensive retinal detachment occurs, a scarring phase ensues within 1 or 2 months, and ultimately leads to blindness. This occurs in approximately 25% of infants with retinal vasospasm during early oxygen therapy. Thus, during the period of oxygen therapy, the only perceptible retinal change is vasoconstriction. Ideally, then, an ophthalmologist should examine the fundi periodically, and vigorous efforts should be exerted to reduce the dose of oxygen to a minimum if vasospasm is noted. Although the best practice is to maintain arterial P_{O_2} between 50 and 70 mm Hg, there is nevertheless no documented level of toxicity, nor are there data to indicate the length of time after which high levels become dangerous.

Bronchopulmonary dysplasia (BPD). When administered in high concentrations, oxygen is also injurious to the lungs. Lung damage is not related to blood oxygen tension but is a direct result of a high F_{IO_2}, and perhaps other factors as well. Histologic damage is characterized by thickening and eventual necrosis of alveolar walls, basement membranes, and bronchiolar epithelial lining layers. Atelectasis and fibrosis are also present. Presumably these changes impair diffusion of oxygen from alveolar lumens to capillaries. Respiratory dysfunction is thus prolonged, and the resultant abnormal radiologic appearance of the lungs may not resolve for several months.

Bronchopulmonary dysplasia (BPD) is a progressive chronic lung disease that follows protracted periods of mechanical ventilation with high concentrations of oxygen by means of an endotracheal tube. The clinical, pathologic, and radiologic features of the disease were first reported in 1967. In the vast majority of instances, hyaline membrane disease precedes the onset of BPD, but other acute pulmonary disorders may play similar roles. Whether preceded by hyaline membrane disease or some other pulmonary disorder, BPD is virtually always associated with the administration of high concentrations of oxygen by mechanical ventilation through an endotracheal tube; the relative etiologic significance of each of these factors has yet to be defined satisfactorily.

RADIOLOGIC CHARACTERISTICS. The radiologic abnormalities of BPD are well delineated in several reports. *Moderate BPD is sometimes characterized by dif-*

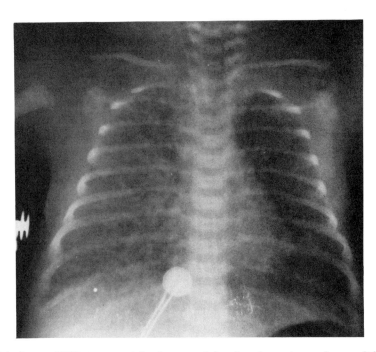

Fig. 8-7. Moderate BPD: interstitial edema and focal atelectasis produce a diffuse density in both lungs. A few small, round radiolucencies represent early regional emphysema.

fuse, virtually homogeneous opacification of the lungs, which obscures cardiac margins. This pattern is not always the first indication of moderate BPD. Frequently, the first indication is replacement of the early x-ray changes seen in mild disease by coarse, irregularly shaped densities that are often confluent and that occasionally contain very small vacuolar radiolucencies (Fig. 8-7). The areas of density are apparently cast by interstitial and septal edema and by atelectasis due to obstruction of small bronchioles by luminal debris. The small vacuolar radiolucencies represent early foci of emphysema.

In the *severe* form of BPD, the lucent vacuoles have expanded and are now identifiable as air cysts among dense patches, which themselves have become smaller than previously described. The cysts are evidence of progressive multifocal emphysema. The dense patches, compressed by expanding air cysts, are largely indicative of collapsed alveoli, edema and fibrosis of the interstitium, and distention of lymphatics.

In *advanced* BPD the lungs appear bubbly on x-ray films, as air cysts continue to enlarge. Opacities are further reduced in size to strands, streaks, and small patches. Overall, the lungs are extensively hyperinflated; emphysema has progressed considerably (Fig. 8-8). The presence of cardiomegaly usually portends right heart failure.

CLINICAL COURSE. The incidence of BPD varies from about 20% to 30% among infants with hyaline membrane disease who require ventilation with oxygen. In a report of a 12-year experience, advanced BPD was identified in 21% of 299 infants who required at least 24 hours of ventilation with oxygen. The incidence of moderate and advanced BPD

has decreased by 50% since the application of distending pressure during ventilatory assistance. End-expiratory pressure usually lowers F_{IO_2} requirements.

About 30% of affected infants are dead by 7 to 8 months of age. In a recent reported experience, a mortality of 38.7% (24 of 62 babies) was noted at all ages. Nineteen of these babies died during their original hospitalization between 1 and 7 months of age. The remaining five died of cardiopulmonary failure after discharge from the initial hospitalization, between 3 months and 3½ years of age.

The onset of BPD may be marked by an increase in oxygen and ventilatory pressure requirements shortly after recovery from hyaline membrane disease has begun, or it may become apparent when there is continued need for such support at a time (between 5 and 10 days

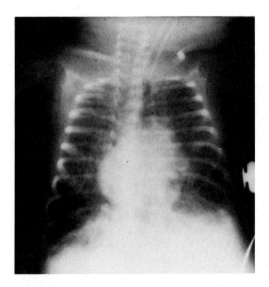

Fig. 8-8. Radiologic appearance of bronchopulmonary dysplasia in advanced stage. White strands are seen throughout both lung fields, representing fibrosis. Lungs are overexpanded in the extreme; diaphragms are at a very low level, and intercostal spaces bulge.

of age) when signs of recovery should have developed. Retractions and diminished breath sounds persist, and crepitant rales become audible. This early phase of the clinical course is associated with an x-ray appearance of moderate disease. During the ensuing days or weeks, oxygen concentrations and ventilatory pressures must be increased to maintain satisfactory arterial blood gas levels. As emphysema progresses, barrel-chest becomes obvious; on the x-ray films, the diaphragms are severely flattened and the lungs are increasingly overexpanded (severe and advanced disease). Oxygenation is more difficult and CO_2 retention increases. Respiratory acidosis results; renal conservation of bicarbonate eventually compensates partially for the imbalance. Right heart failure occurs as pathologic changes in pulmonary vasculature progress. In a reported autopsy series, right heart failure was considered the immediate cause of death in 30% of the infants studied. Even in the absence of cardiac failure, right ventricular hypertrophy is almost universal.

In those infants who recover, decrements of inspired oxygen are feasible only at a very slow rate; room air is eventually tolerated after a course of weeks or months. Survival beyond 7 or 8 months of age is associated with normal cardiopulmonary function by 5 to 6 years of age. During this period, recurrent episodes of pulmonary infections and wheezing are characteristic of the disease; some infants experience repeated bouts of acute pulmonary edema as well.

Most of the reported experience concerning the incidence and mortality of BPD is in babies who received oxygen and ventilatory assistance during the years preceding widespread use of continuous distending pressure. Recent observations are more encouraging in that the frequency of BPD seems to have declined by more than half since that time.

ETIOLOGIC CONSIDERATIONS. In the original description of BPD, high concentrations of inspired oxygen was considered the most likely cause. Affected infants had been given concentrations of 80% or greater for at least 6 days. Although high F_{IO_2} was considered the primary cause, it was nevertheless speculated that intermittent positive pressure ventilation and endotracheal intubation may have also played a role. Now, more than a decade after the appearance of that original description, the speculations are unchanged. The individual roles of oxygen, intermittent positive pressure ventilation, and endotracheal intubation have yet to be defined precisely in spite of a bountiful literature on the subject. Although the contemporary consensus is that all three of these factors are of etiologic significance, there are proponents for the predominant importance of trauma from mechanical ventilation, and for the overwhelming significance of oxygen toxicity. In each instance supporting data is noteworthy.

In the years that have passed since BPD was first described, there has been an interesting downward spiral in the oxygen concentration and the duration of therapy that has been considered toxic. As early as 1969, BPD was reported in babies who had received rather low oxygen concentrations for less than 24 hours. In 1975, the appearance of BPD at oxygen concentrations over 40% for over 72 hours was reported. Later on, in the analysis of data from a 12-year experience with BPD, another report concluded that the duration of therapy with over 40% oxygen was the best predictor of BPD but nevertheless, the concentration of inspired oxygen mattered little because if given over a sufficiently long time, BPD will follow. BPD was diagnosed in babies who were exposed to oxygen concentrations as low as 22% to 30%, but for as long as 53 days.

The importance of peak inspiratory pressure during mechanical ventilation has been emphasized. Apparently there is a statistically significant correlation between pressures over 35 cm H_2O and appearance of severe BPD.

It is thus not surprising that there are no magic numbers. The clinician can only guess the risk for BPD based on a varied reported experience. At best such estimates are as artful as they are scientific. The importance of lung trauma from high pressures during mechanical ventilation and the significance of oxygen concentrations are difficult to separate. The implication of endotracheal intubation is generally agreed on, but the mechanism of involvement is conjectural. Yet another factor to consider is the vulnerability of lungs with hyaline membrane disease to all three of these therapeutic insults. The most seriously ill infants receive high concentrations of oxygen with necessarily high peak pressure by means of an endotracheal tube. If mechanical ventilation must be used, the incidence of BPD will probably be minimized by using the lowest possible F_{IO_2} and airway pressures associated with prolonged inspiratory times and slow rates.

In summary, oxygen therapy may be life-saving but blinding and damaging to lungs. Assiduous monitoring is required to ascertain the presence of effective arterial tensions and the absence of toxic ones. Oxygen must be administered in the smallest possible dose for the shortest possible time.

Methods of oxygen administration. The route of oxygen administration is determined by the infant's needs. If he breathes spontaneously and diminished lung volume (atelectasis) is not a prominent problem, oxygen may simply be given in a head hood. If atelectasis is a major problem, as in hyaline membrane disease, but the baby can breathe spontaneously nevertheless, oxygen is given through a system that maintains some degree of positive pressure throughout the respiratory cycle. CPAP is an example of such a system. If the baby is unable to maintain respiration on his own, if apnea recurs frequently, or if adequate ventilation is not possible while the infant is breathing independently, oxygen must be administed by means of a mechanical ventilator.

Incubator and head hood. Concentrations of oxygen in an incubator cannot generally be raised beyond 60% to 70%. An imperfectly fitting plastic lid may allow significant escape of oxygen to further limit ambient concentrations. Opening portholes to gain access to the baby also depletes ambient oxygen concentration rapidly.

If environmental oxygen concentration must be raised, a plastic head hood should be used. When a hood is used in an incubator, the portholes may be opened without affecting oxygen concentration in the hood. The head box is obviously essential when infants are treated on an open table supplied with radiant heat from an overhead source. Oxygen delivered to a hood must usually be warmed to 87.8° to 93.2° F (31° to 34° C) and must always be humidified. A constant blast of cold gas to the infant's face produces the responses to cold stress, even though the remainder of the body is in a thermoneutral environment, since thermal sensors of the face are more responsive than the skin sensors in any other part of the body.

Continuous positive airway pressure (CPAP). The application of CPAP has considerably diminished the morbidity and mortality of hyaline membrane disease.

Normally, intrathoracic pressure at end-expiration is equal to atmospheric pressure. When alveolar stability is established, the lung remains expanded at end-expiration. In hyaline membrane disease, alveolar collapse is the rule

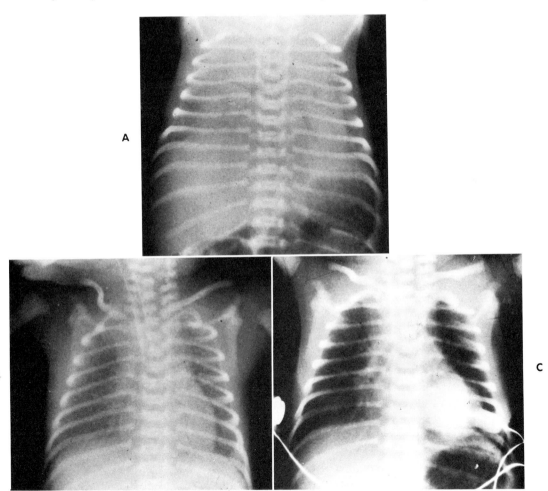

Fig. 8-9. Effect of CPAP on radiologic appearance of lungs. **A,** Before CPAP. Infant had severe hyaline membrane disease. Lungs are dense, with air bronchograms visible. Right cardiac border is obscured. **B,** Twenty minutes after CPAP application. Lungs are not as dense, more air is retained, and the right cardiac border is clearly visible. With better aeration, air bronchograms are not discernible. **C,** One hour after CPAP was applied. Lungs appear normally aerated. Note bulging intercostal spaces indicating some overdistention resulting from CPAP. Cleared x-ray film on CPAP does not indicate disappearance of disease.

(Figs. 8-3 and 8-4). CPAP provides varying degrees of alveolar stability (functional residual capacity) by maintaining positive pressure at end-expiration, thus keeping alveoli expanded when they would otherwise collapse; CPAP forces the alveoli to retain air. The results are often dramatic (Fig. 8-9). Increased ventilatory capacity is provided by virtue of the newly expanded alveoli. Respirations, if disorganized beforehand, become regular within several minutes thereafter. They increase in rate and depth, and the result is a rapid elevation of Pa_{O_2}. Often there is also diminution of Pa_{CO_2}, but at a slower rate. Recurrent apnea usually disappears. Normal levels of Pa_{O_2} are attainable at a lower $F_{I_{O_2}}$. Results are not as beneficial if hypoperfusion of the lung remains severe in spite of increased alveolar stability. Ventilating alveoli cannot be functional without adequate blood supply to take up oxygen and to deliver carbon dioxide for elimination. A number of studies have demonstrated that use of CPAP for hyaline membrane disease increases survival.

CPAP is effective for any disorder that requires therapeutic maintenance of alveolar stability, including hyaline membrane disease, pulmonary edema from any cause, pulmonary hemorrhage, and postoperative thoracotomy. CPAP, as well as any other form of positive end-expiratory pressure, is dangerous if lung compliance is normal. Normally compliant lungs permit transmission of positive pressure to blood vessels in the lung itself and to the large veins that empty into the heart (inferior and superior venae cavae). In these circumstances the transmitted pressure diminishes pulmonary blood supply and impairs venous return to the heart. In the extreme, the heart is smaller on x-ray films. Cardiac output diminishes, and with less blood in the systemic circulation, there is a measurable fall in systemic blood pressure. On the other hand, when lung compliance is poor ("stiff lungs"), as in hyaline membrane disease or pulmonary edema, positive end-expiratory pressure is contained within the airway; it is not significantly transmissible to other intrathoracic structures.

Continuous positive airway pressure is also referred to as *continuous distending pressure (CDP)*. It has been applied by means of a number of devices, all of which provide positive pressure at end-expiration and thus increased lung volume. CPAP was first administered through an endotracheal tube. Several variations have since been introduced; all of them apply positive pressure directly into the respiratory tract. Nasal CPAP is widely utilized instead of the endotracheal tube. By applying a tightly fitted adapter to the external nares, and thus avoiding the necessity of tracheal intubation, nasal CPAP exploits the fact that the neonate is an obligate nose breather. Pressures and oxygen mixtures are administered in the same manner as by the endotracheal route. A positive-pressure hood and also a face mask for transmission of pressure through the nose have been used to avoid the endotracheal tube.

Positive end-expiratory pressure can also be achieved by maintaining continuous negative pressure (CNP) to the thorax. The devices that mediate this approach are designed to envelop the chest or the entire body below the neck. Sustained negative pressure expands the thorax and prevents its usual collapse at end-expiration. The net effect of this system is to maintain a continuous "pull" on the alveoli, preventing their collapse at end-expiration. This is in contrast to the methods that apply positive pressure directly into the respiratory tract and thus maintain alveolar distention by a constant "push." Continuous negative pressure eliminates the need for an endotracheal tube. The infant's head must be in an oxygen hood at an atmospheric pressure that is constantly higher than intrathoracic pressure. F_{IO_2} is regulated in the hood.

All methods of applying distending pressure have their undesirable side effects. They all produce pneumothorax, but with considerably less frequency than mechanical ventilation. There is some evidence that the incidence of pneumothorax due to CNP for hyaline membrane disease is no higher than that caused by the disease itself. The incidence of pneumothorax with endotracheal CPAP is 5% to 10%; with nasal CPAP it is somewhat lower.

Other noteworthy side effects are of an operational nature. The critical factors in the development of complications from endotracheal tubes include trauma during intubation, impaired mucus transport by ciliary action, duration of intubation, size of the tube, trauma from friction while the tube is in place and while the baby moves or is manipulated frequently, introduction of infection, and occurrence of lobar atelectasis after extubation. The endotracheal tube is obviously irritating to the trachea. It virtually eliminates ciliary activity, and secretions accumulate. It is also a source of respiratory tract infection. It frequently becomes displaced downward into the right main bronchus, causing atelectasis of the left lung (Fig. 8-10). Tube position must be monitored assiduously. The danger of laryngeal (subglottic) stenosis is small but real. There seems to be little doubt that the devel-

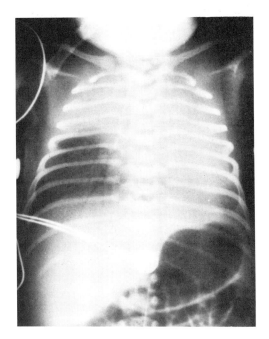

Fig. 8-10. Displacement of endotracheal tube into right main bronchus causes collapse of left lung. In this case, bronchus to right upper lobe is also occluded, causing atelectasis there. Note position of tube deep into right main bronchus.

opment of subglottic stenosis is primarily related to an inappropriately large tube. We use the smallest available tubes (2.5 mm) in babies who weigh below 1250 to 1500 grams and 3 mm tubes for babies between 1500 and 2500 grams. If on insertion, the operator believes that the fit is too tight, the tube is withdrawn and replacement is made with one of smaller diameter.

Atelectasis after extubation is not an uncommon event. Careful and thorough suction just before withdrawal of the tube has been shown to considerably diminish the incidence of lobar collapse. Nasal CPAP has caused infections of the nose an disfigurement of the external nares, but these complications are rare. CNP also has disadvantages. Use of a positive pressure hood with a tight-fitting neck seal has caused transient unilateral Erb's palsy. The CNP body chamber does not permit free access to the infant without interrupting therapy, and the tight fit required around the infant's neck causes abrasion and troublesome cellulitis.

We have been impressed with the discomfort that nasal CPAP causes in a number of infants. The struggle that ensues may predispose them to pneumothorax. Prescribed pressures are sometimes difficult to stabilize. Sedation using chloral hydrate (50 mg/kg of body weight) is usually successful. Nasal CPAP is not usually effective if pressures higher than 10 cm H_2O are required. The infant's open mouth is a natural blowoff valve at this pressure.

At the onset of therapy with CPAP, nasal or endotracheal, we administer the same F_{IO_2} that failed to oxygenate the baby in a head hood (usually 0.60 to 1.00), with a distending pressure of 3 to 4 cm H_2O. In the extreme, pressures are increased to 10 cm H_2O (using tracheal intubation) in an F_{IO_2} of 1.00. When the Pa_{O_2} is 70 or 80 mm Hg, the pressure is lowered to 10 cm H_2O in decrements of 1.0 cm every hour. F_{IO_2} is then diminished by 10 percentage points periodically, depending on the height of the Pa_{O_2}. At an F_{IO_2} of 0.40, pressure is then gradually decreased. There can be no rigid procedures to raise or lower oxygen or pressure. Decisions must be based on arterial blood gas results.

What are the criteria for the initiation of CPAP? They vary from one center to another, virtually all of them using a designated Pa_{O_2} at a given F_{IO_2}. Generally, if the Pa_{O_2} is below 50 mm Hg in an F_{IO_2} of 0.70 or 0.60, CPAP is considered necessary. Recurrent apnea is another indication, regardless of the oxygen tension achieved at a prescribed F_{IO_2}. Apnea often disappears or is considerably diminished after the onset of CPAP therapy.

The nursing skill and close observation required for CPAP are no less demanding than for mechanical ventilation. The nursery that cannot maintain mechanical ventilation, cannot administer CPAP either.

Mechanically assisted ventilation; the use of respirators. In general, the infants who require prolonged ventilatory assistance are severely depressed after perinatal asphyxia. It is indicated in babies with hyaline membrane disease who do not have sufficient vigor to breathe independently or who are repeatedly apneic for prolonged periods and do not respond to CPAP or CNP. These babies generally accumulate CO_2, with resultant severe respiratory acidosis. Administration of sodium bicarbonate is contraindicated in severe respiratory acidosis in which P_{CO_2} exceeds 60 mm Hg. Bicarbonate generates CO_2, which such babies cannot blow off. The result of sodium bicarbonate therapy is a heightened CO_2 and a worsened respiratory acidosis. Mechanical ventilation is the only effective treatment for hypercarbia. Infants whose P_{CO_2} is over 70 mm Hg are in need of mechanical ventilation.

Respirator therapy is a formidable undertaking that should not be attempted unless proper facilities, equipment, and trained personnel are on hand. The technical problems are numerous; they increase as the baby's size decreases, but they are not insurmountable. Scrupulous attention to detail is mandatory, and the major responsibility for these particulars belongs to the neonatal nurse. The endotracheal tube must be maintained in proper position. Once in place, it should not be allowed to slip into the trachea even for a distance of less than 1 cm, since it may then enter the right mainstem bronchus and occlude the left one in bypassing it (Fig. 8-10). The respirator must be observed repeatedly for proper settings. Respiratory difficulties in an infant with hyaline membrane disease are dynamic. Lung compliance may worsen rapidly or improve gradually, requiring adjustments in pressure or volume settings. Bronchial toilet and correct humidification of delivered oxygen must be maintained. Monitoring of blood gases and pH is essential at frequent intervals—so frequent in fact, that small, simple blood transfusions may be required periodically to replace the sampled blood.

Several types of apparatus are available. Positive-pressure respirators are used extensively. One type controls the volume of administered gas by limiting the inspiratory pressure created in the respiratory tract during its delivery; another type directly limits the volume of gas delivered and can be pressure restricted as well. It can provide a calculated volume of tidal air while ensuring that preset pressure limits are not exceeded.

Negative pressure respirators have been used successfully at some centers. However, they are apparently unsatisfactory for the most severely affected and the smallest infants. This type of respirator encloses the body from the neck down and moves gas in and out of the lungs by intermittently creating negative pressure around the trunk. Its great advantage is that it does not require endotracheal intubation. The oxygen content of inspired gas is determined by controlling its ambient concentration in the head chamber.

Bronchopulmonary dysplasia is rare in babies treated with a negative-pressure ventilator.

Acid-base balance; fluid therapy. Metabolic acidosis inevitably develops in infants who are moderately or severely ill from hyaline membrane disease. Insofar as pulmonary function is concerned, the most direct deleterious effect of acidosis is constriction of pulmonary arterioles. Lung perfusion is thus diminished, and the right-to-left shunt increases. Serial measurements of pH and P_{CO_2} provide a basis for infusion of intravenous sodium bicarbonate on the rare occasions when this is indicated. Base deficits less than 8 mEq/L do not generally require treatment. The dose of alkali is calculated and administered as described in Chapter 7.

Intravenous fluid is administered from the time of admission. It is given through the umbilical artery catheter if insertion was essential for blood gas monitoring. Umbilical artery catheters should not be used for the primary purpose of fluid administration except in the smallest babies. If the artery catheter has not been inserted, we use peripheral veins. The umbilical vein is used only in an emergency for short time intervals. Infection, thrombosis, cirrhosis and portal hypertension later in life are reported from protracted fluid therapy through the umbilical vein. Discussion of fluid and electrolyte therapy is presented in Chapter 7.

Provision of proper thermal environment. The deleterious effects of hypothermia are discussed in Chapter 4. Cold stress increases the need for oxygen in a baby who is already having difficulty with his intake. Furthermore, the increased metabolic rate that occurs in response to cold stress enhances metabolic acidosis in the presence of hypoxia by requiring overproduction of lactic acid. In aggravating hypoxia and enhancing acidosis, and by release of norepinephrine, cold stress causes increased pulmonary vasoconstriction, which probably also impairs the production and activity of surfactant. It is therefore crucial that proper temperature of incubator air and walls is maintained.

Maintenance of blood pressure and hematocrit. Systemic blood pressure is low in many infants with hyaline membrane disease. Because hypoxemia and acidemia have an early tendency to increase blood pressure, the hypotensive state is sometimes not detectable until they are corrected. Systemic hypotension increases right-to-left shunt through the ductus arteriosus, especially in the presence of inordinately high pulmonary artery pressure. Infants who are hypotensive cannot be oxygenated optimally. The diminished tissue perfusion and hypoxemia associated with shock cause oxygen deprivation of tissues. As a consequence, anaerobic glycolysis occurs, and lactic acid production casuses severe metabolic acidosis. Ventilatory support is thus ineffective in optimal oxygenation if shock exists. Blood samples persistently demonstrate a low Pa_{O_2} and a high base deficit. Sodium bicarbonate administration has little effect on the metabolic acidosis that accompanies shock.

Hypovolemia is often difficult to identify in the neonate. When blood pressure is low, the issue is straightforward. However, peripheral blood pressure does not decline until circulating blood volume is diminished by 25% to 40 % of normal. Thus, many infants are hypovolemic despite normal peripheral blood pressure readings. In these circumstances, hypovolemia may be suggested by a rapid heart rate (over 160 beats/min).

We monitor blood pressure in the brachial or posterior tibial arteries with a Doppler ultrasound apparatus. Normal blood pressure varies with birth weight. The lower limit of normal mean blood pressure in babies whose birth weight is between 1001 and 2000 grams is 30 mm Hg; between 2000 and 3000 grams, it is 35 mm Hg; and between 3000 and 4000 grams, 43 mm Hg. In low birth weight babies we have found that these differences are not sufficiently large to be significant clinically. We therefore attempt to maintain *systolic* blood pressure at approximately 50 mm Hg. In babies weighing over 2500 grams, 60 mm Hg is our lowest acceptable level.

Having identified hypovolemia by clear-cut blood pressure readings or surmised that it is present because of tachycardia even though blood pressure readings are normal, we immediately administer plasma as a volume expander. Packed red blood cells are ordered from the blood bank at the same time. Plasma is given rapidly in a dose of 10 ml/kg of body weight. Packed red blood cells are given in the same dose as soon as they are delivered to the nursery. If blood pressure remains low after the first dose of plasma, another dose is administered. Blood pressure is monitored at least every hour in the sickest babies.

Hematocrit must also be followed periodically. Most often, it is normal for the first 1 to 3 hours postnatally, even if hypovolemia is present. It falls, however, as the baby attempts to compensate for diminished blood volume by the transfer of tissue fluid into the vascular compartment; hemodilution ensues. We attempt to maintain the hematocrit at 45 to 50 vol%. It is determined at least twice daily during acute illness, and more often if indicated.

Blood sampling for laboratory data is

an important and frequent cause of lower hematocrit readings. A record of the amount withdrawn should be kept at the incubator. When 10% of calculated blood volume (85 ml/kg) is withdrawn, a transfusion of packed cells is given.

Umbilical vessel catheterization

Umbilical artery. The risks of umbilical arterial catheterization are well known and very real. In spite of them, most neonatologists do not hesitate to employ these catheters *if the benefits derived significantly outweigh the risks entailed.*

The placement of arterial catheters is a surgical procedure that requires strict aseptic technique. Proper maintenance of the catheter, once it is in place, depends on the skills and knowledge of the nurse.

The safest location for the cateter tip in the aorta is below the origins of the renal arteries. If the tip is between the third and fourth lumbar vertebrae by x-ray films, it is situated below the renal arteries and above the aortic bifurcation. The catheter should have an end hole, rather than side holes, since the dead space at the tip of the latter type of catheter promotes thrombus formation. Furthermore, the catheter should be radiopaque so that its position can be ascertained by x-ray examination immediately after placement. If it is located above the desired level, it can be withdrawn an appropriate distance. If the tip is too low, *the catheter should not be inserted farther after the sterile insertion procedure has been terminated.*

Maintenance requires careful, constant attention to avert infection, to prevent hemorrhage because of loose fittings or accidental withdrawal, and to identify thromboembolic phenomena.

Infection. The incidence of infection varies from one report to another. The clinical significance of positive cultures from withdrawn catheter tips is questionable; yet a number of available reports cite such data. There is sound basis for applying antibacterial ointment at least once daily to the umbilical stump and to joints in the tubing system. Tubing and stopcock attached to the catheter should be changed daily. After withdrawal of blood from the stopcock, the open portal should be plugged with a sterile insert of some type. We use a syringe. The injection of medication through the stopcock should be meticulous. Care must be exercised to avoid contamination of the syringe tip that is inserted into the stopcock. Inadvertent contact of the syringe tip with contaminated objects (including fingers) prior to its insertion is a common occurrence. The futility of prophylactic antibiotics for infants with umbilical vessel catheters has been well documented.

Hemorrhage. Massive hemorrhage from the umbilical catheter is a real danger if fittings are loosened. Hemorrhage may also occur from the umbilical stump when the catheter is accidentally displaced from its insertion. Aortic blood pressure is high, and considerable blood loss may therefore occur rapidly. This possibility obviously makes constant attention and surveillance by the nurse imperative. Massive hemorrhage into the pelvis has been reported after inadvertent perforation of an artery during the catheterization procedure. We have experienced one such instance.

Thrombosis. Thromboembolic phenomena are the most frequent complications. Varying percentages (as high as 95%) are reported for the incidence of thrombi. In the vast majority of cases they have had no apparent clinical significance; their danger is not negligible, however. Thrombi that encase the catheter or are implanted onto the aortic wall are a potential source of embolization. Emboli are dislodged from these thrombi and released to the lower body, distal to the catheter tip. If they are of substantial size, they obstruct blood flow distal to the vessel they occlude. Necrosis of toes is the most frequent embolic phenomenon. The toes may become progressively cyanotic and ultimately gangrenous. If cyanosis persists for more than 15 minutes, the catheter should be withdrawn. Necrotic ulceration of the skin in the gluteal and perineal regions has been reported in a few infants.

The position of the catheter tip is critical. If the catheter is too high, thrombi may occlude the superior mesenteric artery or, more commonly, the renal arteries, causing infarction of intestines and kidneys, respectively. Hypertension in the neonate has been repeatedly reported as a complication of umbilical artery catheters that may impair renal circulation. The high blood pressure persists for months or years and, if untreated, rapidly leads to cardiac failure. Approximately 80% of cases of neonatal hypertension have been associated with previous umbilical artery catheterization. Opinion differs as to whether thrombi are more likely to occur as the duration of catheterization increases. Thrombosis is more likely in profoundly ill babies.

Vasospasm. The most common manifestation of interrupted blood flow is blanching, which may involve part of a toe, or both lower extremities in their entirety. It is attributed to arterial spasm, and it disappears promptly when the catheter is removed. There is no justification for the past practice of applying moist heat to the uninvolved extremity to relieve spasm of the opposite member.

Infusions. Hypertonic solutions are probably tolerated, if they are infused at a slow rate, because the aorta is large and blood flow through it is rapid. The infused solution is therefore quickly diluted. Sodium bicarbonate should be diluted with equal parts of water or glucose solution and injected at a rate not exceeding 2 ml/min. Rapid injection of any material causes increased turbulence at the catheter tip and predisposes to thrombogenesis. Continuous infusion must be regulated by an automated pump. As a rule, we encounter backflow of aortic blood if the rate of infusion is less than 2 ml/hr.

Umbilical artery catherization is indicated primarily for sampling in monitoring blood gases and pH. It should never be instituted for the sole purpose of fluid administration.

Umbilical vein. We use umbilical vein catheters only for exchange transfusion or for emergency administration of drugs, fluid, or volume expanders when no other route is immediately available. It is also used to monitor central venous pressure. The incidence of complications from protracted periods of catheterization is unacceptably high. Infection is more common in the vein than in the artery. Hepatic necrosis and thrombosis of the portal vein have also been reported. Portal hypertension at a later age has been attributed to portal vein thrombosis from umbilical vein catheterization during the newborn period.

Prevention

Hyaline membrane disease is a developmental disorder that centers about the maturation of metabolic pathways to surfactant production. Until prematurity itself can be prevented, the most promising approach seems to lie in attempts to stimulate the elaboration of surfactant in utero. Thus far, trials of corticosteroids (betamethasone and dexamethasone) given to mothers between 24 hours and 7 days before delivery have yielded promising results. In this group of mothers, if offspring were less than 32 gestational weeks, the incidence of hyaline membrane disease was significantly reduced from that in controls. Mortality from the disease and the incidence of intraventricular hemorrhage were also reduced in babies of the same gestational age. However, even in the group that benefited from betamethasone, hyaline membrane disease occurred in 21%. In addition, betamethasone was ineffective for infants whose gestational age was 32 weeks or more. The betamethasone trial is not in itself a completely successful therapeutic effort, but the results are an encouraging indication that fetal medication is a promising approach to the problem.

Hydrocortisone has been administered postnatally to infants with hyaline membrane disease in a well-controlled trial. A beneficial effect was not demonstrated.

Outcomes

A few years ago we were frustrated spectators who could only observe hyaline membrane disease as it progressed along a predetermined, irrevocable course. Supportive therapy was meager. Those infants who survived had only minimal or moderate involvement. Many of them were afflicted with permanent brain damage and blindness. The most severely affected could only be offered very limited aid. They tired, with deepening cyanosis, from the struggle to expand their noncompliant ischemic lungs. Today our therapeutic regimens are still no more than supportive, but they are effective because they are directed against specific pathophysiologic mechanisms. It is the advent of newborn intensive care units and their concepts of neonatal care that must be credited with the encouraging results that have been recorded.

Neonatal survival. Compilation of the recent results from a number of centers indicates impressive improvement in the survival rate. The disease is, of course, still a serious, life-threatening process, but among infants who did not require mechanical support and who were given only constant distending pressure (CPAP), 93% survived. Of those who received only mechanical support, 47% survived. Among infants who were unsuccessfully treated with distending pressure and required subsequent mechanical support, 49% survived. A few years ago, survival for all infants with the disease, regardless of type of treatment, with or without assisted respiration was 61%. More recently, an overall mortality of only 11% was reported for 153 infants who were treated with various modalities of support.

Increased survival of mechanically ventilated babies has been well documented as more effective manipulation of ventilators has evolved. In Britain, for instance, survival of mechanically ventilated infants increased from 11% to 49% in recent years, and this figure represents the most severely affected group of infants. Intraventricular hemorrhage persists as a major problem. It is the most important cause of death among ventilated infants.

Postneonatal outcomes. Long-term developmental assessment is complicated by the possible role of intrauterine misadventure. Results vary from one institution to another, but overall, the majority of infants are developmentally normal. There are specific data to indicate that impaired development is not related to mechanical ventilation, but rather to gestational age, in the infants who were studied. The high degree of variability among neurologic follow-up studies is a result of numerous uncontrollable factors. It is virtually impossible to compare the results from one center with those of another. Differing populations in respect to gestational age are an important consideration for comparison. Probably of even greater importance is the place of birth of the study infants. Outcomes among referred babies (outborn) are far more likely to be abnormal than among inborn infants. Furthermore, at the same birth weight and gestational age, black infants regularly have a higher survival rate than white babies. Follow-up studies have rarely dealt with these racial differences in terms of neurologic sequelae. The age of follow-up also varies among reports, as well as the date of intensive care. Infants who have been treated more recently have survived intact in greater numbers. Results of treatment in 1977-1979 are superior to those of 1970-1974, for example.

The incidence of neurologic defects in reports of ventilated babies has varied from 11% to 29%. These studies have involved babies whose birth weights were below 1500 grams to those with mean birth weights as high as 2319 grams. Mortality of ventilated babies also differed widely—from 51% in 1974-1975 to 79% in 1966-1973. The neurologic defects are primarily hydrocephalus or cerebral palsy, presumably as a result of intracranial hemorrhage. Deficits in intellectual function usually accompany these neurologic lesions.

Pulmonary sequelae can be divided mainly into lower respiratory tract infections and bronchopulmonary dysplasia

(p. 220). Readmission to the hospital for lung infection increases in frequency when birth weight and gestational age are low. Whether or not hyaline membrane disease predisposes to even higher frequencies of infection cannot be determined from existing studies. Furthermore, in the absence of bronchopulmonary dysplasia, pulmonary infection after discharge from the nursery does not seem to occur more frequently in babies who were mechanically ventilated.

Sequelae of trauma from the ventilatory process are considerably less frequent than lung infections and bronchopulmonary dysplasia. When nasotracheal intubation is used, ulceration of the nares heals with scar formation and stenosis of the involved nostril or nasal vestibule. Midline clefts of the hard palate have been noted among infants who had orotracheal tubes for a protracted period. The mechanism of cleft formation has not been delineated with certainty, but it is doubtful that the cleft is simply the result of pressure exerted by the endotracheal tube. These tubes are constantly moving about, yet in all the affected infants, the clefts have been located precisely in the midline, suggesting that a disorder of palatine growth has resulted from prolonged intubation.

Damage to vocal cords causes hoarseness and stridor that often disappear or improve but are not uncommonly persistent. Subglottic stenosis occurs rather rarely. It requires tracheostomy because it occludes the airway at the level of the larynx.

PATENCY OF THE DUCTUS ARTERIOSUS (PDA)

In premature infants, persistent patency of the ductus arteriosus gives rise to hyperperfusion and edema of the lungs when a significant left-to-right shunt has developed. The ductus remains patent in 50% to 85% of preterm infants under 1200 grams of birthweight; the incidence diminishes as birth weight increases. This discussion is concerned with the syndrome of ductal left-to-right shunting in premature infants, which commonly gives rise to life-threatening pulmonary insufficiency and occasionally to congestive heart failure. It most often appears at 5 to 10 days of age, when ventilatory support for hyaline membrane disease is in the process of gradual withdrawal because of improved lung function. As recovery from hyaline membrane disease progresses, pulmonary vascular pressure decreases hour by hour, until it falls below aortic pressure. The new gradient thus established, blood now flows from aorta to pulmonary artery through the patent ductus arteriosus. The quantity of blood shunted may be as high as 40% of left ventricular output. The result of this redistribution of blood flow is hyperperfusion of lungs with capillary engorgement followed by pulmonary edema. Furthermore, the large amount of aortic blood that is shunted to the pulmonary circuit leads to a correspondingly diminished perfusion of those organs supplied by postductal blood from the aorta. Hypoperfusion of the intestinal tract is thought to be responsible for a higher incidence of necrotizing enterocolitis in babies with significant left-to-right shunts.

It is our experience that an elevation of Pa_{CO_2} is the most frequent early sign of significant ductal shunting in premature infants under treatment for hyaline membrane disease. Recurrent apnea (if the infant is not on a ventilator) and need for an increased $F_{I_{O_2}}$ are also frequent manifestations. These findings are impressive because they appear abruptly when recovery from hyaline membrane disease seems imminent—when $F_{I_{O_2}}$ requirements and ventilator pressures have been confidently decreased to their lowest levels.

The elevation of Pa_{CO_2} usually occurs as end-expiratory pressure (CPAP or PEEP) is lowered. With less end-expiratory pressure in alveoli to oppose it, transudation of fluid occurs from engorged capillaries; pulmonary edema appears. Decreased compliance of the edematous lung develops and exhalation of CO_2 is therefore impaired. This is very soon reflected as an elevated Pa_{CO_2}. With very few exceptions, the Pa_{CO_2} can be lowered by increasing CPAP or PEEP back to its immediately preceding level. This raises alveolar pressure, and fluid transudation is halted. Much of the interstitial fluid probably re-enters the capillaries. Eventually, $F_{I_{O_2}}$ can be lowered again. In some instances, one is confronted with a bizarre situation in which CPAP or PEEP remain indispensable for the control of pulmonary edema, but only room air is needed for normal oxygenation.

In addition to the changes in blood gases and the typical response to elevations of end-expiratory pressure, significant ductal shunts are suggested by several physical signs. The murmur that is so often described as characteristic of patent ductus arteriosus is not particularly significant because the presence and intensity of that murmur are poorly correlated to the seriousness of the left-to-right shunt. On the other hand, a heaving precordial impulse (hyperactive precordium) is a certain indication of an overactive, overloaded left ventricle that must supply blood to a significant ductal shunt. Bounding pulses are also a most reliable indication. If pulmonary edema is advanced, and fluid from capillaries has entered the alveoli from interstitial tissue,

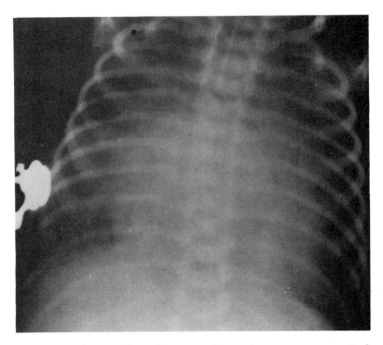

Fig. 8-11. Pulmonary edema and moderate cardiac enlargement are typical radiologic signs of patent ductuc arteriosus associated with a significant left-to-right shunt.

crepitant rales are audible and are particularly profuse over the baby's back.

The chest film often reveals slight or moderate enlargement of the heart and irregular, fluffy lung densities that characterize pulmonary edema (Fig. 8-11). The lung densities diminish considerably when CPAP or PEEP are increased to minimize the pulmonary edema.

The echocardiogram is considered the most reliable diagnostic modality. It demonstrates left atrial enlargement, which occurs because large quantities of blood return to the left atrium from hyperperfused lungs. On the echocardiogram, measurements are made of the diameters of the left atrium and the aortic root. This is called the LA/AO ratio. If it exceeds 1.0 to 1.2, a significant ductal shunt is considered to be present.

Ventilatory support is the most effective immediate treatment. Adjustment of end-expiratory pressure to minimize pulmonary edema and augmentation of F_{IO_2} both exert a rapid salutary effect. Elimination of lung fluid is even better effected by administering, in addition, a diuretic such as furosamide at 1 to 2 mg/kg in a single intravascular dose. Some centers give digitalis; most are not impressed with its effectiveness. We have used it extensively and were unimpressed with its effect. Because fluid overload is thought to precipitate large left-to-right shunts, it is advisable to restrict fluids to the smallest volume that can be tolerated.

The place of surgical ligation in the treatment of affected infants is controversial and varies among centers. If medical therapy, as described above, fails after 48 hours, some units resort to ligation. Others observe for longer periods before resorting to surgery.

The recent use of indomethacin has added a significant therapeutic approach. Indomethacin is a prostaglandin synthetase inhibitor (p. 204). Reports on the extent of its effectiveness have varied somewhat, but there is general agreement that it is effective in most babies if given before 14 to 16 days of postnatal age. The ductus generally closes permanently within 24 hours of the last dose of indomethacin. The drug is given as 0.2 mg/kg per dose for 3 doses at 12-hour intervals. Oral administration has been used, but an intravenous preparation is now available. Contraindications to the use of indomethacin include bleeding diathesis (low platelets, coagulopathy), renal dysfunction (serum creatinine > 1.2 mg/100 ml, BUN > 25 mg/100 ml), suspicion of necrotizing enterocolitis, and gastrointestinal bleeding from any cause. Urine output diminishes significantly in most infants who are given indomethacin. In some babies who were given indomethacin, the ductus reopens within days of closure. Another 3-dose course of treatment is indicated.

PERSISTENT PULMONARY HYPERTENSION (PERSISTENT PULMONARY VASOSPASM; PERSISTENT FETAL CIRCULATION)

Persistent pulmonary hypertension in the immediate postnatal period is due to pulmonary arteriolar constriction. This phenomenon is identifiable as a component of a number of clinical entities; it is also a clinical entity in its own right. Pulmonary vasoconstriction causes pulmonary artery pressure to rise above aortic pressure; a right-to-left shunt across the patent ductus arteriosus results. In addition, pressure in the right atrium may be higher than pressure in the left atrium; right-to-left shunting thus occurs at the atrial level as well. Furthermore, vasoconstriction results in pulmonary hypoperfusion, and the total quantity of oxygenated blood leaving the lungs (destined for the left atrium) is regularly diminished. These pulmonary vascular phenomena are components of a variety of clinical entities: hyaline membrane disease, RDS II, pneumonia (especially group B streptococcal), aspiration of milk, diaphragmatic hernia, and cold stress. Vasoconstriction often follows injudicious decrements in F_{IO_2} in babies receiving oxygen therapy. This is called "flip-flop," and it may be so severe as to be irreversible, even if treated with an F_{IO_2} of 1.0 on a mechanical ventilator.

Pulmonary vasospasm causes hypoxemia and cyanosis. Depending on the tenaciousness and extent of vasoconstriction, amelioration may be possible with simple hood oxygen, or this failing, with mechanical ventilation. Treatment with tolazoline or with hyperventilation to produce respiratory alkalosis may be urgently required in the most severe cases. Any of these approaches is appropriate when hypoxemia is attributable to pulmonary vasospasm, whether it exists by itself or is a component of one of the clinical entities listed above.

Pulmonary vasospasm in the immediate postnatal period is a response to intrauterine or extrauterine asphyxia. When pulmonary vasospasm is identified in the absence of other disorders, and particularly in the absence of parenchymal lung disease, the diagnosis of *persistent pulmonary hypertension* is justifiable. The disorder occurs in infants who are at or near term. In the vast majority of them, there is a history of perinatal asphyxia.

Apgar scores are usually 5 or below at 1 or 5 minutes. The onset of clearly abnormal respiration may be delayed for as long as 12 hours, but in most instances this is discernible within an hour after birth. Tachypnea is the rule; retractions are usually minimal or moderate. Cyanosis occurs soon after delivery. Auscultation of the lungs indicates good air exchange and there are no blatant signs of cardiac abnormality. Systemic blood pressure is normal. Response to oxygen enrichment may be satisfactory at first, but soon hypoxemia eventuates even in pure oxygen.

The chest film is most often normal. Occasionally, slight cardiomegaly is observed, and not uncommonly, dense streaks emanate from the hilar regions to the peripheral lung fields. Occasionally the lungs are overexpanded.

Arterial oxygen tensions are low. With rare exception, the postductal Pa_{O_2} is at least 15% lower than in the preductal sample. The Pa_{CO_2} is normal or low. Elevated Pa_{CO_2} is a rarity because in this disorder there is no significant parenchymal lung involvement.

Low concentrations of serum calcium and glucose have been described, as well as high hematocrit levels (polycythemia). These have been considered of etiologic significance by some authors. Correction of the calcium and glucose abnormalities is, however, unlikely to relieve pulmonary vasospasm. Correction of a high hematocrit level may occasionally be of some benefit. It is noteworthy that these aberrations have also been described as sequelae of fetal asphyxia in numerous publications; it is more plausible to regard them, and the pulmonary vasospasm itself, as neonatal consequences of fetal asphyxia.

If a response to an $F_{I_{O_2}}$ of 1.0 in a hood is inadequate, we do not hesitate to administer tolazoline; it has been lifesaving on numerous occasions. Emphasis must be placed on accurate selection of infants in whom pulmonary vasospasm is virtually the sole cause of severe hypoxemia. In our experience, at least 90% of infants so selected respond dramatically to fairly rapid infusion of 2 mg/kg of tolazoline. We add the drug to 10 ml/kg of plasma volume expander. We have also obtained good results with hyperventilation to a Pa_{CO_2} of 25 to 30 mm Hg, which usually raises arterial pH to approximately 7.5. We consider that tolazoline administration *in these specific infants* is less hazardous than endotracheal intubation and mechanical ventilation. In most cases, a single bolus injection suffices. In others we repeat the dose. In the few resistant infants, we administer tolazoline by continuous infusion. Tolazoline is also given for the disorders that involve lung parenchyma (meconium aspiration, pneumonia, hyaline membrane disease) in addition to pulmonary vasospasm, but with less success.

A note of caution is in order regarding the use of PEEP in babies whose lung parenchyma is not abnormal. In these circumstances, CPAP or PEEP usually worsens the hypoxemia. If mechanical ventilation is used for oxygenation, it should be used without PEEP.

SYNDROMES DUE TO ASPIRATION OR FLUID RETENTION

Among the multiple causes of neonatal respiratory distress, there is a spectrum of abnormalities presumably caused by aspiration of amniotic fluid and its contents into the respiratory tract or by retention of fetal lung fluid. The actual event of aspiration is believed to occur in utero or during delivery—undoubtedly a valid concept. However, in some infants the clinical signs of distress may be due to impaired evacuation of fetal lung fluid that would normally be absorbed into the pulmonary circulation during the first few breaths (p. 200). In either case, the end result is similar: the flow of air is obstructed in varying degrees by the presence of fluid, particulate matter, or both in the respiratory tract.

Most of the clinical signs that characterize these entities can be explained by two simple obstructive phenomena that may occur at any level of the respiratory tract. Fig. 8-12 illustrates both mechanisms: partial obstruction (check-valve, or ball-valve) and complete obstruction (stop-valve). The ball-valve mechanism permits entry of air past the obstruction during inspiration while obstructing its complete egress during expiration. This is possible because the calibers of bronchi and bronchioles become larger during inspiration and smaller during expiration. When bronchioles enlarge, air passes around the obstruction, but when they diminish in caliber during expiration, the lumen becomes completely occluded and air is trapped peripheral to the obstruction. By this mechanism progressive accumulation of trapped air may produce diffuse or regional overexpansion of the lungs (emphysema). On the other hand, a complete obstruction (stop-valve) does not permit entry of any air, and as a result, the portions of lung peripheral to it are collapsed. Both amniotic fluid, with its contents (principally vernix and meconium), and fetal lung fluid are capable of producing either or both of these obstructive phenomena. The spectrum of abnormalities is thus characterized at one end by diffuse emphysema of both lungs without collapse and at the other end by collapse of large areas of the lungs. The clinical entity in which emphysema predominates has been called transient tachypnea of the newborn, respiratory distress syndrome type II, or obstructive emphysema of the newborn. The clinical condition in which occlusion and collapse are more prominent is

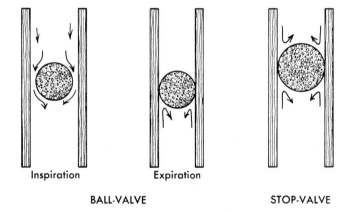

Inspiration   Expiration

BALL-VALVE   **STOP-VALVE**

Fig. 8-12. Mechanisms of airway obstruction. The ball-valve type allows entry of air peripheral to it but blocks air egress, resulting in emphysema. The stop-valve variety allows neither entry nor egress of air, resulting in atelectasis beyond the obstruction. (Modified from Caffey, J.: Pediatric x-ray diagnosis, ed. 5, Chicago, 1967, Year Book Medical Publishers, Inc.)

known as meconium aspiration, or the massive aspiration syndrome.

Respiratory distress syndrome, type II (RDS II; transient tachypnea of the newborn)

Affected infants are at or near term. Respiratory distress begins at birth or shortly thereafter and is characterized by tachypnea, retractions, flaring of the nostrils, and expiratory grunt. Usually there is little or no difficulty with the onset of breathing. Rales are not heard. Cyanosis in room air may be noted, but usually clears in relatively small increments of ambient oxygen concentration. Grunting and retractions may resolve within 24 to 48 hours, or they may persist for several days. As a rule, the duration of the clinical course is 2 to 4 days.

The roentgenogram is characterized by generalized overexpansion of the lungs, which is identifiable principally by a flattened contour of the diaphragm, in contrast to the distinctly domed configuration that is seen in normal infants. Dense streaks radiate from the hilar regions. Only occasionally are patches of density evident, representing areas of collapse and/or large fluid accumulations.

The blood pH is moderately depressed, arterial P_{CO_2} is somwhat elevated, and the base deficit is usually 10 mEq/L or less. Alkali therapy is seldom required, since these infants, depite respiratory dysfunction, seem to manage their alveolar gas exchange sufficiently well to maintain normal blood gas tensions. They rarely require assisted ventilation of any type.

The clinical appearance of these babies suggests hyaline membrane disease, but RDS II is a distinctly different abnormality with a far brighter prognosis. As a rule, affected babies recover, and there

has thus far been no evidence of chronic lung disease among those who were followed to 5 or 6 months of age.

The grunting that occurs in this syndrome requires comment because it apparently serves a purpose that differs from the expiratory grunt of hyaline membrane disease. Since transient tachypnea involves diffuse emphysema (air trapping), the expiratory grunt probably represents an attempt to eject as much of the trapped alveolar air as possible. In hyaline membrane disease the grunt attempts to retain as much air as possible in an effort to maintain alveolar expansion.

RDS II primarily involves retention of fetal lung fluid. Presumably, the infant's lungs are sufficiently mature to function postnatally, save for failure to evacuate this fluid. The syndrome is frequently called "wet lung," but this is an unfortunate designation because fluid is retained in any lung that fails to expand normally after the first few breaths. Thus, the immature lungs of an infant at 32 weeks of gestation are also "wet," as are those affected by hyaline membrane disease. RDS II should be designated in infants who are at or near term, whose respiratory distress is predominantly attributable to the presence of retained lung fluid. With clearance, clinical signs disappear.

Meconium aspiration (massive aspiration syndrome)

Meconium aspiration is a consequence of fetal asphyxia (Fig. 8-13). It rarely occurs in preterm infants. The asphyxial episode in utero apparently increases intestinal peristalsis and relaxes the anal sphincter to release meconium. It also stimulates fetal gasping. The amount of meconium aspirated in utero is quite variable. In most instances, the major por-

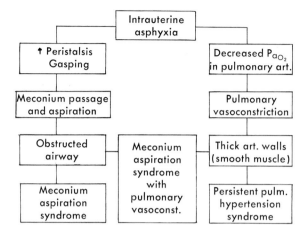

Fig. 8-13. See text.

tion is aspirated postnatally during the first few breaths. The airway is thus completely or partially obstructed at various levels, and alveolar ventilation is either severely decreased in the emphysematous areas or entirely eliminated in the atelectatic areas.

In addition to obstructive phenomena, the airway is also affected by an inflammatory response to meconium—chemical pneumonitis. In animals, inflammation has been demonstrated 48 hours after the instillation of meconium into the trachea. Thickened alveolar walls and interstitial tissue now pose a barrier to the passage of oxygen from alveoli to alveolar capillaries. Thus, the diffusion of oxygen is impaired, in addition to the aforementioned obstruction to its inflow.

Pulmonary vasospasm is another important component of the meconium aspiration syndrome. Vasoconstriction of arterioles occurs in response to intrauterine asphyxia and is sustained postnatally in a substantial number of infants. Persistence of pulmonary vasospasm redirects blood through fetal channels (see Fetal circulation, p. 4), thus maintaining a

right-to-left shunt. In such circumstances, mechanical ventilation fails to oxygenate the infant with meconium aspiration. In the extreme, uncorrectable hypoxemia results in death. Treatment with *tolazoline,* a powerful vasodilating drug, is often lifesaving. In our experience, it is most effective when there is less airway involvement; it is least successful when parenchymal involvement is extensive. Furthermore, because it dilates blood vessels throughout the body, a moderate, sometimes extreme, fall in blood pressure follows its intravascular administration. Tolazoline must be used with extreme caution in carefully selected babies. The most frequent indications for its use are (1) failure to oxygenate by mecahnical ventilation and (2) a significantly higher Pa_{O_2} from the right radial artery (preductal) than from the descending aorta (postductal). The second indication is evidence of pulmonary vasospasm if there is no systemic hypotension. Pulmonary artery pressure is higher than aortic pressure in the presence of pulmonary arteriolar vasoconstriction. Venous blood is shunted from the pulmonary artery across the ductus to the aorta where venous admixture occurs. The Pa$_{O_2}$ in the postductal blood sample, collected from the descending aorta, is thus lower than in the right radial artery where venous admixture is not as extensive. The reader is referred to the description earlier in this chapter of the fetal circulation and the changes that occur in it during the first breath and also to the discussion of persistent pulmonary hypertension on p. 237.

Meconium aspiration syndrome is thus a neonatal consequence of fetal asphyxia. Its postnatal manifestations are due to obstructed airways and often pulmonary vasospasm as well. Both of these factors are responses to a single antecedent event—fetal asphyxia.

Meconium is passed into amniotic fluid in approximately 10% of all pregnancies; it is a sign of fetal distress. Some fetuses aspirate particles of meconium, which, during the first few breaths, may be inspired more deeply toward the alveoli, if this has not already occurred in utero. In contrast to transient tachypnea, affected infants often have difficulty establishing respiration. In some, respiratory distress may be delayed. It has been

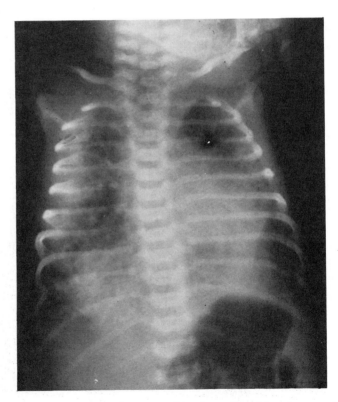

Fig. 8-14. Meconium aspiration is severe in this chest film. Broad areas of density represent atelectasis and interstitial fluid. Regional emphysema is seen in the remaining radiolucent areas. The overall effect of diffuse airway obstruction is overexpansion of the lungs, as indicated by the low position of the diaphragms.

shown in puppies that delayed symptoms are associated with gradual progress of small particles toward the more peripheral airways with each breath. Presumably the same process operates in human infants. At least this explanation for the delayed distress observed in these babies is plausible. The signs of respiratory distress are similar to those described for transient tachypnea, except that the rales are often present.

The radiologic appearance of the lungs is characterized by multiple patches of density, interspersed areas of emphysema, and thick streaks that emanate from the hilar regions (Fig. 8-14). The patchy densities represent relatively large areas of atelectasis that are produced by complete obstruction (stop-valve). They are considerably more prominent and extensive than in transient tachypnea. In most instances, overdistention of the lung is predominant, even in the presence of widespread atelectasis. The x-ray film thus also shows flattened diaphragms and bulging intercostal spaces.

Respiratory abnormalities usually subside in a few days although they may persist longer. Death has been reported in 28% of affected infants. Pneumomediastinum and pneumothorax may complicate the course (see later).

Blood gas and pH determinations indicate varying degrees of mixed respiratory and metabolic acidosis.

We have managed a substantial number of very seriously ill infants with this syndrome. The intensity of respiratory and other types of support is often equal to that required for hyaline membrane disease. With rare exception, these infants are born at term; often they are postterm. In most, there is evidence of some sort of intrauterine distress. Apgar scores at 1 and 5 minutes are usually below 5.

Pneumothorax and pneumomediastinum are not infrequent, though they appear in a minority of infants.

Meconium aspiration syndrome is a serious and frequent pulmonary disorder. Recent data demonstrate that *much of the morbidity and virtually all the mortality is avoidable by appropriate management in the delivery room.* Thus, in one inquiry among meconium-stained infants whose tracheas were suctioned immediately, the incidence of respiratory distress was less than half of that in nonsuctioned infants. Death occurred in approximately 1% of the suctioned infants and 28% of the nonsuctioned infants.

In a prospective investigation involving tracheal aspiration of all cases of meconium-stained amniotic fluid, meconium was removed from the trachea in 57% of the babies. Abnormal x-ray films were noted in half of them. Postnatal respiratory distress was noted in every baby who had both an abnormal x-ray film and tracheal meconium. If either of these factors was absent, the infant's subsequent course was uneventful. Other babies, who were admitted from outlying hospitals and had not been suctioned, had an impressively higher morbidity rate. They also required assisted ventilation more often, and the incidence of pneumothorax and pneumomediastinum was higher. In our own experience, 91 babies were admitted with the diagnosis of meconium aspiration syndrome in the most recent calendar year. Of the 23 who were referred to us from other hospitals, six died (26%); of the remaining 68 who were inborn, only one baby died (1.5%).

The best management of meconium aspiration syndrome requires aspiration of the trachea in all babies who emerge from stained amniotic fluid with any degree of respiratory difficulty. At the moment of birth, tracheal aspiration must be performed by application of gentle suction from the masked mouth of the operator, through an endotracheal tube. Use of a catheter is inadequate for this purpose because large particles cannot be evacuated. Mouth suction is maintained while the endotracheal tube is withdrawn so that if larger meconium masses are adherent to the tip of the tube, they are removed. Intubation is repeated until meconium is no longer in evidence. After arrival in the nursery, physical therapy to the chest, followed by suction, is repeated as often as indicated. Oxygen mixtures must be warm and well humidified. Mechanical ventilation (with or without PEEP) is often essential. The use of steroids has been advocated in the past, purportedly to minimize the inflammatory response to meconium. A well-controlled study has demonstrated that hydrocortisone does not diminish the need for assisted ventilation, nor does it reduce mortality. It does however, prolong morbidity; compared with untreated babies, infants who receive hydrocortisone require a significantly longer period to wean to room air.

EXTRANEOUS AIR SYNDROMES (AIR LEAK)

Extraneous air syndromes are a group of clinically recognizable disorders produced by alveolar rupture and the subsequent escape of air to tissues in which air is not normally present. Table 8-1 lists the sites in which extraneous air has been reported. Although most of these syndromes have long been known to occur spontaneously, their incidence increased as the use of ventilatory support became widespread, particularly since the advent of PEEP. Air leak syndrome now constitutes the most frequent life-threatening complication of ventilatory assistance. The capacity for instant recognition, evaluation, and relief of these disorders is a primary requisite for personnel who assume responsibility for sustained neonatal ventilatory support.

Incidence varies according to type and severity of disease, gestational age, mode of therapy, and expertise of personnel. Complications are most frequent during treatment for hyaline membrane disease. Interstitial emphysema and pneumothorax, for example, are observed more often in babies with hyaline mem-

Table 8-1. Extraneous air syndromes

Site of extraneous air	Syndrome
Pulmonary interstitium (perivascular sheaths)	Interstitial emphysema
Alveoli-trabeculae-visceral pleura	Pseudocysts
Pleural space	Pneumothorax
Mediastinum	Pneumomediastinum
Pericardial space	Pneumopericardium
Perivascular sheaths (peripheral vessels)	Perivascular emphysema
Vascular lumens (blood)	Air embolus
Subcutaneous tissue	Subcutaneous emphysema
Retroperitoneal connective tissue	Retroperitoneal emphysema
Peritoneal space	Pneumoperitoneum
Intestinal wall	Pneumatosis intestinalis
Scrotum	Pneumoscrotum

brane disease than in infants with other disorders. Frequency is also significantly influenced by the vigor of ventilatory assistance, which itself is usually a reflection of the severity of disease. Interstitial emphysema, pneumothorax, and pneumomediastinum have been reported to occur twice as often with the use of PEEP (39.7%) than without it (20.7%). In babies with hyaline membrane disease, the frequency of pneumothorax increases as therapy becomes more vigorous. Pneumopericardium was described as a "very rare condition" in neonates in 1970; there were descriptions of only seven cases. In 1976 one study described six babies with pneumopericardium in as short a time as 6 months. The authors found 57 cases in their review of the literature. Pneumopericardium, a "very rare condition" in 1970, is now not so rare. Most reports allude to a relationship between the increased frequency of this syndrome and the vigor of ventilatory therapy. A similar course of events has been noted for pneumoperitoneum.

Pathogenesis

All air leaks are caused by high intra-alveolar pressure that results from the inhalation, insufflation, or retention of inordinately large volumes of air. The resultant pressure gradient from affected alveoli to adjacent tissue space may be of sufficient magnitude to rupture alveoli where they overlie capillaries. Air escapes through disruption within the meshes of capillaries. It enters perivascular sheaths and migrates toward the hilum. Pulmonary interstitial emphysema is thus primarily characterized by extraneous air in perivascular sheaths. Often, extrusions of air occur in contiguous connective tissue, and at times in trabeculae through which air migrates to pleura to form blebs. Perivascular sheaths stretch considerably as air accumulates and the enveloped vessels are ultimately compressed. The associated circulatory impairment is an important component of interstitial emphysema.

Fig. 8-15 depicts the migration of air from alveolar rupture through lung interstitium into the pleural and pericardial cavities. The chest films in Fig. 8-16 correspond to these diagrams.

Air in perivascular sheaths dissects toward the hilum, invades the mediastinum, and thus causes *pneumomediastinum*. Air bubbles may accumulate at the hilum to form large blebs, which sometimes compress hilar vessels. The blebs are situated where visceral pleura reflects onto parietal pleura. As pressure mounts, rupture of blebs at this location releases air into the pleural space to give rise to *pneumothorax*. Apparently, air also passes from other points in the mediastinal wall to the pleural cavity. The pathway of extension to the *pericardial space* is still conjectural.

Far-flung dispersion of air may occur after alveolar rupture. *Pneumoperitoneum* is thought to result from extension of mediastinal air along the great vessels and esophagus into the peritoneal cavity. We have observed *pneumoscrotum* associated with *pneumoperitoneum*. Presumably migration of air occurred from the peritoneal cavity through the processus vaginalis into the scrotum. *Air embolism* occurs when extremely high pressures are used for ventilatory assistance; air is injected directly into pulmonary capillaries at the time of alveolar rupture. The application of very high peak inspiratory pressure to a lung of low compliance may also lacerate parenchyma, allowing passage of air under a high head of pressure into blood vessels.

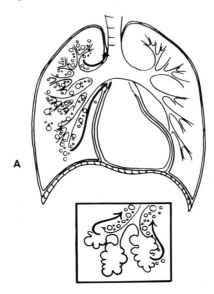

Interstitial emphysema

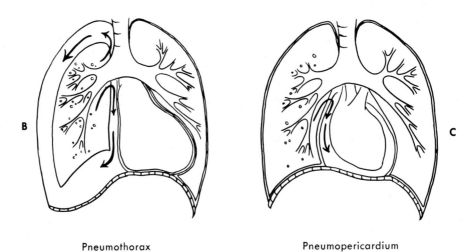

Pneumothorax   Pneumopericardium

Fig. 8-15. A, Air in interstitial lung tissue. Ruptured alveoli are indicated in framed alveoli at bottom. Air dissects from alveoli along vascular sheaths to hilus and thence to pleural space. (See x-ray film in Fig. 8-16, *A.*) **B,** Pneumothorax, indicating origin of air in lung tissue and its pathway to inflate pleural space. Heart shifts to left because of high pressure created in right chest. (See x-ray film in Fig. 8-16, *B.*) **C,** Course of air from lung to pericardial space. Distended pericardial space causes cardiac tamponade, small heart. (See x-ray film in Fig. 8-16, *C.*)

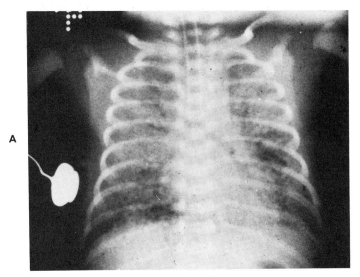

Interstitial emphysema

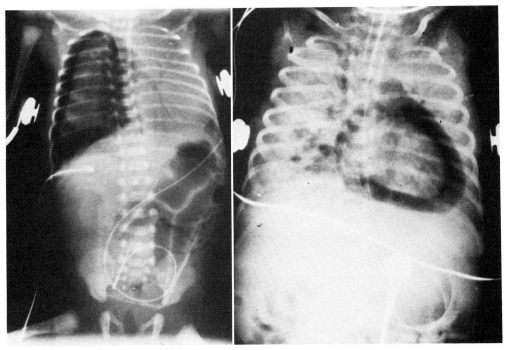

Pneumothorax   Pneumopericardium

Fig. 8-16. A, Interstitial emphysema. Multiple lakes of radiolucency (air), varying in size, impart a spongy appearance to lungs. (See Fig. 8-15, *A.*) **B,** Tension pneumothorax, right pleural cavity. The dense right lung is collapsed by pressure in pleural space created by air accumulation. Air-filled pleural cavity is darkest area that envelops right lung. (See Fig. 8-15, *B.*) **c,** Pneumopericardium. Dark halo of air fills pericardial space, outlining the heart itself. Note interstitial emphysema in right lung, indicated by large lakes of air. (See Fig. 8-15, *C.*)

The appearance of extraneous air, regardless of its location, always begins with alveolar rupture. Migration of escaped air ensues through tissue planes that offer the least resistance, thus giving rise to a spectrum of clinical syndromes that ranges from interstitial emphysema and pneumothorax to air embolism and pneumoscrotum (Table 8-1).

Clinical aspects

Of the twelve syndromes listed in Table 8-1, pneumothorax and pneumopericardium are the only ones that require instant remedial action lest death or brain damage ensue. On rare occasions, pneumomediastinum requires the same urgency. Interstitial emphysema is a serious manifestation of air leak that is associated with a high rate of mortality, but effective treatment is not available. Air embolus is a fatal event, for which there is also no effective therapy.

Pulmonary interstitial emphysema. The migration of air through vascular sheaths regularly precedes the appearance of extraneous air in sites outside the lung. Transient presence of air in the interstitium is most often not evident radiologically. When air accumulates, pulmonary interstitial emphysema is the result. The onset of abnormal clinical signs is relatively gradual. Most infants develop interstitial emphysema during administration of mechanical ventilatory support. Oxygen requirements increase and CO_2 retention may be relentless. Death is eventually caused by failure to adequately ventilate the baby. The extent to which death is attributable to vascular compression, particularly at the hilum, is unknown. The extent to which gas exchange is impaired by the interposition of air between alveoli and blood vessels is also unknown.

Progression of interstitial emphysema to pneumothorax is a frequent event. Approximately 50% of pneumothoraces are associated with interstitial emphysema. A high incidence of interstitial emphysema has been observed during the first 24 hours of life among infants who later developed BPD.

Interstitial emphysema can only be diagnosed radiologically. It is characterized by two basic features: radiolucencies that are linear and those that are cyst-like. The linear radiolucencies vary in width; they are coarse and do not branch. They are seen in the peripheral as well as the medial lung fields. The cyst-like radiolucencies vary from 1 to 4 mm in diameter. In some instances they are oval or lobulated. They may be so numerous that they impart a spongy appearance (Fig. 8-16, A). Interstitial emphysema may involve only one lobe, one lung, or more frequently both lungs. It appears within 96 hours after birth in babies who are receiving ventilatory assistance. There is no adequate therapy for this syndrome. Attempts should be made to minimize peak inspiratory and distending pressures, but usually the development of interstitial emphysema itself imposes a need for more vigorous therapy.

Unilateral interstitial emphysema can be treated effectively by selective intubation. Fig. 8-17 demonstrates the sequence of events that follows this type of intubation. The first film (Fig. 8-17, A) depicts severe involvement of the right lung and selective intubation of the left lung. We were able to ventilate this infant for 30 hours with an inactivated right lung. Fig. 8-17, B shows complete collapse of the previously emphysematous right lung. This occurred within 1 to 2 hours. Fig. 8-17, C shows reexpansion of the right lung after the tube was partially withdrawn back to the trachea. Note that the interstitial emphysema cleared completely; it did not recur.

Pneumothorax. Pneumothorax can occur spontaneously (no iatrogenic factors implicated), as a result of ventilatory assistance, or rarely as a complication following certain procedures.

Spontaneous pneumothorax usually occurs during the first few breaths after birth. The vast majority of infants are asymptomatic. Radiologic surveys have demonstrated an incidence of 1% to 2% of all livebirths, but symptomatic pneumothorax has been noted in only 0.05% to 0.07% of livebirths. Most investigators have found the highest incidence of spontaneous pneumothorax in term rather

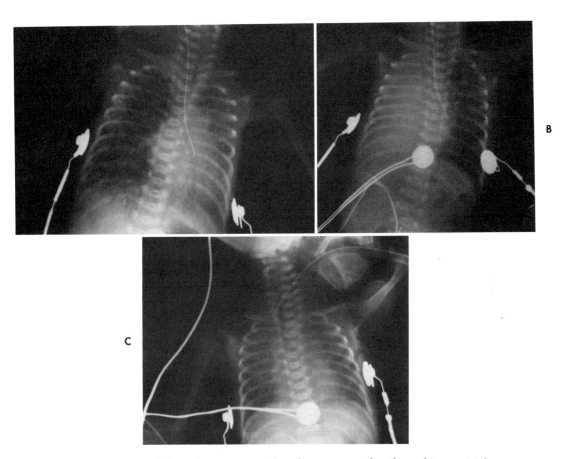

Fig. 8-17. Sequence of films depicting results of treatment of unilateral interstitial emphysema by selective intubation. **A,** Severe involvement of the right lung required intubation of the left main stem bronchus. The baby was successfully maintained only on the left lung for 30 hours. **B,** The desired complete collapse of the right lung was evident approximately 6 hours after intubation of the left lung. **C,** Withdrawal of the endotracheal tube to its usual position in the trachea 30 hours after selective intubation of the left lung reveals complete disappearance of interstitial emphysema on the right.

than preterm infants. Postmature infants are particularly vulnerable.

Distress is generally evident in the delivery room or soon after arrival in the nursery. Tachypnea (to 130 breaths per minute) is a universal occurrence. A prominent chest bulge on the involved side is characteristic. Grunting, retractions, and cyanosis in room air have been noted in virtually all symptomatic infants. As a rule, they have abnormal chest findings attributable to an underexpanded lung and to displacement of the heart away from the affected hemithorax. Restlessness and irritability are frequent. Spontaneous pneumothorax is sometimes a manifestation of serious lung disease; it has long been reported in association with meconium aspiration, hyaline membrane disease, pneumonia, pulmonary hypoplasia with renal anomalies, and diaphragmatic hernia. We have also encountered it in infants who had RDS II. Although spontaneous alveolar rupture is sometimes a worrisome portent of serious underlying pulmonary disease, most infants have otherwise normal lungs. Approximately 80% to 90% are mildly ill, requiring no therapy other than an oxygen-rich environment.

Pneumothorax during ventilatory assistance is common. Mild courses are exceptional; tension pneumothorax is the predominant form of the disorder, particularly in babies who are on mechanical ventilators with PEEP. Vigilance by expert nurses is effective for early detection; better yet, a significant number of pneumothoraces are predictable. Short gestational age, hyaline membrane disease, and high ventilatory pressures are the most significant predisposing factors. Their presence imposes a high risk for air leak. The role of gestational age and hyaline membrane disease can be appreci-

ated from the example of our own experience. In a 12-month period, pneumothorax occurred in ten of 28 infants (35.7%) whose gestational age was 26 through 28 weeks, yet only one out of twelve (8.3%) was involved when gestational age was 35 to 36 weeks. Pneumothorax was 3.5 times more frequent in the presence of hyaline membrane disease than in other abnormalities. The predictive value of these factors is helpful but not specific. Predictions based on chest films are more specific because interstitial emphysema is a frequent precursor, preceding pneumothorax in up to 50% of cases. Pneumothorax follows the appearance of interstitial emphysema within 2 to 72 hours. Pneumomediastinum is another predictor of pneumothorax.

Identification and relief of pneumothorax can be accomplished within a few minutes by detection of abnormal signs. Tension pneumothorax produces abrupt duskiness or cyanosis. There may be significant declines of arterial blood pressure, heart rate, respiratory rate, and pulse pressure before the expected abnormal chest signs. Detection of diminished breath sounds, bulging of the affected hemithorax, and mediastinal shift to the unaffected side are nevertheless valuable indications. We use transillumination of the chest. Prior to availability of transillumination, we proceeded to aspirate air from the pleural cavity on the basis of abnormal physical signs. If the infant's status permits, the presence of pneumothorax is first verified radiologically (Fig. 8-16, *B*).

Immediate evacuation of air is urgent. We insert a rubber catheter (no. 12 to no. 14) for attachment to continuous suction. One should be cautioned against the use of a needle for aspiration of air. At autopsy needle tracts have been demonstrated in the myocardium of the left ventricle, presumably as a result of the resumption of normal cardiac position as tension pneumothorax was relieved by the aspiration of air.

The definitive treatment for tension pneumothorax is placement of a chest tube and application of continuous suction (10 cm H_2O), particularly if end-expiratory pressure is used for ventilatory assistance. Recurrence of pneumothorax during chest drainage is rather frequent. In such circumstances the existing tube must be replaced if it is demonstrably occluded; if the tube is not blocked, a second one must be inserted. The most difficult pneumothorax we have ever treated was a bilateral one that ultimately required 28 tube insertions. At 1 year of age this child is normal.

Pneumothorax as a result of certain procedures is a rare occurrence. Several reports describe pneumothorax after birth of babies whose mothers had an amniocentesis shortly before. In one instance, attention was called to the pneumothorax during the baby's bath when a nurse palpated subcutaneous emphysema in the chest wall. Spontaneous resolution was complete 7 days later. These pneumothoraces may be due to entry of the amniocentesis needle into the fetal chest. Three infants have been described to have developed pneumothorax following perforation of bronchi by suction catheters.

Of the three etiologic groups of pneumothorax described here (spontaneous, during ventilatory assistance, following certain procedures), the most significant are those that occur during ventilatory assistance. These account for increased incidence, for protracted morbidity, and for most of the mortality attributable to pneumothorax.

Pneumopericardium. Pneumopericardium usually occurs in association with one or more of the other extraneous air syndromes. It is uncommon in the absence of mechanical respiratory support. In most instances very high ventilatory pressues are required for adequate therapy. The first sign of its onset is often a sudden appearance or deepening of cyanosis. Heart sounds are muffled; in the most severe cases, heart sounds are inaudible though reduced voltage cardiac activity is evident on the oscilloscope or EKG. If sufficient air accumulates in the pericardial space, pressure within it rises, and eventually stroke volume diminishes. Arterial blood pressure falls and, in the extreme, peripheral pulses are not palpable. As hypoxia worsens, bradycardia becomes evident. Metabolic acidosis develops in response to hypoxemia and to the generally diminished tissue perfusion that results from low cardiac output due to tamponade. The most distinctive features that suggest the onset of tamponade are the abrupt appearance of cyanosis, hypotension, inaudible heart sounds but, with cardiac activity, visible on EKG or oscilloscope, and persistent pulsations of fluid in the umbilical artery catheter. Diagnosis by x-ray film is definitive. A broad radiolucent halo completely surrounds the heart, including the diaphragmatic surface (Fig. 8-16, *C*). In the lateral projection a broad area of radiolucency separates the anterior surface of the heart from the sternum and, to a lesser extent, from the diaphragm as well. We have also identified pneumopericardium by transillumination.

Pneumopericardium varies widely in severity. We have made the diagnosis accidentally on a routine chest film from a baby who had no abnormal cardiac signs. The pericardial air disappeared sponta-

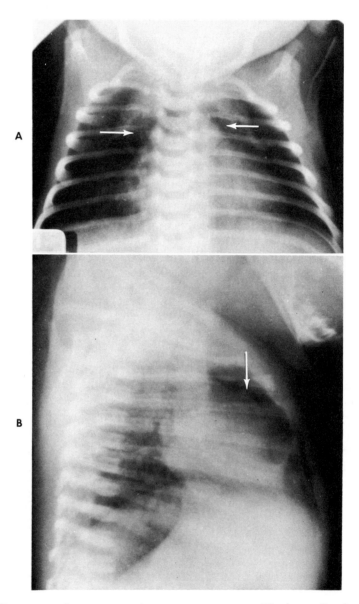

Fig. 8-18. Pneumomediastinum. **A,** Anteroposterior view. The butterfly-shaped shadow of the thymus is above mediastinal air. The air (arrows) separates the thymic shadow and the cardiac shadow beneath it. **B,** Lateral view. Mediastinal air (arrow) is visible in the darkest area immediately beneath the sternum. Since air is situated between the heart and the anterior chest wall, the intensity of heart sounds is substantially diminished.

neously 6 hours later. A review of the literature up to 1976 revealed 63 cases. Approximately 60% survived. Of those infants who were treated with pericardiocentesis, 79% survived. Conservative management (no needle aspiration) was associated with 32% survival. These authors make a case for aggressive management with needle aspiration or catheter insertion. On the other hand, two other reports advocate conservative management. They would not aspirate until cardiac tamponade appears, as indicated by a fall in aortic blood pressure.

Treatment usually consists of multiple pericardial taps as indicated for accumulation of air. The incidence of reaccumulation after initial pericardiocentesis is said to be 53%. The authors of a recent article reported insertion of a no. 14 French Bardex catheter into the pericardial space after two episodes of reaccumulation of air following needle aspirations. The infant recovered. They advocate management of pneumopericardium with tamponade according to the same underlying principles by which tension pneumothorax is managed.

Pneumomediastinum. This is a common isolated disorder when it occurs spontaneously in otherwise healthy infants by the same mechanisms described for spontaneous pneumothorax. It also occurs in hyaline membrane disease spontaneously, after resuscitation immediately following birth, and during ventilator therapy. Spontaneous pneumomediastinum has been observed to occur at a rate of 25 per 10,000 livebirths. As in spontaneous pneumothorax, postmature infants were more vulnerable than others, presumably for the same reason—a higher incidence of meconium aspiration.

Pneumomediastinum, when it occurs in otherwise normal infants at birth, is generally asymptomatic. In other circumstances it produces mild to moderate abnormal clinical signs. Tachypnea, bulging sternum, muffled heart sounds, and cyanosis occur with varying frequencies. The chest film is diagnostic in the lateral projection. Anteroposterior projections often appear spuriously normal. In the lateral view air is seen as a radiolucent area behind the sternum, in the superior portion of the mediastinum if the infant is upright. Occasionally the thymus is visible above the heart. In the anteroposterior view a halo is seen around the heart; sometimes it is quite broad so that it extends toward the lateral reaches of the lungs. The "spinnaker sail sign" is commonly apparent in this projection. It is produced by lifting of the thymus from the heart by the interposed air (Fig. 8-18). Pneumomediastinum resolves spontaneously with rare exceptions. Careful observation is essential; nothing more aggressive is indicated.

Pneumoperitoneum. Free air in the peritoneum usually suggests perforation of an abdominal viscus, requiring immediate surgery. In recent years several reports have shown pneumoperitoneum to be secondary to air leak. Air migrates through the diaphragm to the retroperitoneal space and then to the peritoneal cavity. Fig. 8-19 demonstrates the development of a pneumoperitoneum by extension of air from the posterior mediastinum through the diaphragm and then into the peritoneal space. These films were taken over an interval of 8 hours. The thoracic collection of air on the left side of the vertebral column is in the posterior mediastinum, instead of the more common anterior accumulation shown in Fig. 8-18. The principal difficulty in this

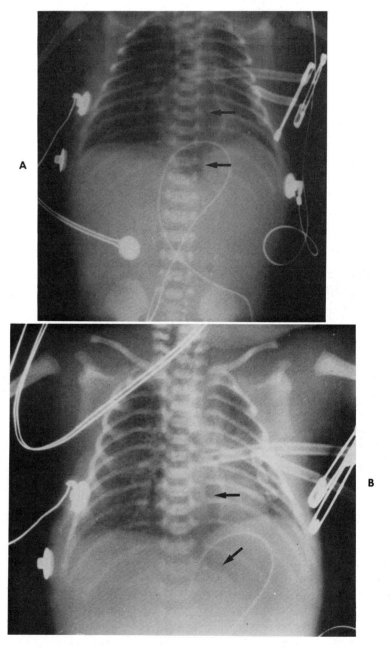

Fig. 8-19. Sequence of three films demonstrating extension of pneumomediastinum through the diaphragm with resultant pneumoperitoneum. The upper arrow in each film indicates collection of air in the posterior mediastinum. The lower arrow of each film indicates the extension of air. Pneumoperitoneum is fully developed in **C.**

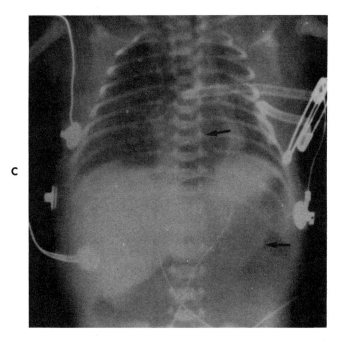

C

Fig. 8-19, cont'd. For legend see opposite page.

situation is exclusion of a serious surgical disorder. The simultaneous presence of aberrant air in the chest is good evidence that the situation is nonsurgical. Absence of peritoneal fluid, normal thickness of bowel wall, and absence of air fluid levels in the intestine are additional evidence of the nonsurgical nature of the pneumoperitoneum. Fig. 8-20 demonstrates the curious extension of a pneumoperitoneum through the processus vaginalis into the scrotum.

Air embolus. This rare condition is the most sinister of the extraneous air syndromes. It occurs when extremely high pressures are required to ventilate extremely stiff lungs. As a result, it is thought that parenchymal lacerations occur and that air is injected into the pul-

monary vasculature. In most infants with air embolus, inflation pressures up to 55 cm H_2O were necessary to provide satisfactory tidal volume.

The clinical presentation of infants with air embolus is a catastrophic event. Sudden cyanosis and circulatory collapse become evident. The heart slows, but with each beat the air-blood mixture is heard to crackle and pop. Withdrawal of blood from the umbilical artery catheter yields alternating segments of air and blood, similar to what one would expect if a stopcock connection were loose. The x-ray film reveals a bizarre picture of intracardiac and intravascular air. Fig. 8-21 shows air in the portal vessels as well as in the heart. There is no effective treatment for massive intravascular air.

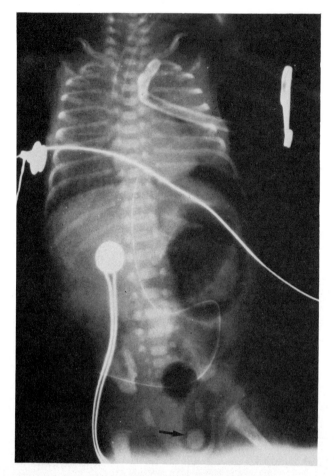

Fig. 8-20. Extension of air in peritoneal space (pneumoperitoneum) through the processus vaginalis and into the scrotum. Arrow at bottom of film indicates the pneumoscrotum.

PNEUMONIA

Infection of the lungs may be acquired in utero (congenital pneumonia) or after birth. The congenital disease is more often lethal. Pneumonia is a common serious perinatal infection. It has a number of attributes that are unique to the neonate and is thus presented in Chapter 12 as a part of the general problem of perinatal infections.

CONGENITAL ANOMALIES

Malformations of the respiratory tract are numerous. A few of the major anomalies are discussed here.

Choanal atresia

The choanae are the posterior nares that open into nasopharynx. Atresia or stenosis is an uncommon malformation that produces dramatic symptoms and re-

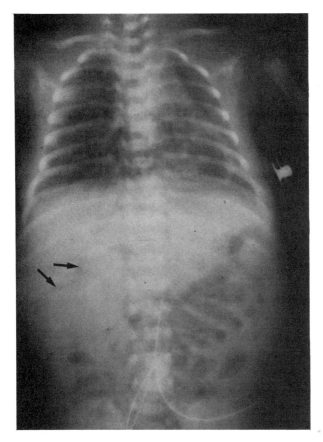

Fig. 8-21. Massive air embolus as a result of high pressures on mechanical ventilator. The heart is filled with air. The arrows indicate air in the portal vasculature.

quires immediate recognition. Complete or partial obstruction of one or both apertures is caused by a membranous or bony structure covering them. Since the neonate can breathe only through his nose, catastrophic respiratory distress may result from obstruction. The first breath is usually normal because it is taken through the mouth. Cyanosis and severe retractions appear as the infant subsequently attempts to breathe through the nose. Thick mucoid secretions characteristically fill the nose. The anomaly can be demonstrated by failure to pass a catheter or probe through the nose into the nasopharynx. If a membrane covers the choanae, it can be punctured to open the airway. Most often this is not the case. An oral airway should be inserted to accommodate mouth breathing pending ultimate surgical correction of the obstruction. Occasionally respiration is possible only after endotracheal intubation. Choanal obstruction may impede the exhalation of carbon dioxide, and as a consequence, diffuse emphysema and an elevated arterial P_{CO_2} develop.

Tracheoesophageal fistula

Among the congenital malformations that cause neonatal respiratory distress, tracheoesophageal fistula is the most common. Several variations have been recognized (Fig. 8-22). The most frequent form of this anomaly is atresia of a segment of the esophagus, which is thus divided into an upper blind pouch and a lower separated portion that communicates with the stomach in a normal fashion. A fistula connects this lower esophageal segment with the trachea. This lesion is present in 85% of infants with esophageal atresia. In another variety, which is far less common, esophageal atresia is the only malformation, the tracheobronchial tree being intact. A third type is characterized by a fistulous connection between an otherwise normal trachea and esophagus, the so-called H type of fistula. The other variations are extremely rare.

A distinctive triad of clinical signs is usually recognizable in the most common variety of tracheoesophageal fistula: (1) accumulation of secretions in the mouth and hypopharynx, often requiring urgent and frequent suction, (2) continuous or sporadic respiratory distress, and (3) repeated regurgitation of feedings. The first two signs should immediately suggest this diagnostic possibility to the nurse. A trial feeding should not be necessary; it could be dangerous because of aspiration. In affected infants, the mouth is full of bubbling saliva, and some degree of respiratory distress is clearly apparent. Often the abdomen is quite distended because air continually enters the stomach through the fistulous connection between the trachea and the lower esophageal segment. Pneumonia and atelectasis, particularly in the right upper lobe, are also rather frequent signs. The nurse should attempt to pass a catheter into the esophagus of any infant with these signs. The obstruction is not always perceived because the catheter may curl on itself in the esophageal pouch while it seems to pass with ease. One or 2 cc of air should be injected into the catheter while the nurse listens over the stomach for gurgling to indicate that the catheter tip is in the stomach. Listening for gurgling is not consistently reliable.

A chest film usually reveals the blind pouch filled with air. Instillation of dye

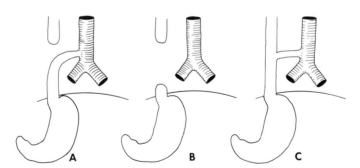

Fig. 8-22. Three most common types of tracheoesophageal fistula. **A,** Esophageal atresia with fistulous connection between the lower esophageal segment and the trachea. This is the most common variety. **B,** Esophageal atresia with normal respiratory tract. **C,** Normal esophagus and trachea connected by a fistula (H type of malformation).

contrast medium into the pouch, although frequently performed, is not necessary for the diagnosis because the air-filled pouch is plainly visible. If air is also present in the intestinal tract and esophageal atresia has been demonstrated, a tracheoesophageal fistula is undoubtedly present. We use two techniques to demonstrate the pouch by x-ray film. The pouch is dramatically visible if

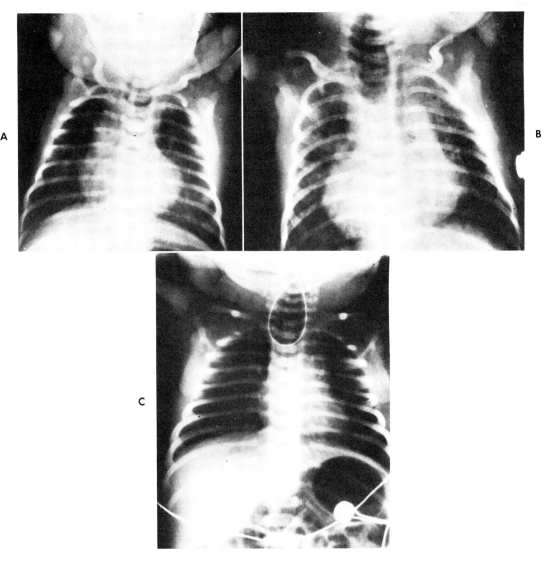

Fig. 8-23. A, Tracheoesophageal fistula with esophageal atresia. Routine chest x-ray film. The radiolucent pocket overlying the vertebrae just superior to the heart is the air-containing esophageal pouch. **B,** Inflated pouch during bagging with mask. **C,** Umbilical artery catheter looped in esophageal pouch.

it can be inflated with air at the moment the x-ray film is taken. The nurse uses bag and mask, insufflating five or six times. Then, with the next squeeze of the bag, the x-ray technician takes the film. Even more diagnostic is the passage of an umbilical artery catheter. It is radiopaque, and it loops within the blind pouch. Fig. 8-23 shows three films of a tracheoesophageal fistula. The first is routine chest film in which the air-filled esophageal pouch is visible. Our clinical nurse supervisor suspected pathology from this film. The second is an x-ray film taken while the pouch was inflated by bag and mask. The third demonstrates the position of an umbilical artery catheter within the pouch.

Infants whose only anomaly is esophageal atresia (without a fistulous connection) have pooling of secretions and feeding difficulties. Respiratory symptoms, if they are present, are a consequence of aspirated secretions.

The H type of fistula is well known but rare; it is often suspected but seldom demonstrated early in the course. Respiratory distress is typically at its worst when the baby is fed, since milk enters the lung from the esophagus through the fistula. Tachypnea may persist between feedings, and pneumonia is almost a constant accompaniment. The tract must be demonstrated by feeding contrast medium while the baby is in a prone and somewhat oblique position. Fluoroscopic visualization is usually possible, but repeated attempts are often necessary because the fistula does not always fill with dye.

We diagnosed a case of H type fistula by measuring changes of intragastric oxygen concentration in response to insufflating the lungs alternately with 100% oxygen and room air. After passing a nasogastric tube, the exterior end was attached to an oxygen analyzer to register fluctuaions of intragastric oxygen concentrations. An endotracheal tube was passed just below the vocal cords. The tip of the tube was thus above the tracheal aperture of the H fistula. The baby was gently insufflated with 100% oxygen, which crossed the fistula into the stomach and resulted in an increased intragastric oxygen concentration. This was registered on the oxygen analyzer to which the outside end of the nasogastric tube was attached. Oxygen concentration was observed to fall when insufflation was continued, but with room air. The fistula was successfully repaired.

All forms of tracheoesophageal fistula must be repaired surgically. As technical surgical problems have been surmounted, pneumonia, septicemia, and associated anomalies have emerged as the major causes of death. For term infants without other anomalies or pneumonia, a 100% survival rate can be expected. Overall survival of term babies is approximately 70%, and for premature infants, 52%. From available data, it has been surmised that improved management of pneumonia and septicemia would substantially diminish mortality. The later the diagnosis is made, the more hazardous are the procedure and postoperative course. Surgery can be delayed with impunity only if optimal supportive care is available. As a rule, the nurse is the infant's first attendant and thus can best direct initial attention to suspicious signs.

Diaphragmatic hernia

Incomplete embryonic formation of the diaphragm results in a congenital defect that allows displacement of abdonimal organs into the thoracic cavity. Severe respiratory distress occurs at birth or shortly thereafter. The left side is involved five to ten times more frequently than the right side. Herniation occurs through one of several possible defective segments of the diaphragm; the most common is at the posterolateral segment (foramen of Bochdalek). Defects at the anterior portion directly beneath the sternum (foramen of Morgagni) and at the esophageal hiatus are considerably less frequent.

In left-sided involvement the intestine, stomach, and spleen compress the lung. The gastrointestinal tract, distended with air, occupies most of the space preempted from the lung, and the mediastinum is dislocated to the right. In right-sided involvement the liver and/or intestine are the herniated abdominal organs; they displace the mediastinum to the left.

The severity of symptoms is related to the amount of lung compressed by the dislocated abdominal organs. The pattern of respiratory distress is no different from that caused by other neonatal disorders. The most severely affected babies gasp a few times at birth, never establishing respiration. If respiratory distress is not particularly severe at birth, it frequently progresses alarmingly as the intestine in the chest expands with the normal entry of swallowed air (Fig. 8-24).

The diagnosis can sometimes be anticipated before birth if there is a history of polyhydramnios. Polyhydramnios occurs in over half of affected infants because the thoracic location of intestine is ob-

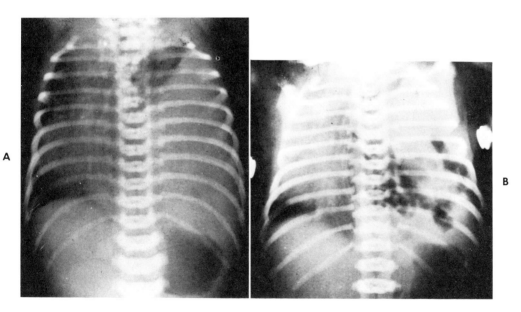

Fig. 8-24. A, Left diaphragmatic hernia immediately after birth. The left chest is opaque, filled with gasless intestine. The heart is displaced to the right chest. **B,** Intestine in left chest has begun to fill with air. The heart is now farther to the right. Fortunately, the infant was bagged with mask for only a short time. Longer periods fill the intestine to produce more tension in left chest, as seen in Fig. 8-25.

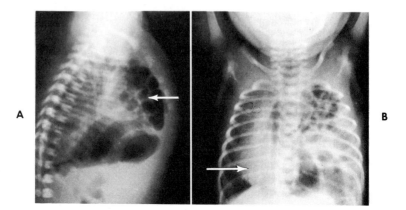

Fig. 8-25. Diaphragmatic hernia. **A,** Lateral view. The cystic appearance in the chest (arrow) is caused by air-filled loops of intestine. **B,** Anteroposterior view. Gas-filled intestinal loops fill the left chest, displacing the heart (arrow) into the right chest. Heart sounds are thus heard in the right chest, and breath sounds in the left chest are virtually absent. (Courtesy Webster Riggs, M. D., LeBonheur Children's Hospital, Memphis, Tenn.)

structive to intrauterine flow of amniotic fluid. The presence of a diaphragmatic hernia is invariably suggested by difficult respiration. Displacement of the cardiac impulse to one side of the chest is the most telling indication of the diagnosis, but pneumothorax can produce the same displacement. If the cardiac impulse is shifted to one side or the other, there should be an immediate realization that one is not dealing solely with the type of perinatal asphyxia in which resuscitative measures would be expected to alleviate much of the difficulty. The abdomen is sometimes sunken (scaphoid), but this condition depends on the displacement of a considerable amount of intestine. More often, the abdominal contour is normal. Diminished breath sounds are the rule in the involved hemithorax.

A chest film confirms the diagnosis. The diaphragmatic margin is absent on the defective side, and the presence of inappropriate thoracic structures is readily discerned. The gas-filled intestines may impart a multicystic appearance to the left chest (Fig. 8-25). If the right side is affected, the liver casts a homogeneous density in the area it occupies. Absence or diminution of the normal liver shadow in the abdomen is another revealing radiologic sign.

The case fatality rate is high, being influenced by the rapidity of diagnosis and surgical correction. Even with optimal management, death is quite frequent because severe pulmonary hypoplasia precludes effective ventilation. Surgery is the only effective treatment, and it must be done with dispatch. Some infants expire before surgery can be initiated.

RESPIRATORY DISTRESS OF EXTRAPULMONARY ORIGIN

Respiratory distress may be the most prominent sign of a number of disorders of extrapulmonary origin. They fall into four broad categories: (1) congenital heart disease, (2) depression due to drugs, (3) metabolic acidosis of nonpulmonary origin, and (4) central nervous system disorders.

Congenital heart disease

In most instances, by the time respiratory difficulty appears in infants with major cardiac anomalies, congestive failure is well developed. In our experience, patent ductus arteriosus in small premature infants is the most common condition associated with congestive failure and pulmonary edema. A high mortality rate during the neonatal period among these infants is well documented. Of the many types of lesions involved in cardiac anomalies, approximately eight of them account for most deaths. Three of these eight anomalies are responsible for almost half the deaths: hypoplastic left heart syndrome (hypoplasia of the left ventricle, aortic atresia, and mitral atresia), coarctation of the aorta, and transposition of the great vessels. The remaining five conditions that are most frequently lethal in the first month of life include hypoplastic right heart syndrome with pulmonary arterial atresia or stenosis, tetralogy of Fallot, truncus arteriosus, endocardial cushion defect, and ventricular septal defect.

Respiratory distress of cardiac origin usually can be identified with the aid of a few simple observations. Breathing is rapid, but not often labored or obstructed. Heart sounds are loud and rapid. A gallop rhythm is particularly indicative of heart failure. Enlargement of the liver (more than 3 cm below the right costal margin), when present, is also a valuable sign. Enlargement of the heart can be seen on the chest film of almost all infants in congestive heart failure. These signs indicate primary cardiac dysfunction, and with few exceptions the electrocardiogram is abnormal in their presence.

Effects of drugs

Respiratory distress due to drugs is characterized by depressed function rather than the rapid, facile breathing associated with heart disease or the rapid, labored breathing so typical of intrinsic lung disorders. Drugs that depress neonates are adminstered to their mothers during labor; they are usually anesthetics and analgesics. Almost all these agents are known to cross the placenta. Affected infants usually initiate respiration, but the breathing that follows is shallow and slow. If depression is sufficiently deep, generalized cyanosis may be prominent. Cardiac activity is normal, unless hypoxemic bradycardia occurs as a result of depressed ventilation. The breath sounds are diminished, but only because respiration is shallow, thus reducing air intake. Painful stimuli cause little response in depressed infants, and, at best, the cry is feeble.

Barbiturates are notorious depressive agents. They cross the placenta rapidly. Infants who are born a few hours after maternal barbiturate administration have significant blood levels of the drug for several days after birth. Liberal use of barbiturates during labor and delivery has been curtailed.

Inhalational agents are often used in combination with other drugs during labor, and their individual effects are difficult to evaluate. Anesthetic concentrations of nitrous oxide over 75% generally produce asphyxiated infants. Maternal overdosage with any of these agents will cause depressed respiratory function in the neonate.

Narcotic analgesics are used extensively during the management of labor and delivery. Meperidine is most commonly employed, and its administration in doses that depress the infant is widespread. If it is given intramuscularly between 1 and 3 hours before delivery, some degree of neonatal depression is almost inevitable. If it is administered intramuscularly within an hour of birth in appropriate dosage, significant depression does not usually occur. The effects of meperidine are potentiated if barbiturates are used in combination with it.

Metabolic acidosis of extrapulmonary origin

Rapid respiration is stimulated by an abnormally low pH; if the lungs are normal, increased carbon dioxide excretion occurs and the arterial P_{CO_2} is reduced. Metabolic acidosis of extrapulmonary origin is most often caused by renal disorders, diarrhea, infection, and a peculiarity of protein metabolism in premature infants called "late metabolic acidosis." The respiratory rate usually subsides after proper alkali therapy for correction of the blood pH.

Central nervous system disorders

Intracranial hemorrahge occurs most frequently in premature infants in whom it is usually of intraventricular or subarachnoid origin. In term infants, subdural and intracerebral hemorrhages are more common. These episodes severely depress respiratory function. Sporadic apnea and irregular breathing are characteristic. Blood gas and pH alterations are identical to those of perinatal asphyxia.

SUMMATION

Respiratory problems are the most frequent cause of neonatal mortality and morbidity. Although most often attributable to intrinsic lung disease, some form of abnormal respiration is inevitable in any type of serious illness; the diagnostic possibilities suggested by breathing difficulties are thus numerous. Several situations require immediate diagnosis and therapy; such optimal management is often lifesaving. No one can better make the first discovery of serious respiratory dysfunction than the nurse, nor is anyone else better equipped to ascertain that therapy is proceeding effectively and without jeopardy to the infant.

REFERENCES

Adams, F. H., Yanagisawa, M., Kuzela, D., and Martinek, H.: The disappearance of fetal lung fluid following birth, J. Pediatr. **78**:837, 1971.

Auld, P. A. M.: Oxygen therapy for premature infants, J. Pediatr. **78**:705, 1971.

Auld, P., Hodson, A., and Usher, R.: Hyaline membrane disease: a discussion, J. Pediatr. **80**:129, 1972.

Avery, M. E., and Said, S.: Surface phenomena in lungs in health and disease, Medicine **44**:503, 1965.

Avery, M. E., Gatewood, O. B., and Brumley, G.: Transient tachypnea of newborn, Am. J. Dis. Child. **111**:380, 1966.

Bancalari, E., and Berlin, J. A.: Meconium aspiration and other asphyxial disorders, Clin. Perinatol. **5**:317, 1978.

Berg, T. J., Pagtakhan, R. D., Reed, M. H., et al.: Bronchopulmonary dysplasia and lung rupture in hyaline membrane disease: influence of continuous distending pressure, Pediatrics **55**:51, 1975.

Berman, W., Dubynsky, O., Whitman, V., et al.: Digoxin therapy in low-birth-weight infants with patent ductus arteriosus, J. Pediatr. **93**:652, 1978.

Black, I. F. S., Kotrapu, N., and Massie, H.: Application of Doppler ultrasound to blood pressure measurement in small infants, J. Pediatr. **81**:932, 1972.

Boddy, K., Dawes, G. S., and Robinson, J.: Intrauterine fetal breathing movements. In Gluck, L., editor: Modern perinatal medicine, Chicago, 1974, Year Book Medical Publishers, Inc.

Briggs, J. N., and Hogg, G.: Perinatal pulmonary pathology, Pediatrics **22**:41, 1958.

Butler, J. N., and Claireaux, A. E.: Congenital diaphragmatic hernia as a cause of perinatal mortality, Lancet **1**:659, 1962.

Capitanio, M. A., and Kirkpatrick, J. A.: Roentgen

examination in the evaluation of the newborn infant with respiratory distress, J. Pediatr. **75:**896, 1969.

Chernick, V.: Continuous distending pressure in hyaline membrane disease: of devices, disadvantages, and a daring study, Pediatrics **52:**114, 1973.

Chernick, V.: Fetal breathing movements and the onset of breathing at birth, Clin. Perinatol. **5:**257, 1978.

Chernick, V., and Reed, M. H.: Pneumothorax and chylothorax in the neonatal period, J. Pediatr. **76:**624, 1970.

Cifuentes, R. F., Olley, P. M., Balfe, J. W., et al.: Indomethacin and renal function in premature infants with persistent patent ductus arteriosus, J. Pediatr. **95:**583, 1979.

Comroe, J. H., Jr.: Physiology of respiration, ed. 3, Chicago, 1974, Year Book Medical Publishers, Inc.

Corbet, A., and Adams, J.: Current therapy in hyaline membrane disease, Clin. Perinatol. **5:**299, 1978.

Cotton, R. B., Stahlman, M. T., Kova, I., and Catterton, W. Z.: Medical management of small preterm infants with symptomatic patent ductus arteriosus, J. Pediatr. **92:**467, 1978.

Cowett, R. H., et al.: Foam-stability test on gastric aspirate and the diagnosis of respiratory distress syndrome, N. Engl. J. Med. **293:**413, 1975.

Cumarasamy, N., Nussli, R., Vischer, D., et al.: Artificial ventilation in hyaline membrane disease: the use of positive end-expiratory pressure and continuous positive airway pressure, Pediatrics **51:**629, 1973.

Daily, W. J. R., and Smith, P. C.: Mechanical ventilation of the newborn infant. I and II. In Gluck, L., editor: Current problems in pediatrics, Chicago, 1971, Year Book Medical Publishers, Inc.

Dawes, G. S.: Fetal circulation and breathing, Clin. Obstet. Gynecol. **1:**139, 1974.

De Leon, A. S., Elliot, J. H., and Jones, D. B.: The resurgence of retrolental fibroplasia, Pediatr. Clin. North Am. **17:**309, 1970.

Drummond, W. H., Peckham, G. J., and Fox, W. W.: The clinical profile of the newborn with persistent pulmonary hypertension: observations in 19 affected neonates, Clin. Pediatr. **16:**335, 1977.

Duc, G.: Assessment of hypoxia in the newborn, suggestions for a practical approach, Pediatrics **48:**469, 1971.

Emery, J. L., and Mithal, A.: The number of alveoli in the terminal respiratory unit of man during late intrauterine life and childhood, Arch. Dis. Child. **35:**544, 1960.

Farrell, P. M., and Hamosh, M.: The biochemistry of fetal lung development, Clin. Perinatol. **5:**197, 1978.

Fenner, R., Muller, H. G., Busse, M., et al.: Transcutaneous determination of arterial oxygen tension, Pediatrics **55:**224, 1975.

Fitzhardinge, P. M.: Follow-up studies in infants treated by mechanical ventilation, Clin. Perinatol. **5:**451, 1978.

Fox, W. W., et al.: Pulmonary hypertension and the perinatal aspiration syndromes, Pediatrics **59:**205, 1977.

Fox, W. W., Gutsche, B. B., and DeVore, J. S.: A delivery room approach to the meconium aspiration syndrome (MAS), Clin. Pediatr. **16:**325, 1977.

Friedman, W. F., Heymann, M. A., and Rudolph, A. M.: Commentary: new thoughts on an old problem—patent ductus arteriosus in the premature infant, J. Pediatr. **90:**338, 1977.

Friedman, W. F., Fitzpatrick, K. M., Merritt, T. A., and Feldman, B. H.: The patent ductus arteriosus, Clin. Perinatol. **5:**411, 1978.

Gershanik, J. J.: Neonatal pneumopericardium, Am. J. Dis. Child. **121:**438, 1971.

Gersony, W. M.: Commentary: patent ductus arteriosus and the respiratory distress syndrome—a perspective, J. Pediatr. **91:**624, 1977.

Goldman, H. I., Maralit, A., Sun, S., and Lanzkowsy, P.: Neonatal cyanosis and arterial oxygen saturation, J. Pediatr. **82:**319, 1973.

Gregory, G. A., Gooding, C. A., Phibbs, R. H., and Tooley, W. H.: Meconium aspiration in infants: a prospective study, J. Pediatr. **85:**848, 1974.

Gregory, G. A., et al.: Treatment of the idiopathic respiratory distress syndrome with continuous positive airway pressure, N. Engl. J. Med. **284:**1333, 1971.

Hall, R. T., and Rhodes, P. R.: Pneumothorax and pneumomediastinum in infants with idiopathic respiratory distress syndrome receiving continuous positive airway pressure, Pediatrics **55:**493, 1975.

Harned, H. S.: Fetal physiology, In Barnett, H. L., editor: Pediatrics, New York, 1968, Appleton-Century-Crofts.

Harned, H. S., Jr., and Ferreiro, J.: Initiation of breathing by cold stimulation: effects of change in ambient temperature on respiratory activity of the full-term fetal lamb, J. Pediatr. **83:**663, 1973.

Harrison, V. C., Heese, H. de V., and Klein, M. B.: The significance of grunting in hyaline membrane disease, Pediatrics **41:**549, 1968.

Harrod, J. R., L'Heureux, P., Wangensteen, O. D., and Hunt, C. E.: Long-term follow-up of severe respiratory distress syndrome treated with IPPB, J. Pediatr. **84**:277, 1974.

Hartmann, A. F., Jr., Klint, R., Hernandez, A., and Goldring, D.: Measurement of blood pressure in the brachial and posterior tibial arteries using the Doppler method, J. Pediatr. **82**:498, 1973.

Indyk, L.: P_{O_2} in the seventies, Pediatrics **55**:18 1975.

Johnson, J. D., Malachowski, N. C., Grobstein, R., et al.: Prognosis of children surviving with the aid of mechanical ventilation in the newborn period, J. Pediatr. **84**:272, 1974.

Karlberg, P.: The adaptive changes in the immediate postnatal period, with particular reference to respiration, J. Pediatr. **56**:585, 1960.

Karlberg, P.: The first breaths of life. In Gluck, L., editor: Modern perinatal medicine, Chicago, 1974, Year Book Medical Publishers, Inc.

Kattwinkel, J., Fleming, D., Cha, C. C., et al.: A device for administration of continuous positive airway pressure by the nasal route, Pediatrics **52**:131, 1973.

Kitterman, J. A., Phibbs, R. H., and Tooley, W. H.: Aortic blood pressure in normal newborn infants during the first 12 hours of life, Pediatrics **44**:959, 1969.

Klaus, M. H.: Respiratory function and pulmonary disease in the newborn. In Barnett, H. L., editor: Pediatrics, New York, 1968, Appleton-Century-Crofts.

Klaus, M. H.: Cleansing the neonatal trachea, J. Pediatr. **85**:853, 1974.

Koop, C. E., Schnaufer, L., and Broennie, A. M.: Esophageal atresia and tracheoesophageal fistula: supportive measures that affect survival, Pediatrics **54**:558, 1974.

Krauss, D. R., and Marshall, R. E.: Severe neck ulceration from CPAP head box, J. Pediatr. **86**:286, 1975.

Kuhns, L. R., Bednarek, F. J., and Wyman, M. L.: Diagnosis of pneumothorax or pneumomediastinum in the neonate by transillumination, Pediatrics **56**:355, 1975.

Leonidas, J. C., Hall, R. T., Holder, T. M., and Amoury, R. A.: Pneumoperitoneum associated with chronic respiratory disease in the newborn, Pediatrics **51**:933, 1973.

Levy, R. J.: Persistent pulmonary hypertension in a newborn with congenital diaphragmatic hernia: successful management with tolazoline, Pediatrics **60**:740, 1977.

Liggins, G. C.: The prevention of RDS by maternal steroid therapy. In Gluck, L., editor: Modern perinatal medicine, Chicago, 1974, Year Book Medical Publishers, Inc.

Liggins, G. C., and Howie, R. N.: A controlled trial of antepartum glucocorticoid treatment for prevention of the respiratory distress syndrome in premature infants, Pediatrics **50**:515, 1972.

Marriage, K. J., and Davies, P. A.: Neurological sequelae in children surviving mechanical ventilation in the neonatal period, Arch. Dis. Child. **52**:176, 1977.

Merenstein, G. B., Dougherty, K., and Lewis, A.: Early detection of pneumothorax by oscilloscope monitor in the newborn infant, J. Pediatr. **80**:98, 1972.

Merritt, T. A., DiSessa, T. G., Feldman, B. H., et al.: Closure of the patent ductus arteriosus with ligation and indomethacin: a consecutive experience, J. Pediatr. **93**:639, 1978.

Morrow, G., III, Hope, J. W., and Boggs, R., Jr.: Pneumomediastinum: a silent lesion in the newborn, J. Pediatr. **70**:554, 1967.

Northway, W. J., Jr., Rosan, R. C., and Porter, D. Y.: Pulmonary disease following respirator therapy of hyaline-membrane disease: bronchopulmonary dysplasia, N. Engl. J. Med. **276**:357, 1967.

Oski, F. A., and Delivoria-Papadopoulos, M.: The red cell, 2,3-diphosphoglycerate, and tissue oxygen release, J. Pediatr. **77**:941, 1970.

Outerbridge, E. W., Roloff, D. W., and Stern, L.: Continuous negative pressure in the management of severe respiratory distress syndrome, J. Pediatr. **81**:384, 1972.

Philip, A. G. S.: Oxygen plus pressure plus time: the etiology of bronchopulmonary dysplasia, Pediatrics **55**:44, 1975.

Reynolds, E. O. R., and Taghizadeh, A.: Improved prognosis of infants mechanically ventilated for hyaline membrane disease, Arch. Dis. Child. **49**:505, 1974.

Rhodes, P. G., Hall, R. T., and Leonidas, J. C.: Chronic pulmonary disease in neonates with assisted ventilation, Pediatrics **55**:788, 1975.

Robert, M. F., Neff, R. K., Hubbell, J. B., et al.: Maternal diabetes and the respiratory distress syndrome, N. Engl. J. Med. **294**:357, 1976.

Rooth, G.: Transcutaneous oxygen tension measurements in newborn infants, Pediatrics **55**:232, 1975.

Rowe, R. D.: Abnormal pulmonary vasoconstriction in the newborn, Pediatrics **59**:318, 1977.

Rudolph, A. M.: Congenital diseases of the heart, Chicago, 1974, Year Book Medical Publishers, Inc.

Stahlman, M.: Recovery from the respiratory distress syndrome, Pediatrics **52**:280, 1973.

Stahlman, M. T., and Gray, M. E.: Anatomical development and maturation of the lungs, Clin. Perinatol. **5**:181, 1978.

Stahlman, M., Hedvall, G., Dolanski, E., et al.: A six-year follow-up of clinical hyaline membrane disease, Pediatr. Clin. North Am. **20**:433, 1973.

Stern, L.: The use and misuse of oxygen in the newborn infant, Pediatr. Clin. North Am. **20**:447, 1973.

Stevenson, D. K., et al.: Refractory hypoxemia associated with neonatal pulmonary disease: the use and limitations of tolazoline, J. Pediatr. **95**:595, 1979.

Stiehm, E. R., and Rich, K.: Recognition and management of shock in pediatric patients. In Gluck, L.: Current problems in pediatrics, vol. 3, Chicago, 1973, Year Book Medical Publishers, Inc.

Strang, L. B.: Onset of breathing and its control in the neonatal period. In Neonatal respiration: physiological and clinical studies, Philadelphia, 1977, Blackwell Scientific Publications, Ltd.

Strong, R. M., and Passey, V.: Endotracheal intubation, Arch. Otolaryngol. **103**:329, 1977.

Sundell, H., et al.: Studies on infants with type II respiratory distress syndrome, J. Pediatr. **78**:754, 1971.

Thibeault, D. W., Lachman, R. S., Laul, V. R., and Kwong, M. S.: Pulmonary interstitial emphysema, pneumomediastinum, and pneumothorax, Am. J. Dis. Child. **126**:611, 1973.

Ting, P., and Brady, J.: Tracheal suction in meconium aspiration, Pediatr. Res. **7**:398, 1973.

Tyler, D. C., Murphy, J., and Cheney, F. W.: Mechanical and chemical damage to lung tissue caused by meconium aspiration, Pediatrics **62**:454, 1978.

Walsh, S. Z., Meyer, W. W., and Lind, J.: The human fetal and neonatal circulation, Springfield, Ill., 1974, Charles C Thomas, Publisher.

Weller, M. H.: The roentgenographic course and complications of hyaline membrane disease, Pediatr. Clin. North Am. **20**:381, 1973.

Workshop on bronchopulmonary dysplasia, J. Pediatr. **95**:815-920, 1979.

Yeh, T. F., Vidyasagar, D., and Pildes, R. S.: Neonatal pneumopericardium, Pediatrics **54**:429, 1974.

Yeh, T. F., Srinivasan, G., Harris, V., and Pildes, R. S.: Hydrocortisone therapy in meconium aspiration syndrome: a controlled study, J. Pediatr. **90**:140, 1977.

Yu, V. Y. H., Liew, S. W., and Roberton, N. R. C.: Pneumothorax in the newborn: changing pattern, Arch. Dis. Child. **50**:449, 1975.

Hematologic disorders

Perplexing hematologic problems are more frequent during the neonatal period than at any other time in childhood. The most common manifestations of neonatal blood disorders are anemia, hemorrhage into tissues, hyperbilirubinemia, and polycythemia. Anemia may be the end result of hemolysis, blood loss, or impaired red cell production. Hemorrhage into tissues is produced by disorders of the clotting mechanism. Hyperbilirubinemia follows intravascular hemolysis or the degradation of extravasated blood. Polycythemia is the result of an oversupply of blood to the fetus.

HEMOGLOBIN IN NORMAL NEONATAL BLOOD

The normal neonate's blood volume at birth is somewhat influenced by the quantity of blood allowed to flow from the placenta before the cord is clamped. The placental circulation contains approximately 75 to 125 ml at term, comprising one fourth to one third of total fetal blood volume. The infant's blood volume may be increased significantly by allowing the placenta to empty. At birth, infants held at levels below the placenta tend to acquire blood, and those held above it may lose some. In normal circumstances approximately 25% of the placental blood is transfused into the infant within 15 seconds after birth; at the end of 1 minute 50% of blood is transferred. If a term infant is held below the level of the placenta and clamping of the cord is delayed several minutes, blood volume can be increased by 40% to 60%. The increase is greater in a premature infant. Whether this added volume has a salutary effect on the baby's subsequent course has not been well defined. Thus some studies indicate a lower incidence of respiratory distress if cord clamping is delayed, whereas others do not demonstrate such an association. In any event, during the first few days of life, hemoglobin concentrations are higher in babies whose cords are clamped late, but there is no evidence that the additional hemoglobin is of any particular benefit.

Hemoglobin and hematocrit determinations may vary according to sampling site. At birth and for several days thereafter, hemoglobin concentration is higher in capillary than in venous blood. Normal hemoglobin concentration in cord blood ranges from 16 to 19 grams/100 ml (mean, 16.8 grams/100 ml), whereas capillary values may be 2 to 8 grams/100 ml higher. Even higher capillary levels may result from peripheral circulatory stasis, in which slowed blood flow causes stasis of the red blood cells, thereby increasing their concentration.

Normally, hemoglobin concentrations rise up to 6 grams/100 ml during the first few hours of life, particularly if the cord is clamped late. This rise is due to shifts of fluid that result in decreased plasma volume. After 24 hours they decline slightly, and by the end of the first week hemoglobin levels are at least equal to or greater than that of cord blood. In normal term infants, there is ordinarily no significant decrease in hemoglobin during the first week of life. A drop during this period usually indicates blood loss or hemolysis. Venous values below 13 grams/100 ml or capillary hemoglobin less than 14.5 grams/100 ml are indicative of anemia. A normal decrease continues after the first week. At birth the reticulocyte count is

between 4% and 7%, but by the end of the first week it is 1% or less.

ANEMIA DUE TO HEMOLYSIS

An abnormally rapid rate of red cell breakdown causes anemia and hyperbilirubinemia. Ordinarily, erythropoiesis increases in response to hemolysis, thus augmenting the number of reticulocytes and nucleated red cells in circulating blood. The hallmarks of hemolysis are anemia, hyperbilirubinemia, reticulocytosis, and increased numbers of nucleated red cells. The most common causes of fetal and neonatal hemolysis are isoimmunization (maternofetal blood incompatibility) and infection. Less frequently, hemolytic anemia is due to toxic drug effects, erythrocyte enzyme defects, or abnormal red cell morphology.

Isoimmunization: Rh incompatibility (erythroblastosis fetalis)

Erythroblastosis fetalis is also known as hemolytic disease of the newborn. Before the widespread use of anti-Rh gamma globulin to prevent fetal disease, approximately one third of all cases of isoimmunization involved Rh incompatibility; this form of the disease is often serious. Most cases of isoimmunization are now due to ABO incompatibility, which is generally mild, occasionally severe.

Antigens and blood group factors. The terms *blood group antigens* and *blood group factors* are used interchangeably. There are a number of blood group systems, of which the Rh and ABO systems are the most significant. Other antigenic systems are only rarely involved in maternofetal blood incompatibilities. An antigen is a substance that stimulates the production of antibodies. Thousands of discrete patches of red cell antigens are situated on or in the covering cell membrane. The Rh system is comprised of six factors: C,c, D,d, and E,e. Although the terms *Rh positive* and *Rh negative* strictly indicate the presence or absence of any Rh factor, in common usage these terms refer to the D factor, which is involved in 95% of Rh incompatibilities.

Pathogenesis. In the pathogenesis of Rh disease, fetal red cells pass across the placenta to an Rh-negative mother, who produces antibodies to Rh antigen on fetal red cell surfaces. These antibodies are transmitted across the placenta to the fetus; they become attached to fetal red cells, and hemolysis follows. This course of events requires maternal antibody production, which can occur only in the presence of incompatibility between mother and fetus (Rh-negative mother, Rh-positive fetus). *The mother produces antibodies to fetal antigens only if her own cells lack these antigens.* This is the basis of Rh incompatibility. Thus an Rh-negative mother (whose cells lack D factor) is the recipient of erythrocytes from her Rh-positive fetus. She responds by generating anti-D antibodies, which pass across the placenta and become attached to the D antigen on fetal red cells, causing their eventual dissolution.

During normal pregnancy, small quantities of fetal blood (0.1 to 0.2 ml) may cross the placenta into the maternal circulation, whereas larger amounts are transferred during placental separation. During a first pregnancy, initial sensitization to D antigens does not occur prior to the onset of labor because at least 0.5 to 1 ml is required for a sensitizing maternal immune response. Thus the minute leakage of fetal blood before labor is insufficient to sensitize a primigravida, but the larger amount of blood transferred during placental separation is sufficient to cause sensitization. During the second

pregnancy with an Rh-positive fetus, the usual small amount of fetal blood leakage now acts as a booster dose because the mother has been previously sensitized, and her antibody production increases remarkably. Offspring of this and all subsequent pregnancies may thus be affected. Firstborn babies may be erythroblastotic if maternal sensitization has occurred after past transfusion of Rh-positive blood or if there was previous abortion of an Rh-positive fetus, but these events are unusual.

Clinical manifestations. The disease begins in utero, at which time its severity can be estimated by analysis of amniotic fluid (p. 11). In response to hemolysis, the rate of erythropoiesis is accelerated, and immature red cells (erythroblasts) appear in the fetal circulation. Red cell destruction releases hemoglobin, thus increasing the formation of bilirubin, which is largely, although not entirely, excreted across the placenta into the maternal circulation. At birth most affected infants have slightly elevated bilirubin levels, but jaundice is rarely evident. Anemia is present in proportion to the severity of hemolysis.

If amniocentesis has not been performed, the first visible indication of the severity of the disease may be the color of amniotic fluid at the time of membrane rupture. Straw-colored fluid is usually associated with mild or absent fetal disease; deep yellow fluid indicates a severely involved fetus. Intrauterine death may be associated with green- or brown-tinted fluid.

Most mildly affected infants appear to be normal at birth, although the liver and spleen may be somewhat enlarged. If the fetus is profoundly affected, pallor is obvious because of anemia.

The hemolytic process that originated

in utero continues after birth. Bilirubin production increases as a function of hemolysis, and now it accumulates in the infant because placental excretion is precluded. Anemia is progressive and the number of nucleated red cells increases. Although jaundice is usually not apparent at birth, it may appear 30 minutes later in the most severely affected babies. As a rule, it is evident within 24 to 36 hours. The liver and spleen may be enlarged so extensively as to reach well below the level of the umbilicus.

Hydrops fetalis is the most severe expression of Rh disease. Progressive anemia due to intense hemolysis leads to fetal hypoxia, cardiac failure, generalized edema, and effusion of fluid into the pleural, pericardial, and peritoneal spaces. Hydrops is a frequent cause of intrauterine death among infants with Rh disease. It generally appears between the thirty-fourth and fortieth gestational weeks. Intrauterine transfusion apparently supports some of these infants until an exchange transfusion can be performed after delivery. At birth, the most striking findings of hydrops fetalis include universal edema (anasarca) and alarming pallor. The edema may be so extensive that the infant is almost twice the expected birth weight for gestational age. Respiratory distress is sometimes severe. Jaundice is usually not apparent until later. Immediate exchange transfusion is urgent, but hydropic infants seldom survive.

Laboratory diagnosis. Fetal diagnosis of the disease and an accurate estimate of its severity are accomplished by analysis of amniotic fluid for bilirubin (p. 11). Repeated amniocentesis is usually essential to monitor the extent of fetal involvement. Erythroblastosis can also be anticipated by demonstrating a rising titer of anti-D antibodies in maternal serum during pregnancy, but this is not as reliable as amniotic fluid studies. These antibodies are produced by the mother in response to D factor on fetal cells that leaked through the placenta into her circulation. In the infant, the diagnosis is made postnatally by demonstrating these same antibodies on the surface of red blood cells. These maternal antibodies crossed the placenta to enter the fetal circulation. The diagnosis is accomplished by the direct Coombs' test. If anti-D antibody has become attached to D antigen on the infant's erythrocytes, the addition of Coombs' reagent causes visible agglutination of the cells, thus establishing the diagnosis of erythroblastosis. The diagnosis can be excluded if the Coombs' test is negative.

Treatment: exchange transfusion. The most effective treatment is exchange transfusion. Details of this procedure are well described in monographs devoted to erythroblastosis. Although the indications for exchange transfusions can be complex and equivocal, they are generally performed when bilirubin concentrations reach 20 mg/100 ml in term infants, 15 mg/100 ml in larger premature infants, and lower levels in smaller ones. The goal of treatment is to prevent the most sinister complication of the disease, kernicterus (p. 293), and to eliminate the possibility of progressively severe anemia. A "two-volume" exchange is utilized. This term refers to the exchange of an amount of donor blood that is twice the infant's blood volume. Donor blood is thus given at 170 ml/kg of body weight. This volume replaces 85% of the infant's blood. Fresh Rh-negative blood is used, either type O or the infant's own type. The transfusion is given through a catheter in the umbilical vein by alternately removing 7 to 20 ml of blood, depending on the size of the infant, and infusing like amounts of donor blood. The procedure should be completed in little over an hour. Careful attention to thermal balance is essential. The procedure thus should be performed under a source of radiant heat. In experienced hands the mortality rate from the complications of exchange transfusion is less than 1%.

The nurse must keep scrupulous records of the amount of blood transfused. Constant attention to cardiac and respiratory rates is essential, and this is greatly facilitated by the use of heart rate and apnea monitors. The nurse must be familiar with the potential hazards of an exchange transfusion.

Hazards of exchange transfusion. The possibilities for misadventure during exchange transfusion are numerous. *Heart failure* may occur as a result of transfusion overload if the infused blood volume is miscalculated. *Cardiac arrest due to hyperkalemia* may follow the use of old donor blood (over 4 days) because its serum potassium content is considerably higher than normal. Recent reports have demonstrated that the traditional practice of administering calcium gluconate after each 100 ml of exchanged blood may be neither necessary nor effective. Reduction of ionized calcium during exchange transfusion is related to binding of calcium by citrate in the ACD solution that is generally used as an anticoagulant in donor blood. Calcium levels do indeed fall gradually and considerably during the procedure. They return to normal a very short time later, sometimes within 10 minutes. The infants studied (term and premature) had no symptoms that could be related to hypocalcemia. Occasionally the nurse may encounter repeated bursts of *irregular cardiac rhythm* caused

by contact of the catheter tip with myocardium or by rapid injection of blood directly into the heart when the catheter is inserted too deeply. *Air embolus* may occur when large amounts of air are sucked into an open-ended catheter if the infant gasps deeply. The catheter should be filled with saline solution and attached to a stopcock before insertion. *Perforation of the umbilical vein* during vigorous attempts to force catheter passage may cause hemorrhage into the liver. Negligent technique adds to the hazard of *bacterial infection. Acidemia* may be severe during the exchange transfusion and for some time thereafter because the pH of donor blood is often 6.8 or less. At some centers, alkali is added to donor blood to avert acidemia, which is increased in the presence of cold stress, for want of an external heat source. *Hypoglycemia* occurs in Rh disease independently of exchange transfusion, but it may be aggravated by the procedure (Chapter 11). It is more frequent in severe than in mild erythroblastosis. Blood sugar determination, or a screening test such as Dextrostix, should be part of the overall evaluation of these babies before exchange transfusion. Dextrostix testing should be done every hour after the procedure for 2 to 4 hours. The treatment of hypoglycemia is described in Chapter 11.

Perforation of the intestine, primarily the colon, occurs in 1% to 2% of infants. The symptoms are those of a perforated gut or peritonitis. They include abdominal distension, bloody stools, bilious vomiting, gastric retention, respiratory distress, hypotension, pallor, and cyanosis. Abdominal distension appears first, usually within 48 hours of the last exchange transfusion. X-ray examination reveals free air in the peritoneal space in most instances, but perforation of the intestine often occurs without this sign. Intestinal dilatation and peritoneal fluid are also visible on x-ray films. Most infants require surgery, and postoperative recovery has been reported in 90% of infants. Intestinal perforation after exchange transfusion is attributed to ischemia of the gut. Blood flow to the intestine may be profoundly disrupted during the procedure as a result of back pressure created in the portal venous sytem during the injections of blood. Whereas the catheter tip should pass through the ductus venosus into the inferior vena cava, in fact this maneuver is not possible in the majority of cases. As the catheter passes through the umbilical vein in the liver, it is deflected into the portal vein. Blood is thus exchanged directly in and out of this vessel. Since the portal vein drains blood from the intestine, disruption of normal vascular pressure during exchange transfusion precludes normal blood flow to and from the intestinal wall. Diminished blood supply causes ischemia and necrosis. Perforation of the wall is the result of this process.

Phototherapy. The use of intense fluorescent lights for reduction of serum bilirubin levels is discussed in Chapter 10. Phototherapy is not recommended for treatment of Rh disease because the rate of hemolysis usually exceeds the rate of bilirubin diminution brought about by phototherapy.

Prevention. Erythroblastosis has recently become a preventable disease. Maternal sensitization can be prevented by the administration of high-titered, anti-D gamma globulin to unsensitized mothers (primigravidas) within 48 hours after delivery or abortion. The effectiveness of this vaccine is based on the fact, previously described, that fetal red cells enter the maternal circulation in greatest quantity at the time of delivery. In the presence of injected anti-D antibody, fetal cells passing into the maternal circulation are destroyed before they can exert their immunogenic effect. In essence, the mother is temporarily immunized against her fetus' invading red cells, and she is thus protected from sensitization. Administration of anti-Rh gamma globulin must be repeated after each delivery. This procedure is effective. The incidence of rhesus disease has declined remarkably.

Isoimmunization: ABO incompatibility

The disorder produced by incompatibility in the ABO groups is usually considerably milder than Rh disease. Group A or B infants of group O mothers are most commonly involved; group B infants of group A mothers are only occasionally affected. Group O infants are never affected, regardless of the mother's blood type.

ABO incompatibility differs from Rh disease in several respects. Preexistent natural anti-A and anti-B antibodies from group O mothers pass to the fetus without previous sensitization by leakage of fetal blood. As a result, firstborn infants are frequently involved, and there is no relationship between the appearance or severity of disease and repeated sensitization from one pregnancy to the next. Stillbirth and hydrops fetalis are rare. Jaundice is common; hepatosplenomegaly occurs inconsistently. Reticulocytosis indicates a hemolytic process, but significant anemia during the neonatal period and later is rare. The direct Coombs' test on the infant's cells may be negative or mildly positive, but the indirect Coombs' test utilizing infant's serum on adult red cells may be strongly positive. Infants whose direct Coombs' test is positive are more likely to be jaundiced, with bilirubin in excess of 10 mg/100 ml. An affected group A infant has demonstrable anti-A antibody in his serum. A blood smear reveals increased numbers of spherical, plump, mature erythrocytes called *spherocytes*. These cells are thicker and smaller in diameter than normal red cells. They are not observed in abnormally increased numbers on smears from infants with Rh disease. The usual indication for exchange transfusion for ABO incompatibility is progressive elevation of serum bilirubin concentration to 20 mg/100 ml in term infants and 15 mg/100 ml in premature infants. The donor blood must be group O; it should never be the infant's own type.

Hemolysis due to infection

Infectious diseases, bacterial and nonbacterial, are associated with hemolytic anemia. Hyperbilirubinemia, and to a lesser extent anemia, are often prominent signs of septicemia and neonatal renal infection. The nonbacterial infections that cause hemolysis are of intrauterine origin. They include cytomegalic inclusion disease, toxoplasmosis, rubella, herpesvirus, and coxsackievirus infections. Congenital syphillis also causes hemolysis. Hyperbilirubinemia during infections is due to hepatocellular damage as well as to hemolysis. Infections are discussed in Chapter 12.

Other causes of hemolysis

A number of enzymatic deificencies in red cells are known to cause hemolytic anemia. *Glucose-6-phosphate dehydrogenase (G-6-PD) deficiency* is the most common. It occurs primarily among blacks, Filipinos, Sephardic (not Ashkenazic) Jews, Sardinians, Greeks, and Arabs. It is genetically transmitted, occurring predominantly in males, rarely in females. The disorder is manifest during the newborn period in only a fraction of affected individuals. Jaundice and anemia are the presenting signs. A large number of drugs have been reported to cause hemolysis in G-6-PD–deficient patients. Most of these substances are rarely, if ever, used in the newborn infant.

Large doses of water-soluble vitamin K analogue (Synkavite, Hykinone) may produce severe jaundice. Doses of 1 mg do not cause such an effect. Vitamin K_1 is generally utilized rather than the water-soluble analogue because it appears to be safer in respect to hemolysis.

Vitamin E deficiency has been demonstrated as a cause of moderately severe hemolytic anemia in premature infants. Reticulocytosis and a tremendous number of platelets (thrombocytosis) are associated with the anemia. The most profoundly affected infants are severely edematous, often in association with cardiovascular difficulties and hypoproteinemia. Administration of vitamin E tocopherol) produces a rapid response. However, administration of alpha-tocopherol is effective only when the infant is chronologically at term. Until then, intestinal absorption is inefficient. Furthermore, simultaneous oral administration of iron preparations or of milk with iron results in impaired absorption of both.

Abnormal morphology of erythrocytes occurs in several varieties; they are uncommon causes of hemolytic anemia. *Hereditary spherocytosis* is the most frequent of these conditions. The red cells are abnormally fragile and thus are predisposed to premature breakdown. The life span of these cells is therefore abnormally short. They are remarkably susceptible to deposition and dissolution in the spleen. The responsible molecular abnormality has not been identified. A substantial number of affected individuals have hemolytic anemia in the newborn period. Jaundice and pallor due to anemia are the outstanding signs of the disease. The blood smear reveals a preponderance of spherocytes. They are small and round, and they stain densely as a result of their spherical configuration. These cells are similar in appearance to those observed in ABO incompatibility. Treatment during the newborn period includes exchange transfusion for high bilirubin levels or simple transfusion if anemia is the only difficulty.

Hemolytic anemia has also been described in the rare entity known as *hereditary elliptocytosis*. Most of the red cells in affected infants are a bizarre elliptical shape, and those of one of the parents have a similar appearance. Treatment during the newborn period is the same as that for hereditary spherocytic anemia.

ANEMIA DUE TO LOSS OF BLOOD

Causes of fetal and neonatal blood loss

I. Cord
   A. Rupture of varices or aneurysms
   B. Traumatic rupture of normal cord
   C. Torn vessels with velamentous insertion
II. Placenta
   A. Incision into fetal side during cesarean section
   B. Placenta previa
   C. Abruptio placentae
   D. Multilobed placenta with interlobar vessels
III. Fetal blood loss
   A. Fetomaternal (acute or chronic blood loss)
   B. Fetofetal (into twin, acute or chronic blood loss)
IV. Enclosed hemorrhage
   A. Intracranial
   B. Ruptured liver
   C. Ruptured spleen
   D. Adrenal hemorrhage
   E. Retroperitoneal
   F. Subaponeurotic (scalp)
   G. Cephalhematoma
   H. Pulmonary (massive)

Prenatal blood loss

The fetus may lose blood before or during parturition. In utero it may bleed into the mother's circulation, into the vessels of a twin, or as a result of mishap during the birth process. The latter is usually due to some factor in the placenta or cord that predisposes to ruptured vessels or to operative complication during cesarean section.

Fetomaternal transfusion is a common phenomenon, but resultant abnormal clinical signs in the neonate are infrequent. Loss of fetal blood presumably occurs at the intervillous spaces. The precise site of placental leak has not been demonstrated. Fetal blood cells in maternal circulation have been detected in as many as 50% of pregnancies; yet in only 1% of them is blood loss sufficient to cause neonatal anemia. Fetal red cells are easily detected in maternal circulation by the acid elution technique. They do not disappear completely for several weeks after delivery.

Fetofetal transfusion occurs in monochorionic (identical) twins through arteriovenous anastomoses in the common placenta. This condition is also known as the *intrauterine parabiotic syndrome*. The effect of blood loss on the donor twin depends on the size of the transfusion and its duration. Clinical signs of acute or chronic blood loss may therefore occur (see later). In the extreme, death occurs in utero early in pregnancy. In approximately 15% of monochorionic twins, or perhaps more, significant anemia occurs in the donor. Hemoglobin has been reported as low as 5 grams/100 ml. Signs of acute or chronic hemorrhage are observed. The donor twin is often considerably smaller than the recipient and may be severely undergrown for dates. All the physical attributes of in utero undergrowth are in evidence. Oligohydramnios and hypotension are also common. Postnatal hypoglycemia occurs as a result of intrauterine malnutrition. Pallor is impressive proportional to the anemia. The recipient twin is polycythemic, with a significantly increased blood volume. Hemoglobin concentration may be 20 to 30 grams/100 ml volume. A deep red complexion contrasts dramatically with the pallor of the donor sibling. Polyhydramnios and hypertension are common. The recipient sibling may be strikingly larger than his twin, often appearing overnourished by comparison. The size of twins differs little if the transfusion occurs late in pregnancy. Thus, gross differences may exist in blood volume and other hematologic attributes in the absence of other discrepancies of size and development. The cardiovascular, pulmonary, and central nervous system signs of polycythemia (see later) are noted in the recipient baby.

Obstetric misadventure may cause life-threatening fetal blood loss. In all instances the signs of acute hemorrhage are in evidence. Placenta previa and abruptio placentae are sometimes associated with fetal as well as maternal hemorrhage. Anomalous vessels at the insertion of the cord (velamentous) are vulnerable to disruption and hemorrhage. Even the normal cord can be torn if it is inordinately short or regardless of length during unattended delivery. Severe acute hemorrhage may complicate cesarean section if the placenta is inadvertently in-

cised during the procedure. In multilobular placentas, the vascular connections between lobes rupture easily, which may result in severe fetal hemorrhage. During cesarean section, delayed clamping of the cord causes anemia *if the baby is above the level of the placenta*. The infant is usually placed on the mother's abdomen, or is held at approximately that level, when the cord is clamped and cut. A significant amount of blood thus passes from fetus to placenta by virtue of gravity if clamping is delayed. Furthermore, unlike the situation in vaginal deliveries, the uterus is not contracted; it is atonic. This enhances backflow of blood to the placenta because low vascular resistance persists. The result is reduction in blood volume, red blood cell volume, and plasma volume. These values are significantly higher, however, if delayed clamping occurs *while the infant is below the level of the placenta*.

Acute hemorrhage may result from any of the conditions listed previously; fetomaternal and fetofetal transfusions are most often chronic. The signs of acute hemorrhage are those of hypovolemia (shock) and anemia. They are generally present at birth and include pallor, cyanosis, tachycardia, feeble or absent pulses, gasping, tachypnea, and retractions. The cry is weak, spontaneous activity is absent or diminished, and flaccidity is severe. Superficially these infants appear to be asphyxiated, but three differentiating clinical signs are helpful. First, babies who are in shock from acute blood loss have a rapid heart rate (over 160 beats/min) unless they are also profoundly hypoxic; infants who are only asphyxiated usually have bradycardia as a result of profound hypoxemia. Second, infants in shock remain cyanotic in spite of oxygen therapy; asphyxiated babies respond to it. Third, infants who are in shock usually breathe rapidly; asphyxiated infants breathe slowly. Acute blood loss should be suspected in the presence of these differentiating signs. Suspicion is the initial step; without it the baby is lost. The diagnosis is more assured if there is knowledge of an obstetric accident. Low hemoglobin and hematocrit values are diagnostic, but they are sometimes misleadingly normal at birth. The hematocrit may remain normal immediately after acute blood loss because often 3 or 4 hours must pass before hemodilution occurs from the influx of interstitial fluid into the circulation in an attempt to maintain blood volume. Hemoglobin values in capillary blood may be a source of error; they can be spuriously high because of severe stasis of peripheral circulation. Venous blood samples are preferable. Immediate transfusion is lifesaving.

Protracted fetomaternal or fetofetal hemorrhage is associated with slowly developing anemia and compensatory adjustment of blood volume. At birth, affected infants are pale and anemic, but misleadingly vigorous. Several reports have described pale babies, otherwise apparently well, whose hemoglobin concentrations were as low as 5 grams/100 ml. After chronic intrauterine blood loss, hemoglobin at birth may range from 5 to 12 grams/100 ml. The temptation to immediately transfuse a chronically anemic baby is often irresistible. If signs attributable to severe anemia (tachycardia, hypoxia) are evident, a packed-cell transfusion is indeed indicated. There is no need to rapidly restore hematocrit or hemoglobin values to normal levels, certainly not to levels higher than 35 vol % or 12 grams/100 ml, respectively. Packed cells should be given as a partial exchange transfusion. The red cell mass required to increase the hematocrit to 35 vol % is calculated, and the packed cells are given in exchange for equal volumes of the infant's blood. This technique avoids volume overload while simultaneously increasing red cell mass. Two characteristics of chronic intrauterine blood loss must be kept in mind for their critical therapeutic implications. Most important is that generally there is no diminution in blood volume in chronic loss that can compare with that of acute loss. Rapid, overzealous transfusion is thus dangerous; it may overload the vascular space and cause failure of a heart that already functions marginally because of severe anemia. Second, chronic blood loss involves iron deficiency. Therefore many of these babies do not require transfusion at all; they need only elemental iron, 5 to 10 mg/kg of body weight daily. The iron therapy should be maintained for a year.

Postnatal blood loss

Postnatal hemorrhage most often occurs into enclosed spaces (see list on p. 275). Defects of the clotting mechanism, also responsible for serious postnatal blood loss, are discussed later. Enclosed hemorrhage is a common cause of anemia during the first 3 days of life. *Intracranial hemorrhage* (subarachnoid, subdural, and intraventricular) may be sufficiently severe to cause a significant drop in hemoglobin, although signs of central nervous system dysfunction are predominant. *Hemorrhage into the scalp* may be extensive, resulting in massive blood loss and a hemoglobin concentration as low as 3 grams/100 ml. The scalp is boggy and thick, obscuring the sutures and fontanelles of the skull, and extending over the forehead to impart a blue suffusion to the skin. Deficiency of vitamin K–dependent and other clotting factors is often present in affected infants. We have encountered severe scalp hemorrhage in an infant with hemophilia. In addition, a high incidence of difficult labor and delivery has been noted. Scalp hemorrhage is first apparent from 30 minutes to 4 hours after birth. Pallor increases as blood continues to accumulate in the scalp, and if hemorrhage is severe, shock ensues. Transfusion is urgent, and intravenous sodium bicarbonate is also necessary because of severe metabolic acidosis. Vitamin K_1 or any other coagulation factor shown to be deficient should be given intravenously.

After traumatic labor, especially in breech deliveries, hemorrhage may occur into the liver, spleen, adrenals, and kidneys. Hemorrhage into the liver is particularly pernicious. It may also follow vigorous external cardiac massage. Blood accumulates beneath the liver capsule for a day or two while the infant appears quite well, although perhaps somewhat pale. When the capsule ruptures and pressure is released, bleeding from the liver becomes copious, and sudden shock ensues. Liver enlargement is easily palpated, and the upper abdomen appears distended, particularly after rupture of the capsule. Rupture of the spleen may occur during traumatic delivery, from severe enlargement in erythroblastosis fetalis, or during exchange transfusion.

Enclosed hemorrhage, in addition to causing shock, often gives rise to hyperbilirubinemia from degradation of the extravasated blood. Treatment first consists of simple transfusion for blood loss, and then if the bilirubin rises to 10 mg/100 ml, phototherapy is indicated (p. 296). Exchange transfusion is necessary if bilirubin continues to accumulate beyond

serum levels of 20 mg/100 ml and at lower levels in preterm infants.

DISORDERS OF COAGULATION

Hemorrhage may result from inherited disorders of the clotting mechanism, from clotting defects created by other disease processes, or from exaggerations of physiologic neonatal clotting deficiencies. Platelet abnormalities are also an important cause of hemorrhage. When trauma is superimposed on coagulation defects, serious hemorrhage may result, as exemplified by massive bleeding into the scalp. A complete presentation of the coagulation defects would not be appropriate here; discussion is thus restricted to the most prominent of these disorders, vitamin K deficiency, and platelet abnormalities.

Hemorrhagic disease of the newborn: vitamin K deficiency

Hemorrhagic disease of the newborn is a bleeding disorder during the first few days of life that is caused by a deficiency of vitamin K, which is in turn responsible for a deficiency of prothrombin and other coagulation factors (factors II, VII, IX, and X). These factors are generated in the liver, and their production is also dependent on normal hepatic function.

Vitamin K–dependent factors are substantially reduced from adult values at birth. In normal infants, particularly those fed cow's milk early, these levels are gradually restored. Hemorrhagic disease is rare in infants who receive cow's milk on the first day of life. Hemorrhage is most common in breast-fed infants. In a few babies (less than 0.5%), hemorrhage occurs as a result of sustained low levels. The babies of mothers who have taken phenobarbital and diphenylhydantoin (Dilantin) are especially at risk for vitamin K deficiency with severe hemorrhagic complications. They should not be treated in a routine fashion with vitamin K but rather should be treated as though actively bleeding; 1 to 2 mg of the vitamin are thus administered intravenously immediately after birth. Coagulation studies are obtained prior to treatment and should be repeated subsequently. As a rule, the hemorrhagic manifestations become apparent on the second or third day. Bloody or black stools (melena), hematuria, and oozing from the umbilicus are the most frequent signs. Hemorrhage from the nose, from the circumcision site, and into the scalp and skin (ecchymosis) is also visible. The most characteristic laboratory feature of the disease is a prolonged prothrombin time.

Prophylactic administration of vitamin K at birth prevents deficiencies of the involved clotting factors. Vitamin K_1 is the preferred preparation. The recommended intramuscular dose in 0.5 to 1 mg. Larger doses do not exert an increased prophylactic effect. Cow's milk contains approximately 6 μg of vitamin K per 100 ml, and breast milk contains only one fourth as much. The consumption of 10 ounces of cow's milk formula during the first 48 hours thus tends to restore the prothrombin time toward normal. In premature infants, the response to vitamin K administration and to early feedings is less pronounced, presumably because of immature liver function.

Vitamin K is effective in the treatment, as well as the prevention, of hemorrhagic disease. Intravenous administration of 1 to 2 mg is preferred to intramuscular injection in bleeding infants because the latter route results in large hematomas. This precaution applies to any bleeding diathesis. The coagulation defect is ordinarily corrected within 2 to 4 hours after vitamin K administration. Bleeding may be sufficiently pronounced to require blood transfusion for correction of diminished blood volume, or fresh-frozen plasma to supply the deficient coagulation factors.

THROMBOCYTOPENIA

Platelets are the smallest cells in the blood. They do not possess nuclei and are normally visible on a routine blood smear in small aggregations. Formed from megakaryocytes in the bone marrow, platelets are indispensable to effective coagulation. They function in the earliest stages of hemostasis by aggregating at points of vascular injury, where they literally act as a plug. They also release substances that are essential for coagulation in its later stages.

Clinical manifestations of platelet deficiency

Petechiae and ecchymoses are the characteristic lesions produced by platelet deficiencies. They are present at birth, or they appear any time therafter. Typically, new lesions continue to form in crops if the deficiency persists. Central nervous system hemorrhage is always a potential hazard in the presence of platelet deficiency, but fortunately it occurs infrequently. Although bleeding can sometimes be massive, it is usually insufficient to cause a significant decline in hemoglobin concentration. However, the breakdown of extravasated blood sometimes results in serious hyperbilirubinemia. The principal disorders that produce thrombocytopenia are infectious, pharmacologic, or immunologic in nature.

Thrombocytopenia due to infection

Thrombocytopenia is a frequent accompaniment of perinatal infection. Among the bacterial infections, septicemia is by far the most prominent. Congenital syphilis also produces platelet deficiency. Thrombocytopenia, petechiae, and ecchymoses are major clinical signs of congenital rubella, toxoplasmosis, cytomegalovirus infection, and herpesvirus infection (Chapter 12). These bacterial and nonbacterial infections may produce a constellation of signs comprised of hepatosplenomegaly, jaundice, anemia, and thrombocytopenia.

Thrombocytopenia induced by drugs

A number of drugs taken by the mother during pregnancy may destroy her platelets and the platelets of her fetus as well. The sulfonamides and quinine are of significance because of their widespread use in the past. These and other drugs stimulate the production of maternal antibodies, which destroy maternal platelets and cross the placenta to exert identical effects in the fetus.

Thrombocytopenia is also produced by the thiazides, a group of diuretics used for the treatment of preeclamptic edema. In these circumstances, platelet antibodies are not produced in the mother; her own platelets remain intact, but those of the fetus are destroyed by toxic effects of the drug. Thrombocytopenia may persist for as long as 3 months after birth in some infants. In a few babies, hemorrhage may be extensive, primarily involving the gastrointestinal tract, brain, and lungs.

Thrombocytopenia induced by immune mechanisms

Fetal platelets may be destroyed by placental passage of antibody from the mother. This destruction is rare, and it is produced by two distinct mechanisms. In one type, antiplatelet antibodies are the result of maternal disease. They destroy her platelets and cross the placenta to destroy those of her fetus. This mechanism is operative in maternal idiopathic thrombocytopenic purpura and systemic lupus erythematosus. In another type of immune mechanism, the mother's platelets are unaffected. This pattern is similar to that described for erythroblastosis fetalis. Platelets are serologically distinct because of the different antigens they possess. When fetal platelets enter the maternal circulation, the mother produces antibodies to them that cross the placenta to destroy fetal platelets. The resultant disease varies widely in severity. Intracranial hemorrhage is apparently more common in this type of thrombocytopenia than in most others. Firstborn infants are frequently affected. The clinical signs are otherwise similar to any other type of platelet deficiency.

Thrombocytopenia and giant hemangioma

Congenital hemangiomas, usually large ones, may reduce the number of circulating platelets considerably. These vascular tumors trap and destroy tremendous numbers of platelets, thereby creating thrombocytopenia, which causes generalized bleeding. The platelet count of blood within the hemangioma is higher than in blood taken from other sites. Generalized hemorrhage is usually preceded by abrupt swelling and tenseness of the hemangioma. Treatment consists of irradiation of the hemangioma, which usually shrinks in several days. Removal of the tumor may be urgent if it compresses the trachea when situated in the neck. Irradiation should be given first, surgical excision may follow a few days later.

Disseminated intravascular coagulation (DIC)

Intravascular coagulation is produced by a diversity of factors that themselves are associated with a multiplicity of disease states. It is therefore the symptom complex that results from a number of serious disorders. It is characterized by inappropriate activation of the clotting process. Inordinately rapid consumption of clotting factors and platelets occurs during intravascular coagulation, and DIC is thus also referred to as *consumption coagulopathy.* The resultant depletion of these factors leads to a paradoxic hemorrhagic diathesis, which constitutes the most serious threat of this syndrome.

Any disorder that introduces a stimulus to clotting into the bloodstream can cause DIC. In the neonate, infections of bacterial and viral origin are the most common sources of such stimuli. Bacterial septicemia due to gram-negative rods, disseminated herpesvirus, and rubella are particularly noteworthy. It has been noted in association with abruptio placentae, presumably in response to the entry of amniotic fluid into the fetal circulation. Severe antigen-antibody reactions, as in Rh disease, also seem to be responsible for triggering this process.

Clinical signs are variable and widespread because bleeding may occur anywhere in the body. Bleeding from venipunctures is a very common initial sign, even from the punctures inflicted 24 hours previously. Life-threatening hemorrhage into vital organs is cause for considerable anxiety when coagulation factors and platelets are extremely depressed.

The presumptive diagnosis can be made by demonstrating prolonged prothrombin time (PT) and partial thromboplastin time (PTT), thrombocytopenia, and a decreased fibrinogen level. Strong evidence for the diagnosis is the presence of fragmentation of red cells on a routine blood smear. Their architecture is disrupted as they pass through the smallest vessels in which fibrin thrombi have formed as a result of intravascular coagulation. The red cells are sheared by the microthrombi. Treatment, to be ultimately effective, must be directed against the underlying disorder. With few exceptions such treatment is too time-consuming; something more immediate must be done to reverse the life-threatening hemorrhagic tendency. Heparin is usually given to interrupt the ongoing coagulation. When effective, it halts consumption of platelets and clotting factors that are being incorporated into the intravascular clots. Bleeding then ceases. Heparin is given intravenously, 100 units/kg/4 hr. Exchange transfusion blood is also effective.

POLYCYTHEMIA AND INCREASED BLOOD VOLUME

Increased blood volume and hematocrit values may arise from four possible sources: (1) prolonged emptying of placental blood into the infant after birth, (2) continuous transfer of maternal blood to the fetus (maternofetal transfusion), (3) transfusion from a donor twin in utero (fetofetal transfusion), and (4) increased red cell production. In the last category are small-for-dates babies, infants who experienced intrauterine hypoxia, and babies with certain chromosomal abnormalities.

The normal, benign upper limits of hemoglobin and hematocrit values are difficult to define precisely. Infants with high levels are often asymptomatic, whereas some are quite ill from less extensively elevated levels. As a rule, difficulties should be anticipated if the hemoglobin concentration exceeds 23 grams/100 ml and the hematocrit is over 70%. Some authors have noted symptoms at 60% or over. Increased blood volume and viscosity seem to be related to several clinical signs. Respiratory distress occurs, and there is some evidence that it is a consequence of diminished pulmonary compliance because engorged vasculature probably stiffens the lungs. Cardiac decompensation may result from an increased blood volume. Convulsions, which have been observed in association with hypervolemia and polycythemia, are presumably caused by suboptimal brain perfusion associated with increased blood viscosity. Finally, hyperbilirubinemia often follows polycythemia at birth because larger amounts of bilirubin are formed by the breakdown of increased numbers of red cells. Treatment requires withdrawal of blood in amounts determined by the extent of plethora and size of the infant. This is accomplished by small exchange transfusion in which plasma replaces blood, volume for volume.

SUMMATION

Most of the blood disorders discussed in this chapter are a threat to the infant's intact survival, although they usually constitute only a transient threat. In the majority of instances, early recognition and rapid treatment can avert tragedy. A nurse's role in the early recognition of difficulty cannot be overestimated. With knowledge of the course of pregnancy and labor she can anticipate many of the described abnormalities before birth. Thus, if a preeclamptic woman has taken thiazides during pregnancy, it is possible that thrombocytopenia will appear in her

offspring. If placenta previa or abruptio placentae were present or if cesarean section was performed, shock due to fetal blood loss is a distinct possibility. If twins are delivered, plethora in one and severe anemia in the other are potential threats. Recognition of abnormal clinical signs, combined with the history of pregnancy, provides the nurse with alertness to the problems that may arise. The most gratifying results of such alertness are realized in instances of acute blood loss, when prompt action is an absolute necessity. The potential danger of this occurrence is suggested by the history; its presence is indicated by clinical signs and confirmed by laboratory results. As in so many other aspects of neonatal disease, the nurse is in a position to initiate appropriate management of blood disorders, if only by calling attention to their presence.

REFERENCES

Allen, F. H., and Diamond, L. K.: Erythroblastosis fetalis, Boston, 1958, Little, Brown & Co.

Barrow, E., and Peters, R. L.: Exsanguinating hemorrhage into scalp in newborn infants, S. Afr. Med. J. **42:**265, 1968.

Bleyer, W. A., Hakami, N., and Shepard, T. H.: The development of hemostasis in the human fetus and newborn infant, J. Pediatr. **79:**838, 1971.

Danks, D. M., and Stevens, L. H.: Neonatal respiratory distress associated with a high hematocrit reading, Lancet **2:**499, 1964.

Gatti, R. A., et al.: Neonatal polycythemia with transient cyanosis and cardiorespiratory abnormalities, J. Pediatr. **69:**1063, 1966.

Gershanik, J. J., Levkoff, A. H., and Duncan, R.: Serum ionized calcium values in relation to exchange transfusion, J. Pediatr. **82:**847, 1973.

Gross, G. P., Hathaway, W. E., and McGaughey, H. R.: Hyperviscosity in the neonate, J. Pediatr. **82:**1004, 1973.

Gross, S., and Melhorn, D. K.: Exchange transfusion with citrated whole blood for disseminated intravascular coagulation, J. Pediatr. **78:**415, 1971.

Gross, S., and Melhorn, D. K.: Vitamin E., red cell

lipids and red cell stability in prematurity, Ann. N.Y. Acad. Sci. **203**:141, 1972.

Hathaway, W. E., Mull, M. M., and Pechet, G. S.: Disseminated intravascular coagulation in the newborn, Pediatrics **43**:233, 1969.

Immunohematology; principles and practice: a programmed instruction course, Raritan, N. J., 1965, Ortho Pharmaceutical Corp.

Maisels, M. J., Li, T., Piechocki, J. T., and Werthman, M. W.: The effect of exchange transfusion on serum ionized calcium, Pediatrics **53**:683, 1974.

Michael, A. F., and Mauer, A. M.: Maternal-fetal transfusion as a cause of plethora in the neonatal period, Pediatrics **28**:458, 1961.

Naeye, R.: Human intrauterine parabiotic syndrome and its complications, N. Engl. J. Med. **268**:804, 1963.

Naiman, J. L.: Current management of hemolytic disease of the newborn infant, J. Pediatr. **80**:1049, 1972.

Orzalesi, M.: ABO system incompatibility: relationship between direct Coombs' test positivity and neonatal jaundice, Pediatrics **51**:288, 1973.

Oski, F. A., and Naiman, J. L.: Hematologic problems in the newborn, ed. 2, Philadelphia, 1972, W. B. Saunders Co.

Queenan, J. T.: Modern management of the Rh problem, New York, 1967, Harper & Row, Publishers.

Sacks, M. O.: Occurrence of anemia and polycythemia in pheno-typically dissimilar single-ovum human twins, Pediatrics **24**:604, 1959.

Saigal, S., O'Neill, A., Surainder, Y., et al.: Placental transfusion and hyperbilirubinemia in the premature, Pediatrics **49**:406, 1972.

Schulman, I.: Anemias due to increased destruction of red cells. In Barnett, H. L., editor: Pediatrics, New York, 1968, Appleton-Century-Crofts.

Sisson, T. R. C., Knutson, S., and Kendall, N.: The blood volume of infants. IV. Infants born by cesarean section, Am. J. Obstet. Gynecol. **117**:351, 1973.

Touloukian, R. J., Kadar, A., and Spencer, R. P.: The gastrointestinal complications of neonatal umbilical venous exchange transfusion: a clinical and experimental study, Pediatric **51**:36. 1973.

Usher, R., and Lind, J.: Blood volume of the newborn premature infant, Acta Paediatr. Scand. **54**:419, 1965.

CHAPTER 10

Neonatal jaundice

According to adult standards, all neonates have hyperbilirubinemia; their serum bilirubin levels exceed 1 mg/100 ml at some time during the first few days of life. These elevations of serum bilirubin levels produce visible jaundice in only half of all newborn infants, and for the majority of these babies the icterus is a normal event; in others it may indicate a number of disorders of diverse etiology (see outline, p. 287).

BILIRUBIN IN THE NORMAL NEONATE
Types of bilirubin (conjugated and unconjugated)

The existence of direct- and indirect-reacting bilirubin has been known for over 50 years, but the chemical differences that characterize them were first demonstrated in the 1950s. Direct-reacting bilirubin is bilirubin glucuronide, which is also referred to as conjugated bilirubin because the free bilirubin molecule undergoes conjugation with a glucuronide radical in the liver. Because the resultant complex is water soluble, it is normally excreted through the biliary tree and also through the kidneys if serum levels are abnormally high. Indirect-reacting bilirubin is unconjugated bilirubin because it has not been converted to the glucuronide form in the liver. Since it is fat soluble and not water soluble, it cannot be excreted in bile or through the kidneys. Because it is fat soluble, unconjugated bilirubin has a high affinity for extravascular tissue, particularly fatty tissue and brain. In plasma it is complexed to albumin. A laboratory report of total bilirubin includes the direct and indirect fractions and does not distinguish between them unless the direct fraction is specifically determined.

Formation of bilirubin

The fetus excretes bilirubin across the placenta into the maternal circulation. Only unconjugated (indirect) bilirubin is discarded by the placental route; conjugated (direct) bilirubin is not. The fetal liver is severely limited in its capacity to conjugate bilirubin. In exceptional circumstances, however, substantial quantities of direct bilirubin are demonstrable at birth. This has been observed in severe Rh disease that is managed by intrauterine transfusions, severe congenital rubella, toxoplasmosis, cytomegalovirus infection, and other severe infections.

Approximately 80% of the body's bilirubin is formed from the breakdown of erythrocytes. The life span of a normal neonatal red cell is estimated at 80 to 100 days by different investigators (adult life span is 120 days); its fragility increases as the cell ages, and it is then sequestered from the blood. Hemoglobin is then split into 2 fragments, heme and globin. The globin fraction is a protein, and it is utilized as such by the body. Unconjugated bilirubin is formed from heme in reticuloendothelial cells that are primarily located in the spleen and liver. One gram of hemoglobin yields 35 mg of unconjugated bilirubin. The normal neonate produces bilirubin at a rate of 6 to 8 mg/kg/24 hr. The remaining 20% of the body's bilirubin is produced by destruction of early red cell forms soon after their release from bone marrow or within the marrow itself and from nonhemoglobin sources that are predominantly in the liver.

Bilirubin in plasma (albumin binding)

Once formed, bilirubin is transported in plasma to the liver, where it is conjugated with glucuronide (see later). In plasms, unconjugated bilirubin is bound to albumin; 1 gram of albumin binds between 8.5 and 17 mg of bilirubin. The albumin molecule has two binding sites for bilirubin. One of them binds bilirubin tightly, the other more loosely. These loosely bound bilirubin molecules tend to migrate to plasma as free (unbound) bilirubin. After complete saturation of "tight" binding sites, there is a relatively abrupt rise in loosely bound or free bilirubin. The level of bilirubin at which saturation occurs is extremely variable. Bilirubin that is complexed to albumin cannot leave the vascular space. A minute amount of the pigment is unbound, in which state it is free to leave the blood and permeate tissues. It is in the unbound state that bilirubin also diffuses into liver cells, where conjugation with glucuronide takes place. When not bound to albumin, bilirubin permeates other extravascular tissues, including the brain. The quantity of unbound bilirubin is increased if albumin-binding capacity is reduced or if the affinity of bilirubin for albumin is diminished. This may occur in several circumstances. Thus, unconjugated bilirubin may accumulate to levels that surpass albumin-binding capacity. This accumulation generally occurs at serum bilirubin levels of 20 mg/100 ml or more, but it is quite variable, depending on maturity and illness of the baby. Furthermore, at any serum level, bilirubin is displaceable from albumin-binding sites by several substances having a greater affinity for these sites. These substances include metabolites such as free fatty acids, or drugs such as sulfonamides, salicylates, and sodium benzoate. Albumin-binding capacity is also reduced in the presence of an acid blood pH. Hypoalbuminemia causes low binding capacity, whereas binding capacity can be increased by giving albumin intravenously. Neonatal serum albumin does not bind bilirubin as effectively as adult serum albumin. Thus, gram for gram, "fetal albumin" has a lower binding capacity than that of the adult. Binding capacity increases with age to approximately adult levels by 5 months. The binding capacity of purified human serum albumin, administered at the time of exchange transfusion to augment bilirubin removal, is half that of circulating serum albumin in adults. Neonatal serum albumin falls between the two.

Bilirubin in the liver; conjugation and excretion

The liver cell is uniquely effective in removing unconjugated bilirubin from blood. Once within the cell, the bilirubin is bound to and transferred by a substance called "Y protein" (ligandin) and also less effectively by "Z protein." These proteins are intracellular carriers of bilirubin and other substances as well. Diminished activity of ligandin contributes to the limited capacity of the neonate's liver to take up and excrete bilirubin.

The conjugation of bilirubin with a glucuronide radical takes place within liver cells through a series of reactions that culminates in the transfer of glucuronic acid from uridine diphosphate glucuronic acid (UDPGA) to bilirubin. This last reaction is catalyzed by the transfer enzyme, glucuronyl transferase. These reactions transpire in the smooth endoplasmic reticulum of the liver cell. The steps that precede the formation of UDPGA require oxygen and glucose. Oxygen deprivation and hypoglycemia may thus impair UDPGA production and contribute to hyperbilirubinemia. Bilirubin glucuronide is passed from the liver cell into the biliary tree and thence into the gastrointestinal tract.

The fetal and neonatal small intestinal mucosa contains a considerable amount of the enzyme beta-glucuronidase. This substance can convert the bilirubin glucuronide that has entered the intestine back to unconjugated bilirubin by splitting off the glucuronide. Bilirubin is now fat soluble once again and is absorbed across the intestinal wall into the portal (enterohepatic) circulation. Meconium contains 0.5 to 1 mg of bilirubin per gram. Delayed meconium passage thus increases the amount of bilirubin reabsorbed across intestinal mucosa because more bilirubin glucuronide is converted to the unconjugated reabsorbable form. This "enterohepatic shunt" contributes significantly to physiologic jaundice: it may explain the high incidence of hyperbilirubinemia in some cases of upper intestinal obstruction. It is the mechanism by which late feeding, because it promotes intestinal stasis, results in higher mean serum bilirubin levels than does early feeding. The old practice of withholding feedings for 48 hours has long been discontinued for this and several other good reasons as well. During the first few days of life the neonate's capacity to excrete bilirubin is only 1% or 2% that of the adult's. This apparently related to deficient activity of glucuronyl transferase, which increases gradually after a few days, probably attaining adult levels at 2 to 4 weeks of age.

Physiologic jaundice

Although a deficiency of glucuronyl transferase has been said to be the major cause of physiologic jaundice, the diminution in activity of this enzyme is not as profound as previously believed. Glucuronyl transferase deficiency is not the sole cause of physiologic jaundice; a number of other immature functional difficulties are accountable. First, *an excessive amount of bilirubin is delivered to the liver* because synthesis is increased and because there is significant reabsorption of the pigment from the intestine via the enterohepatic shunt (see previous discussion). For several reasons, the neonate generates three times more bilirubin per kilogram of body weight than the adult. The number of red cells per kilogram of weight is greater, and these cells have shorter survival times (70 to 90 days versus 120 days in adults). Therefore, senescent red cells are sequestered and dismembered in greater numbers during shorter time intervals to yield a higher rate of bilirubin production. Second, *there is a diminished capacity of the liver to excrete the excessive bilirubin delivered to it* because (1) uptake by hepatic cells is inhibited and (2) there is diminished conjugation of pigment in the liver cell. The inhibited uptake of bilirubin is probably attributable to deficient "Y protein" in the hepatic cell. Hyperbilirubinemia is therefore a regular occurrence in all neonates, but jaundice occurs in only half of them because serum bilirubin levels must exceed 4 to 6 mg/100 ml before it is visible as pigment in the skin. In term infants a peak unconjugated bilirubin level is reached on the third or fourth day of life; in premature infants it is attained on the fifth or sixth day. This is physiologic jaundice. Physiologic jaundice is a useful clinical concept because it implies a normal state that does not require therapy. However, the limitations of functional immaturity may persist, and

bilirubin may accumulate to hazardous levels. As a rule, physiologic jaundice fulfills the following specific criteria: (1) the infant is otherwise well; (2) in term infants, jaundice first appears after 24 hours and disappears by the end of the seventh day; (3) in premature infants, jaundice is first evident after 48 hours and disappears by the ninth or tenth day; (4) serum unconjugated bilirubin concentration does not exceed 12 mg/100 ml, either in term or preterm infants; (5) hyperbilirubinemia is almost exclusively of the unconjugated variety, and conjugated (direct) bilirubin should not exceed 1 to 1.5 mg/100 ml; (6) daily increments of bilirubin concentration should not surpass 5 mg/100 ml. Bilirubin levels in excess of 12 mg/100 ml may indicate either an exaggeration of the physiologic handicap or the presence of disease. *At any serum bilirubin level, the appearance of jaundice during the first day of life or persistence beyond the ages previously delineated usually indicates a pathologic process.*

CAUSES OF NEONATAL JAUNDICE

The following list presents the most prominent disorders associated with neonatal jaundice categorized by the mechanisms involved. Most of these conditions also involve some degree of anemia, particularly in the presence of intravascular hemolysis or blood loss into enclosed spaces.

Causes of pathologic neonatal jaundice*

I. Intravascular hemolysis (unconjugated hyperbilirubinemia)
   A. Hemolytic disease of the newborn (Rh, ABO, others)

*Modified from Odell, G. B.: Postnatal care. In Cooke, R. E., editor: The biologic basis of pediatric practice, New York, 1968, McGraw-Hill Book Co.

B. Polycythemia (large placental transfusion, fetofetal transfusion, maternofetal transfusion)
C. Abnormalities of red cells
   1. Hereditary spherocytosis
   2. Enzyme deficiencies (G-6-PD deficiency and others)
   3. Elliptocytosis
   4. Pyknocytosis
   5. Hemoglobinopathy (Barts, Zurich)
D. Chemical hemolysins (vitamin K analogues, maternal naphthalene ingestion in G-6-PD deficiency)
II. Extravascular hemolysis; enclosed hemorrhage (unconjugated hyperbilirubinemia)
A. Petechiae, ecchymoses
B. Hematoma
C. Hemorrhage
D. Intraventricular hemorrhage
III. Impaired hepatic function
A. Deficient glucuronyl transferase (unconjugated hyperbilirubinemia)
   1. Familial nonhemolytic jaundice, types I, II
   2. Transient familial neonatal hyperbilirubinemia (Lucey-Driscoll syndrome)

B. Infection (conjugated, unconjugated hyperbilirubinemia)
   1. Bacterial (septicemia, syphilis, pyelonephritis)
   2. Nonbacterial
      a. Toxoplasmosis
      b. Cytomegalovirus
      c. Rubella
      d. Herpes simplex
      e. Coxsackievirus
      f. Neonatal hepatitis
C. Metabolic factors (unconjugated hyperbilirubinemia)
   1. Infants of diabetic mothers
   2. Galactosemia
   3. "Breast milk jaundice"
   4. Hypothyroidism
D. Biliary obstruction (conjugated, unconjugated hyperbilirubinemia)
   1. Biliary atresia

Table 10-1 presents the most important clinical and laboratory data that suggest the causes of abnormal jaundice. It is important to understand that jaundice is probably the most common potentially abnormal sign in the immediate postnatal

Table 10-1. Significance of clinical data in diagnosis of neonatal jaundice*

Information	Significance
Clinical data	
Family history	
Parent or sibling with history of jaundice or anemia	Suggests hereditary hemolytic anemia, such as hereditary spherocytosis
Previous sibling with neonatal jaundice	Suggests hemolytic disease due to ABO or Rh isoimmunization
History of liver disease in siblings or disorders such as cystic fibrosis, galactosemia, tyrosinemia, hypermethioninemia, Crigler-Najjar syndrome, or alpha$_1$-antitrypsin deficiency	All associated with neonatal hyperbilirubinemia

*Modified from McMillan, J. A., Nieburg, P. I., and Oski, F. A.: The Newborn. In The whole pediatrician catalog, Philadelphia, 1977, W. B. Saunders Co.

Table 10-1. Significance of clinical data in diagnosis of neonatal jaundice—cont'd

Information	Significance
Clinical data—cont'd	
Maternal history	
Unexplained illness during pregnancy	Consider congenital infections such as rubella, cytomegalovirus, toxoplasmosis, herpes, syphillis, or hepatitis
Diabetes mellitus	Increased incidence of jaundice among infants of diabetic mothers
Drug ingestion during pregnancy	Ingestion of sulfonamides, nitrofurantoins, or antimalarials may initiate hemolysis in G-6-PD–deficient infant
History of labor and delivery	
Vacuum extraction	Increased incidence of cephalhematoma and jaundice
Oxytocin-induced labor	Increased incidence of hyperbilirubinemia
Delayed cord clamping	Increased incidence of hyperbilirubinemia among polycythemic infants
Apgar score	Increased incidence of jaundice in asphyxiated infants
Infant's history	
Delayed passage of meconium or infrequent stools	Increased enterohepatic circulation of bilirubin. Consider intestinal atresia, annular pancreas, Hirschsprung's disease, meconium plug, drug-induced ileus (hexamethonium)
Caloric intake	Inadequate caloric intake results in delay in bilirubin conjugation
Vomiting	Suspect sepsis, galactosemia, or pyloric stenosis; all associated with hyperbilirubinemia
Infant's physical examination	
Small for gestational age	Infants frequently polycythemic and jaundiced
Head size	Microcephaly seen with intrauterine infections associated with jaundice
Cephalhematoma	Entrapped hemorrhage associated with hyperbilirubinemia
Pallor	Suspect hemolytic anemia
Petechiae	Suspect congenital infection, overwhelming sepsis, or severe hemolytic disease as cause of jaundice
Appearance of umbilical stump	Omphalitis and sepsis may produce jaundice
Hepatosplenomegaly	Suspect hemolytic anemia or congenital infection
Optic fundi	Chorioretinitis suggests congenital infection as cause of jaundice

Continued.

Table 10-1. Significance of clinical data in diagnosis of neonatal jaundice—*cont'd*

Information	Significance
Clinical data—cont'd	
Infant's physical examination—cont'd	
Umbilical hernia	Consider hypothyroidism
Congenital anomalies	Jaundice occurs with increased frequency among infants with trisomic condition
Laboratory data	
Maternal	
Blood group and indirect Coombs' test	Necessary for evaluation of possible ABO or Rh incompatibility
Serology	Rule out congenital syphillis
Infant	
Hemoglobin	Anemia suggests hemolytic disease or large entrapped hemorrhage; hemoglobin above 22 grams/100 ml associated with increased incidence of jaundice
Reticulocyte count	Elevation suggests hemolytic disease
Red cell morphology	Spherocytes suggest ABO incompatibility or hereditary spherocytosis; red cell fragmentation seen in disseminated intravascular coagulation
Platelet count	Thrombocytopenia suggests infection
White cell count	Total white cell count less than $5000/mm^3$ or increase in band forms to greater than $2000/mm^3$ suggests infection
Sedimentation rate	Values in excess of 5 during the first 48 hours indicate infection or ABO incompatibility
Direct bilirubin	Elevation suggests infection or severe Rh incompatibility
Immunoglobulin M	Elevation indicates infection
Blood group and direct and indirect Coombs' test	Required to rule out hemolytic disease as a result of isoimmunization
Carboxyhemoglobin	Elevated in infants with hemolytic disease or entrapped hemorrhage
Urinalysis	Presence of reducing substance suggests diagnosis of galactosemia

period but that only a fraction of affected infants require detailed investigation. Diagnostic assessment is necessary for babies in whom:

1. Jaundice appears within the first 24 hours after birth

2. Serum bilirubin is over 12 mg/dl if term, 15 mg/100 ml if premature
3. Serum bilirubin rises more than 5 mg/100 ml in 24 hours
4. Conjugated (direct) bilirubin is more than 2 mg/100 ml

5. Phototherapy is considered necessary
6. Jaundice persists beyond 7 days if term and beyond 10 to 14 days if premature

Intravascular hemolysis

Isoimmune hemolytic disease of the newborn (p. 269). Maternofetal blood group incompatibility (Rh, ABO) is the most frequent cause of pathologic jaundice. Hemolysis is intravascular by virtue of an antigen-antibody reaction on the surface of the red cells.

Polycythemia (p. 281). An increased quantity of erythrocytes results in sequestration of greater numbers of aged cells, which, when broken down, yield excessive amounts of bilirubin. The accumulation of pigment is occasionally sufficiently pronounced to necessitate an exchange transfusion. Hyperbilirubinemia occurs in the absence of maternal blood group incompatibility or any other disorder that accelerates hemolysis.

Intrinsic red cell abnormalities. Enzymatic deficiencies, the most prominent of which is G-6-PD deficiency (p. 274), are responsible for hemolysis and jaundice because of disrupted erythrocyte metabolism; that is particularly noteworthy in premature black infants.

Abnormal contours of erythrocytes also render them vulnerable to early dissolution and the occasional production of jaundice. Hereditary spherocytosis is the most common disorder in this category. Rare abnormalities of red cell morphology that may also cause icterus are hereditary elliptocytosis (p. 275) and pyknocytosis. In pyknocytosis the red cells are small and stain rather deeply; the cell borders are irregular. Their life span is abnormally short, thereby increasing the rate of hemolysis.

Drug toxicity (chemical hemolysins). Excessive doses of vitamin K produce hyperbilirubinemia in premature infants. Hemolysis is more severe and more likely to occur in the presence of G-6-PD deficiency. Hyperbilirubinemia has also been reported in infants whose mothers received large doses of vitamin K to protect the infant from hemorrhagic disease of the newborn. Vitamin K should be administered to the infant, preferably in the form of K_1, only in an intramuscular dose of 0.5 to 1 mg. Ingestion or inhalation of naphthalene is a rare but fascinating example of drug-induced icterus. It has been reported in G-6-PD–deficient infants whose mothers ingested or inhaled fumes from mothballs.

Extravascular hemolysis (unconjugated hyperbilirubinemia)

Degradation of blood in enclosed spaces is relatively rapid. Perhaps the most graphic example is the hyperbilirubinemia that follows the formation of petechiae in the skin from any cause. One gram of hemoglobin is transformed into 35 mg of bilirubin; the added pigment from rapid hemolysis of a small amount of blood thus overtaxes the neonate's limited capacity to conjugate bilirubin. Extensive ecchymosis from traumatic delivery is not uncommon in small premature infants; an inordinately high level of serum bilirubin often occurs as a result. Large cephalhematomas produce the same effect, particularly if they are bilateral.

Impaired hepatic function

Deficient glucuronyl transferase activity. Two rare entities that involve glucuronyl transferase deficiency are worthy of mention. *Familial nonhemolytic jaundice,* (Crigler-Najjar syndrome) is a heritable, permanent deficiency of glucuronyl transferase that does not involve hemolysis. Unconjugated hyperbilirubinemia persists throughout life because of an inability to form bilirubin glucuronide. The syndrome occurs in a serious, often lethal form (type I) and in a milder form that is apparently a partial deficiency of glucuronyl transferase type II. Type I bilirubinemia ranges upward from 20 to 25 mg/100 ml. Numerous exchange transfusions are often required in the neonatal period. In contrast to type II, it resists phenobarbital therapy. Kernicterus and death are common. Serum bilirubin in type II disease is generally under 20 to 25 mg/100 ml, and small amounts of bilirubin glucuronide are in bile. Response to phenobarbital is usually satisfactory. Kernicterus is less likely to occur in the milder expression of the syndrome. Most survivors suffer severe brain damage as a result of bilirubin toxicity. Occasionally kernicterus develops later in childhood.

Transient familial neonatal hyperbilirubinemia (Lucey-Driscoll syndrome) affects all the offspring of one mother. Severe unconjugated hyperbilirubinemia appears during the first few days and subsides during the second or third week. An unidentified factor in the sera of affected mothers and in their infants has been shown to impair glucuronyl transferase activity in vitro.

Infection. Bacterial and nonbacterial infections are often associated with jaundice. Some degree of conjugated (direct) hyperbilirubinemia is frequent, indicating impaired liver function and often actual destruction of hepatic tissue. Septicemia and renal infection produce hemolysis as well. The nonbacterial infections and syphilis probably do likewise; structural liver damage occurs

more frequently in them than in the bacterial diseases.

Metabolic factors

Infants of diabetic mothers. The basis for increased incidence of hyperbilirubinemia in infants of diabetic mothers is unknown. The frequency of prematurity and respiratory distress among these babies is probably the most important factor. Depression, by asphyxia, of hepatic function that is already immature seems plausible. Furthermore, severe illness diminishes intestinal mobility, thereby enhancing reabsorption of bilirubin from the small intestine.

Galactosemia. Protracted bilirubinemia, with either moderately or severely elevated levels, may occur in galactosemia as the only clinical manifestation. Jaundice may persist over 10 days. The bilirubin is unconjugated at first, but later, as liver damage begins, conjugated bilirubin is retained in the blood.

Breast milk jaundice. This syndrome of unconjugated hyperbilirubinemia occurs in 1% to 5% of breast-fed term infants. Two substances in breast milk, a pregnanediol and a free fatty acid, have been suggested as causes of this syndrome. Both are believed to inhibit the activity of glucuronyl transferase in the neonatal liver. Unless the mother has had a previously involved baby, the syndrome cannot be anticipated during the first 3 to 4 days of life because only the normal pattern of physiologic jaundice is discernible. Breast milk does not augment bilirubin levels during the first 3 days of life. If there has been a previous infant with breast milk jaundice, there is a 70% possibility of recurrence in subsequently born siblings. On the fourth or fifth day of life, when physiologic hyperbilirubinemia is expected to subside, bilirubin levels continue to climb until they reach peak concentrations of 10 to 27 mg/100 ml between 10 and 15 days of age. If breast feeding is not interrupted, bilirubin levels gradually decline from peak to normal levels sometime between 3 and 12 weeks of age. If breast feeding is discontinued for 48 to 72 hours, a prompt decline in bilirubin occurs. Resumption of breast feeding is followed by a rise in bilirubin of only 2 or 3 mg/100 ml and a subsequent decline. We prefer to interrupt breast feeding to establish the diagnosis of this benign syndrome and to allay the maternal apprehensions that are inevitable in the face of protracted jaundice. Affected infants are otherwise well. They feed and gain weight normally and their bowel movements are unaffected.

Hypothyroidism. Persistent low-grade hyperbilirubinemia may be, as in galactosemia, the only sign of hypothyroidism in the first 2 to 4 weeks of life. Only unconjugated bilirubin is involved.

Biliary obstruction (biliary atresia)

Obliteration of the biliary tree is not common. It has been noted in congenital rubella infection, but other causes, still unknown, are operative as well. Jaundice appears during the first week or later; half the affected infants are not icteric until the second week. Conjugated hyperbilirubinemia always develops eventually, although some degree of unconjugated bilirubin accumulation also occurs, particularly at the onset of jaundice. The conjugated hyperbilirubinemia progresses relentlessly in the months or few years left of life. Biliary cirrhosis eventually becomes so extensive as to virtually eliminate most of the liver functions.

Currently, biliary atresia is not considered to be a congenital anomaly but a progressive obliteration of the biliary tract of unknown etiology that, in only a few instances, may eventually clear spontaneously. Infection of some sort, as yet undemonstrated, is a favored explanation by many. Obliteration of the bile duct system occurs at any level—from the microscopic canaliculi in liver parenchyma down to the common bile duct. Thus, intrahepatic obstruction is the sole manifestation in a minority of infants, extrahepatic obstruction being far more common. Occasionally, both areas are involved. The obliterative process may begin in utero or in the immediate postnatal period; the disease progresses postnatally. It has not been found in stillborn fetuses, probably indicating that it is not a completely evolved congenital anomaly.

Biliary atresia is preponderantly a disorder of term infants, affecting females twice as often as males. These otherwise well infants become jaundiced in the second week of life or later; the liver, and eventually the spleen, become massively enlarged. Hyperbilirubinemia, at first unconjugated, soon becomes largely conjugated. Stools are clay colored and putty-like in consistency. For several months these infants appear well, except for the jaundice. Later, as hepatic dysfunction progresses, nutrition and severe growth impairment supervene. Ultimately a bleeding diathesis appears. Surgery may help a minority of infants.

KERNICTERUS (BILIRUBIN ENCEPHALOPATHY)

Kernicterus, the most serious complication of neonatal hyperbilirubinemia, is caused by deposition of unconjugated and unbound bilirubin in brain cells.

Neurologic signs appear between the second and tenth days of life. They produce depression (coma, lethargy, diminished or absent Moro reflex, hypotonia, and absent sucking and rooting reflex) followed by excitation (twitching, generalized seizures, opisthotonos, hypertonia, and a high-pitched cry). Occasionally the anterior fontanelle bulges. Many affected infants die in the neonatal period, and those who survive usually have impaired intellectual or motor function. The effects of these neurologic deficits in later childhood may vary from severe to subtle dysfunction. Morphologic changes in affected brain cells suggest that damage from kernicterus impairs learning, memory, and adaptive behavior. In some children perceptual function may be diminished even in the absence of subnormal IQ or motor deficits. Deafness is frequent.

Serum bilirubin concentrations in excess of 20 mg/100 ml in term infants, 15 mg/100 ml in preterm babies, and 10 to 12 mg/dl in the smallest premature infants are generally accepted as the levels at which kernicterus is likely to occur. This rule of thumb has traditionally provided the clinician with a simple guide for deciding whether to perform an exchange transfusion. Actually, the extent to which bilirubin is bound to albumin is even more important than its concentration in the serum. Bilirubin encephalopathy is caused by the migration of unbound bilirubin into brain substance. Therefore it may not occur at high serum bilirubin levels if the pigment is albumin bound. Conversely, it can occur at serum levels considerably below 20 mg/100 ml if significant quantities of bilirubin are not albumin bound. The causes of diminished albumin binding have been described on p. 285. Respiratory or metabolic acidosis, drugs, and hypothermia are impediments to albumin binding. Acidosis impairs the capacity to albumin to hold bilirubin, and some drugs competitively displace the pigment from its binding site. The metabolic response to cold stress releases free fatty acids that dislocate bilirubin from albumin. Kernicterus has been reported in small premature infants at serum bilirubin levels below 10 mg/100 ml, but more often between 10 and 15 mg/100 ml. The factors that increase the vulnerability of these infants are stated by Lucey as follows:

Birth weight less than 1500 grams
Hypothermia
Asphyxia, severe prenatal or postnatal
Hypoalbuminemia
Septicemia
Meningitis
Drugs that affect albumin binding
Serum bilirubin above 10 mg/100 ml

Yet in spite of these variables and the importance of unbound bilirubin, total serum bilirubin determination rather than assessment of albumin-binding capacity is currently the most practical guide for evaluating the need for exchange transfusion. This guide to treatment has been used for decades and is still the most reliable group of parameters. Although several laboratory procedures that asses the status of albumin-binding capacity have been described in recent years, none has been shown to be sufficiently predictive of clinical course to warrant routine application. Should these tests be utilized, results must be interpreted in conjunction with serum bilirubin levels, gestational age, and type and severity of illness. *There is as yet no single test that can identify the bilirubin levels that will produce damage to a neonatal brain.* Table 10-2 presents general

Table 10-2. Recommended maximal total serum bilirubin concentrations (mg/100 ml)*†

Birth weight category (grams)‡	Uncomplicated course	Complicated course§
Less than 1250	13	10
1250-1499	15	13
1500-1999	17	15
2000-2499	18	17
2500 and up	20	18

*From Gartner, L. M., and Lee, K. S.: Jaundice and liver disease. In Behrman, R. E., editor: Neonatal-perinatal medicine: diseases of the fetus and infant, ed. 2, St. Louis, 1977, The C. V. Mosby Co.

†Direct-reacting bilirubin concentrations are not subtracted unless they amount to more than 50% of the total serum bilirubin concentration. Applicable during the first 28 days of life.

‡Equivalent gestational age categories may be used in lieu of birth weight for small-for-gestational age (SGA) infants.

§Complications include: perinatal asphyxia and acidosis, postnatal hypoxia and acidosis, significant and persistent hypothermia, hypoalbuminemia, meningitis and other significant infection, hemolysis, and hypoglycemia.

guidelines for these bilirubin levels according to birth weight and presence of illnesses that are thought to potentiate the toxicity of bilirubin to brain tissue.

THERAPY FOR HYPERBILIRUBINEMIA
Exchange transfusion

Exchange transfusion is the classic therapeutic procedure for hyperbilirubinemia of any etiology. The two-volume exchange removes approximately 85% of the infant's red blood cells. In the case of erythroblastosis the offending cells are thus eliminated. In cases of drug toxicity the circulating drug may be largely removed. Exchange transfusion is less effective for the removal of total body bilirubin, although it remains the most valuable form of therapy for this purpose.

Whereas most of the bilirubin in plasma is indeed eliminated by the procedure, pigment in extravascular tissue rapidly migrates back into the blood after the transfusion. As a rule, serum bilirubin at the end of an exchange transfusion is approximately 50% of preexchange levels. However, as a result of the diffusion of bilirubin from tissues, these levels promptly rise to 70% or 80% of their previous values, and the process may continue so that bilirubin concentrations soon equal or surpass preexisting levels. The rapidity and extent of this rebound phenomenon depend on the amount of pigment stored in tissues and the remaining vigor of the hemolytic process that caused hyperbilirubinemia. Serum bilirubin may thus reaccumulate after the first transfusion, so that one or more additional transfusions are frequently necessary. (Exchange transfusion is also discussed on p. 271.)

Administration of albumin

Since albumin-binding capacity is a crucial determinant of the development of kernicterus, it would seem rational to enhance it. The use of albumin before or during the exchange transfusion does indeed increase binding capacity and therefore results in removal of larger amounts of bilirubin, because the additional circulating protein pulls bilirubin out of extravascular tissue to bind it. Intravenous administration of 1 gram of albumin in a 25% salt-poor preparation 1 or 2 hours before exchange transfusion exerts such a measurable effect. Other investigators have given 6 to 12 grams of albumin during the transfusion by adding it to donor blood. By attracting bilirubin from the tissues into the blood during this procedure, albumin causes higher posttransfusion serum levels of the pigment. However, the resultant values may spuriously indicate the need for another transfusion when this is in fact not the case, since binding capacity has been enhanced by continuous addition of albumin during the exchange transfusion. The issue can be resolved only by determination of albumin-binding capacity, a procedure that is not yet generally available. There has been a recent report of a fluorescent dye method for determination of bilirubin binding capacity of serum albumin that holds promise of widespread application. It is a simple, rapid procedure that requires less serum than is required for routine bilirubin determination. A considerable amount of data, especially long-term follow-up results, will be essential before this test can be applied clinically. For the time being, when albumin is given, most clinicians use serum values somewhat in excess of 20 mg/100 ml as an indication for a repeat transfusion.

Phototherapy

The use of intense fluorescent light to reduce serum bilirubin gained widespread acceptance in the United States after a decade of general use abroad. Blue light decomposes bilirubin by photooxidation. When light is applied to jaundiced infants, shielded skin remains more icteric, which suggests that decomposition transpires in the skin. The products formed in the breakdown of bilirubin are not toxic. There is no doubt that serum unconjugated bilirubin concentrations are reduced by phototherapy. Numerous precautions have been urged by investigators whose experience with lights is extensive. Long-term outcomes have not been completely evaluated, nor have the theoretic effects of intense light on a wide spectrum of biologic processes

been assessed. Many of the objections that have been raised are hypothetical; significant immediate adverse effects have not been demonstrated, nor have any long-term adverse effects. Yet the "light controversy" rages on. The use of lights must be regarded with the same caution as the use of a new drug: the potential dangers of the unknown should not outweigh the benefit expected. However, it will be a rare new drug indeed that can be withheld from the neonate until its long-term effects are totally known. For both patient and physician, life is too short. The etiology of jaundice must be sought before and during therapy. In the presence of a mild hemolytic process, hemoglobin determination is essential at frequent intervals because anemia may develop in spite of diminishing bilirubin levels.

The effectiveness of phototherapy is in the blue segment of the light spectrum. This is 420 to 460 nanometers (nm). The commonly utilized fluorescent bulbs (daylight or cool white) deliver relatively little energy from blue light. Fluorescent bulbs, specially designed for phototherapy (for example, Vitalite) deliver more blue light, while special blue bulbs (designated BB by manufacturers) deliver the most blue light within a narrow spectrum. Incandescent light, delivered through a filter, delivers satisfactory quantities of blue light. Fluorescent lights mounted overhead on a hood over radiant warmers have been shown to be inadequate sources of phototherapy.

The adequacy of blue light intensity can be demonstrated only by measuring energy in the 400 to 500 nm range. Special instruments are available at modest cost for this purpose. The units of energy are expressed as microwatts per square centimeter per nanometer (μW/cm^2/nm).

Footcandle meters are of no value for these energy measurements. Currently, a minimum of 4 μW/cm²/nm is considered necessary for effective phototherapy. This will vary, however, depending on the rate of bilirubin production. It is also generally accepted that there is a linear relationship between effectiveness and dose of light between 4 and 14 μW/cm²/nm.

Phototherapy should not be used for routine prophylaxis against hyperbilirubinemia in any infant, term or premature. In ABO incompatibility, it is useful for infants who are candidates for exchange transfusion but in whom there is as yet no clear indication for its performance. Phototherapy has been utilized for Rh disease, and the data indicate that fewer early (first 12 hours of life) and late transfusions are necessary. One must be mindful that in removing bilirubin with phototherapy, the vulnerable red cells remain in circulation for ultimate hemolysis. The result is progressive anemia at safe levels of serum bilirubin. There is frequent prolongation of hospital stay for close observation of precipitous decline in hemoglobin. In our experience, a need arises for multiple simple transfusions because of progressive anemia. We still believe it best *in Rh disease* to observe for hyperbilirubinemia, perform the first exchange transfusion, and then apply phototherapy.

For hyperbilirubinemia from any cause, lights should never be used to delay an exchange transfusion once the serum bilirubin approaches levels that require it. If indicated, phototherapy should be instituted when the bilirubin concentration reaches 10 mg/100 ml in premature infants and sometimes at even lower levels in smaller babies. The response to phototherapy, assuming delivery of appropriate doses of light, will depend on the rate of bilirubin production. Rapid increases in ABO incompatibility will respond less extensively to the same dose of light than the increments that characterize physiologic hyperbilirubinemia. The effect of lights is probably immediate even though decreases in bilirubin are not evident during the first 24 hours of therapy. Phototherapy minimizes or eliminates any increase in bilirubin that otherwise occurs without it. Rebound elevations of several milligrams per 100 ml are the rule after therapy is discontinued.

In the day-to-day management of infants, the most important immediate untoward effects of phototherapy include increased metabolic rate, hyperthermia, loose stools, and significantly increased loss of water through the skin. Metabolic rate increases, and the caloric requirement thus rises. There may be difficulty in meeting caloric needs if intestinal transit time is increased to cause loose stools. Hyperthermia (and the loose stools) increases water losses, and the daily fluid requirement thus increases. Urine may darken because photodegradation products are water soluble and are thus excreted by the kidneys.

The effect of phototherapy on growth of premature infants during the neonatal period has been assessed, and the data negate the previous conclusion (from the same investigator) that long-term growth is impaired. There is indeed diminished growth during the period of phototherapy, but there is also a catch-up period during the second and third weeks of life. The reason is probably that phototherapy causes increased metabolic demands and decreased intestinal absorption of milk (because intestinal transit time is increased).

That natural light conditions affect serum bilirubin levels has been demonstrated in a study from Finland, where, through the year, seasonal daily duration of daylight varies from 3 to 22 hours. Premature babies born during the "light" half of the year had significantly lower bilirubin levels than those born during the "dark" half of the year. None of them received phototherapy. Environmental light undoubtedly also influences the effect of phototherapy. Factors such as the number of windows in a nursery, the light they admit, the position of the baby in relation to windows, and the geographic location of the hospital all must be considered in evaluating the results of light therapy.

A warning issued by the Federal Drug Administration called attention to the protective effect of a plastic barrier between phototherapy lights and babies. Without a plastic shield, ultraviolet light from fluorescent bulbs has caused skin erythema in two babies. Commercial lights have Plexiglas shields built into the apparatus. The plastic walls of an incubator are also protective. Phototherapy should be used only with plastic interposed between the light and the baby. The erythematous skin caused by ultraviolet light suggests that the retina would also be jeopardized in the absence of a surface that filters out the ultraviolet light.

Because blue light is the effective segment of the spectrum that acts on bilirubin, narrow-spectrum blue lights have been used for phototherapy. Reduction of serum bilirubin levels was greater than with the usual fluorescent bulbs. However, as one might anticipate, it was impossible to detect cyanosis or pallor. Furthermore, we have also noted the reported incidence of nausea and dizziness in a few nurses who care for infants in blue lights.

The "bronze baby syndrome" has received wide attention. It occurs in light-treated babies with liver disease whose hyperbilirubinemia has a significant direct component. A gray-brown discoloration of skin, serum, and urine was observed. The discoloration cleared 3 weeks after therapy was discontinued. "Tanning" of black infants has been also reported. This is distinct from the "bronzing" effect. The skin simply becomes more deeply pigmented during exposure to the lights. A maculopapular rash has also been noted as one of the side effects of therapy.

The infant's eyes are shielded from the intense light he receives during phototherapy. No evidence from human eyes has indicated that the light is injurious, but microscopic injury to retinal cells has been observed in monkeys exposed to phototherapy (without shielding eyes) for 3 to 7 days. The extent of the damage was well correlated with duration of exposure. *There is thus now strong evidence to justify conscientious maintenance of eye patches during treatment.* The nurse should be certain that the lids are closed when the blindfold is applied. It should be removed daily to inspect the eyes for conjunctivitis. Failure to change the eye shields has resulted in unsuspected severe purulent conjunctivitis.

Phenobarbital

Phenobarbital has been shown to lower peak bilirubin levels of physiologic jaundice by approximately 50%. It exerts its effect by increasing activity of glucuronyl transferase and ligandin, thus increasing hepatic capacity to conjugate and take up bilirubin. There was at first widespread hope that phenobarbital therapy would materially diminish the incidence of hyperbilirubinemia. It is now apparent that its beneficial use is quite restricted for several reasons. It is effective when given to mothers several days to 2 weeks before delivery. Thus, large numbers of mothers would receive the drug before anticipated delivery that at best could only be estimated. There would also be no method by which the need for therapy in the neonate could be identified prenatally. Postnatal administration is of limited effect for the term baby and is of little or no benefit to the premature infant. Administered to the mother, phenobarbital may precipitate withdrawal symptoms in the neonate. Thus, the drug is not generally used to diminish bilirubin levels. It is of no value in combination with phototherapy. Its application is rather specific, such as in type II glucuronyl transferase deficiency.

REFERENCES

Anttolainen, I., Simila, S., and Wallgren, E. I.: Effect of seasonal variation in daylight on bilirubin level in premature infants, Arch. Dis. Child. **50:**156, 1975.

Behrman, R. E., et al.: Preliminary report of the committee on phototherapy in the newborn infant, J. Pediatr. **84:**135, 1974.

Boggs, T. R., and Bishop, H.: Neonatal hyperbilirubinemia associated with high obstruction of the small bowel, J. Pediatr. **66:**349, 1965.

Bonta, B. W., and Warshaw, J. B.: Importance of radiant flux in the treatment of hyperbilirubinemia: failure of overhead phototherapy units in intensive care units, Pediatrics **57:**502, 1976.

Broughton, P. M. G.: The effectiveness and safety of phototherapy. In Bergsma, D., Hsia, D. Y-Y, and Jackson, C., editors: Birth defects: bilirubin metabolism in the newborn, vol. VI, no. 2, White Plains, N.Y., June, 1970, National Foundation–March of Dimes.

Cashore, W. J., Gartner, L. M., Oh, W., and Stern, L.: Clinical application of neonatal bilirubin-binding determinations: Current status, J. Pediatr. **93:**827, 1978.

Diamond, L. K.: A history of jaundice in the newborn. In Bergsma, D., Hsia, D. Y-Y, and Jackson, C., editors: Birth defects: bilirubin metabolism in the newborn, vol. VI, no. 2, White Plains, N.Y., June, 1970, National Foundation–March of Dimes.

Food and Drug Administration (HEW): Comment: Hazard of ultraviolet radiation from fluorescent lamps to infant during phototherapy, J. Pediatr. **84:**145, 1974.

Gartner, L. M., and Lee, K.: Jaundice and liver disease. In Behrman, R. E., editor: Neonatal-perinatal medicine: diseases of the fetus and infant, ed. 2, St. Louis, 1977, The C. V. Mosby Co.

Gartner, L. M., Lee, K., Vaisman, S., et al.: Development of bilirubin transport and metabolism in the newborn rhesus monkey, J. Pediatr., **90:**513, 1977.

Gellis, S. S.: Biliary atresia, Pediatrics **55:**8, 1975.

Gitzelmann-Cumarasamy, N., and Kuenzle, C. C.: Commentaries: Bilirubin binding tests: living up to expectations?, Pediatrics **64:**375, 1979.

Hodgman, J. E., and Teberg, A.: Effect of phototherapy on subsequent growth and development of the premature infant. In Bergsma, D., Hsia, D. Y-Y, and Jackson, C., editors: Birth defects: bilirubin metabolism in the newborn, vol. VI, no. 2, White Plains, N.Y., June, 1970, National Foundation–March of Dimes.

Kapitulnik, J., Horner-Mibashan, R., Blondheim, S. H., et al.: Increase in bilirubin-binding affinity of serum with age of infant, J. Pediatr. **86:**442, 1975.

Karp, W. B.: Biochemical alterations in neonatal hyperbilirubinemia and bilirubin encephalopathy: a review, Pediatrics **64:**361, 1979.

Keenan, W. J., Perlstein, P. H., Light, I. J., and Sutherland, J. M.: Kernicterus in small sick premature infants receiving phototherapy, Pediatrics **49:**652, 1972.

Kopelman, A. E., Brown, R. S., and Odell, G. B.: The "bronze" baby syndrome: a complication of phototherapy, J. Pediatr. **81:**466, 1972.

Kwang-sun, L., Gartner, L. M., and Zarafu, I.: Fluorescent dye method for determination of the bilirubin-binding capacity of serum albumin, J. Pediatr. **86:**280, 1975.

Lester, R., Jackson, B. T., and Smallwood, R. A.: Fetal hepatic function. In Bergsma, D., Hsia, D. Y-Y, and Jackson, C., editors: Birth defects: bilirubin metabolism in the newborn, vol. VI, no. 2, White Plains, N.Y., June, 1970, National Foundation–March of Dimes.

Lucey, J. F.: The unsolved problem of kernicterus in the susceptible low birth weight infant, Pediatrics **49:**646, 1972.

Lucey, J. F.: Light: a time for change to "radiant flux," or microwatts per square centimeter (μW/CM^2), Pediatrics **50:**5, 1972.

Lucey, J. F.: Comment: Another view of phototherapy, J. Pediatr. **84**:145, 1974.

Lucey, J. F., Ferreiro, M., and Hewitt, J.: Prevention of hyperbilirubinemia of prematurity by phototherapy, Pediatrics **41**:1047, 1968.

Messner, K. H., Leŭre-Dupree, A. E., and Maisels, M. J.: The effect of continuous prolonged illumination on the newborn primate retina (abstr.), Pediatr. Res. **9**:368, 1975.

Mims, L. C., Estrada, M., Gooden, D. S., et al.: Phototherapy for neonatal hyperbilirubinemia—a dose:response relationship, J. Pediatr. **83**:658, 1973.

Moller, J., and Ebbesen, F.: Phototherapy in newborn infants with severe rhesus hemolytic disease, J. Pediatr. **86**:135, 1975.

Nakai, H., and Margaretten, W.: Protracted jaundice associated with hypertrophic pyloric stenosis, Pediatrics **29**:198, 1962.

Odell, G. B.: "Physiologic" hyperbilirubinemia in the neonatal period, N. Engl. J. Med. **277**:193, 1967.

Odell, G. B.: The distribution and toxicity of bilirubin, Pediatrics **46**:16, 1970.

Odell, G. B., Storey, B., and Rosenberg, L. A.: Studies in kernicterus. III. The saturation of serum proteins with bilirubin during neonatal life and its relationship to brain damage at five years, J. Pediatr. **76**:12, 1970.

Poland, R. L., and Odell, G. B.: Physiologic jaundice: the enterohepatic circulation of bilirubin, N. Engl. J. Med. **284**:1, 1971.

Shennan, A. T.: The effect of phototherapy on the hyperbilirubinemia of rhesus incompatibility, Pediatrics **54**:417, 1974.

Sisson, T. R. C., Kendall, N., Shaw, E., and Kechavarz-Oliai, L.: Phototherapy of jaundice in the newborn infant. II. Effect of various light intensities, J. Pediatr. **81**:35, 1972.

Woody, N. C., and Brodkey, M. J.: Tanning from phototherapy for neonatal jaundice, J. Pediatr. **82**:1042, 1973.

Wu, P. Y. K., Lim, R. C., Hodgman, J. E., et al.: Effect of phototherapy in preterm infants on growth in the neonatal period, J. Pediatr. **85**:563, 1974.

Zuelzer, W. W., and Brown, A. K.: Neonatal jaundice, Am. J. Dis. Child. **101**:113, 1961.

CHAPTER 11

Disorders of glucose, calcium, and magnesium metabolism

GLUCOSE DISORDERS
The fetus: glucose and other sources of energy

The fetus receives glucose continuously across the placenta from maternal blood. At term, neonatal cord blood glucose is 70% to 80% of the maternal level. Glucose is the primary source of fetal energy, but to what extent it predominates among other substances is still unsettled. Investigators have estimated that glucose provides 50% to 100% of fetal energy. From presently available data, it appears that other substances such as amino acids, lactate, and perhaps ketones and free fatty acids also provide fuel, but that glucose is the preponderant factor in total energy requirement. It passes across the placenta by facilitated diffusion, a process that itself requires expenditure of energy. Lactate appears to be normally generated in the placenta and it may well provide 25% of fetal oxidative metabolism.

The fetal uptake of glucose depends on maternal blood glucose levels. Fetal blood glucose is generally 25% to 30% lower than maternal levels. When denied glucose by virtue of maternal deprivation, the fetus may utilize ketones as a substitute. On the other hand, when maternal hyperglycemia exists (as in diabetic mothers), fetal blood glucose is elevated. Early in gestation fetal insulin production is negligible in response to maternal hyperglycemia, but as gestation proceeds, the beta cells in the pancreatic islets respond more vigorously. Fetuses of diabetic mothers who are recurrently hyperglycemic, respond with insulin production with increasing vigor. At term or near term, the insulin-producing islet cells are hyperplastic and have been shown to contain more than normal quantities of the hormone. Normally, however, there is no need for a significant fetal insulin response because glucose is constantly fed and regulated from the mother's blood. Maternal insulin does not cross the placenta. The continuous supply of glucose also eliminates any need for the fetus to synthesize glucose from glycogen or from other noncarbohydrate sources (fluconeogenesis). It also eliminates any need for the fetus to regulate its own blood glucose level since the mother does so by regulating her levels.

While fuel supplied to the fetus is utilized for the ongoing needs of growth and development, it must also be stored for availability during the inevitable exigencies of birth and immediate postnatal life. Once born, the neonate must supply his own fuel until external sources are well established. Thus, something like a neonatal energy crisis transpires when the maternal source of substrate is literally cut off. Now the neonate needs fuel to survive the asphyxia of normal birth, to withstand the cold stress caused by entry into the world of air, to perform the work of initial breathing, and to sustain vigorous muscle activity. Furthermore, fuel stores must be available for unanticipated perinatal asphyxia during which glycogen stores are extravagantly dissipated. In the asphyxiated baby, myocardial survival itself is directly related to the quantity of accumulated cardiac glycogen, for with greater quantities of glycogen in storage, the survival period during asphyxia is known to be more protracted.

Glucose is stored as glycogen in fetal tissues beginning in the ninth or tenth week. Glycogen storage in the liver increases continuously to term, at which time there is about 80 to 120 mg of glycogen per gram of wet hepatic weight. This is approximately twice the adult concentration. Cardiac glycogen is also continuously accumulated so that at term its concentration is ten times that of the adults, whereas in skeletal muscle, three to five times adult concentrations have been demonstrated.

These glycogen stores are also available to the fetus at any time intrauterine stress occurs. During fetal asphyxia, glycogen is rapidly broken down by anaerobic glycolysis with a resultant sizeable accumulation of lactate in blood and tissues.

The fetus synthesizes protein from amino acids that are derived transplacentally. Amino acids are probably not a direct source of energy. Triglycerides are generated from the ongoing input of glucose and are stored in fat depots. Fat deposits are not quantitatively significant until the last trimester, particularly in the latter half. Like glycogen stores, accumulations of adipose tissue serve as energy reservoirs that can be drawn on immediately after birth. As glycogen supplies are depleted and less glucose is generated, the free fatty acids derived from these fat stores become a metabolic fuel.

The neonate: glucose metabolism and the postnatal "energy crunch"

The storage of energy-yielding substrate throughout gestation, particularly during the last trimester, seems directed toward sustaining the neonate during his first postnatal days because at birth an "energy crunch" is created by amputation of the maternal supply line and by an abrupt demand for increased energy. The increased energy requirements are imposed by entry into the extrauterine environment. Specifically, substrate is consumed more rapidly because of the normal asphyxia of birth, the work of initiating extrauterine breathing, the loss of heat on exposure to cold, and the activation of muscle tone and activity. These events are ordinarily well managed by normal term neonates. In abnormal infants who are stressed for a variety of reasons, the instant switch from total maternal nurture to total, but transient, independence is often troublesome and threatening to intact survival.

After birth, the infant's caloric needs must be supplied from external sources, and it may be hours or days before expended glycogen is even partially replenished. In the meantime, there is abrupt diminution of glycogen stores. It follows then that intrauterine malnutrition, and the low stores of glycogen that it involves, poses a serious threat to the asphyxiated infant in terms of depleted carbohydrate. Even in normal infants, approximately 90% of liver glycogen is consumed by the end of the third hour after birth, rising gradually thereafter to attain adult concentrations by the end of the third week. The effects of respiratory distress on energy expenditure are well illustrated by the virtually complete depletion of glycogen stores found in postmortem analysis of the heart, liver, and diaphragm. The normal newborn infant can tolerate a relatively short period of fasting without chemical derangement. Carbohydrate stores are consumed during the first 2 or 3 days; later, fat is probably a principal source of energy.

The first defense against the fall in blood glucose after the cord is cut is activation of *glycogen breakdown (glycogenolysis)*. Within 2 hours the normal neonate's blood glucose falls from its cord blood level of approximately 70 or 80 mg/ 100 ml to 50 mg/100 ml. To prevent further decline, pancreatic islet cells respond to this stimulus by increasing the production of glucagon from alpha cells and diminishing the secretion of insulin from beta cells. Glucagon is one of several factors that promotes glycogenolysis, while the diminished presence of insulin does likewise. Not only is glycogen breakdown increased, but by several changeovers in the activity of hepatic enzymes, glycogen formation is inhibited as well.

The net effect of these activities is an increased release of hepatic glucose and a restoration of blood glucose to near cord blood levels. If restoration of higher levels is not quite accomplished, at the very least, the postnatal decline in blood glucose is reversed for the time being.

Gluconeogenesis is another source of hepatic glucose that first becomes active immediately after birth. This process involves the conversion of noncarbohydrate substances (principally amino acids) to glucose. Gluconeogenesis is not active in the fetus; at birth it is stimulated by appearance of the hormones and hepatic enzymes required for its activation. In sheep, gluconeogenesis is initiated within 3 minutes after birth. It seems likely that in the human neonate, the process also begins very soon after delivery.

The restoration of blood sugar is accomplished at a cost of hepatic glycogen reserves. These are depleted rapidly— hours after birth and more gradually in the ensuing 2 to 3 days. The neonate turns increasingly to fat as a fuel, and as a result, blood glucose is spared. Thus, free fatty acids (FFA) are released to the blood to meet tissue energy requirements. Soon after birth, blood levels of FFA increase threefold as a consequence of the breakdown of fat deposits (lipolysis) that were accumulated in utero largely during the last trimester. Lipolysis is triggered at birth by the release of catecholamines, principally norepinephrine. The most vigorous stimulus to the secretion of norepinephrine is the low temperature of room air that is encountered at birth and perceived by the thermal receptors in the skin. This mechanism, and the effects of norepinephrine secretion, are discussed on p. 89.

The "energy crunch" of the immediate postnatal period is thus temporarily alleviated by release of glucose from the liver (glycogenolysis and gluconeogenesis) and by the use of FFA as an alternative fuel that is derived from the breakdown of fat stores (lipolysis). Ultimately, the provision of external nutrition must maintain adequate energy levels. With these normal events in mind, the reader can appreciate the limited capacity of some infants to cope with the perinatal "energy crunch." The premature infant, for example, stores less hepatic glycogen and less fat than he would had he gone to term. He is thus vulnerable to hypoglycemia. The more immature the infant, the smaller the stores of energy substrate. Similarly, the malnourished fetus cannot accumulate adequate stores of substrate—neither glycogen nor fat. He, too, is vulnerable to hypoglycemia. Whether normal, premature, or undergrown, the fetus who is asphyxiated will rapidly dissipate glycogen stores because he must resort to anaerobic glycolysis as a major source of energy. The effect of asphyxia on energy deprivation is even more profound when it is chronic (placental insufficiency) and when it occurs in immature or malnourished fetuses. These babies also are predisposed to hypoglycemia.

The liver has a unique capacity to convert blood glucose to hepatic glycogen for storage and to convert glycogen back to glucose for release to the blood when levels are low. Blood glucose taken up by skeletal muscle is converted to glycogen and is ultimately utilized as glucose at that site; there is no release of glucose to the blood from any organ except the liver. Adipose tissue takes up blood glucose and converts it to triglycerides; it too does not release glucose to the blood. At any given moment, blood sugar concentration is a reflection of two principal balancing functions: hepatic release of glucose and utilization of glucose by tissues.

In the liver, glucose is primarily produced by breakdown of glycogen and production from noncarbohydrate substances (gluconeogenesis). Normal output of glucose from the liver also depends on adequate glycogen stores and effective activity of enzymes and hormones concerned with its production. Utilization of glucose by tissues is abnormally increased by the metabolic response to cold stress, acidosis, and hypoxia.

Hypoglycemia in the neonate

In term infants, hypoglycemia occurs when whole blood glucose is less than 30 mg/100 ml (serum glucose < 35 mg/100 ml) during the first 3 days of life; thereafter it occurs at 40 mg/100 ml whole blood (48 mg/100 ml in serum). In low birth weight infants, the diagnosis of hypoglycemia during the first week of life is established when whole blood sugar is less than 20 mg/100 ml (serum glucose < 25 mg/100 ml) in two consecutive blood samples. The diagnostic requirement of two low determinations is necessary because blood sugar levels normally fluctuate widely. The restriction of diagnostic criteria to laboratory data is unavoidable because the symptoms associated with hypoglycemia occur with similar frequency in normoglycemic infants with unrelated disorders. After the third day of life, normal blood sugar is at least 40 mg/100 ml. We do not play the "numbers game" with these prescribed normal levels of glucose. With or without symptoms, if blood sugar values are close to the designated low levels in an infant who is at known risk for hypoglycemia, we begin treatment.

The symptoms attributable to hypoglycemia from any cause may also occur in infants with central nervous system

Table 11-1. Causes of neonatal hypoglycemia

Clinical entity	Mechanism	Duration
Intrauterine malnutrition	Low liver glycogen store	Transient
Fetal asphyxia	Glycogen depletion	Transient
Cold stress	Glycogen depletion	Transient
CNS hemorrhage	Unknown	Transient
CNS malformation	Unknown	Transient
Adrenal hemorrhage, insufficiency	Ineffective catecholamine response	Transient
Infants of diabetic mothers	Increased plasma insulin activity	Transient
Erythroblastotic infants	Increased plasma insulin activity	Transient
Maternal tolbutamide, chlorprop-amide	Hyperinsulinism	Transient
Abrupt stop of intravenous glucose, ≥ 10%	Hyperinsulinism	Transient
Glycogen storage disease (types I and II)	Defective glycogen breakdown	Protracted
Galactose intolerance (galactosemia)	Defective conversion of galactose to glucose	Protracted
Islet cell tumor	Hyperinsulinism	Protracted
Cyanotic congenital heart disease with congestive failure	Unknown	Transient
Hypopituitarism	Adrenal insufficiency	Protracted
Septicemia	Unknown	Transient

disorders, septicemia, hypocalcemia, hypomagnesemia, cardiorespiratory disorders, and a multiplicity of other abnormalities. There are no pathognomonic clinical signs of hypoglycemia. The signs associated with low blood sugar include apnea, cyanosis, rapid and irregular respirations, tachypnea, tremors, jitters, twitches, convulsions, lethargy, coma, abrupt pallor, sweating, upward rolling of the eyes, weak cry, and refusal to feed. The etiologic relationship of these signs to hypoglycemia is credible if they clear within a short time after intravenous glucose administration; if they do not clear, a cause other than hypoglycemia is undoubtedly operative.

Blood sugar falls to abnormally low levels if glycogen stores are suboptimal, gluconeogenesis (glucose from lipids and protein) in the liver is diminished, available

insulin is excessive, or carbohydrate-regulating hormones such as cortisol, epinephrine, and glucagon are insufficient. In rare circumstances, enzyme deficiencies in the liver impair the release of glucose, thus causing hypoglycemia.

These pathophysiologic mechanisms are responsible for four broad clinical categories. One category is comprised of small-for-dates infants who were subjected to intrauterine malnutrition. Another category includes infants of diabetic mothers and erythroblastotic infants. Another group includes infants with birth weights below 1250 grams who are subjected to such severe stress that their metabolic requirements exceed their glycogen stores. These infants are often asymptomatic. The last group includes infants with rare developmental and genetic disorders such as glycogen storage disease, galactosemia, and tumors of the pancreatic islets (insulinomas). In any of these clinical groupings an additive hypoglycemic effect may be exerted by severe respiratory distress, hypoxia, and hypothermia. Table 11-1 lists the most important clinical entities associated with hypoglycemia and the mechanisms involved.

Hypoglycemia and intrauterine malnutrition. Hypoglycemia occurs in approximately 20% of infants with intrauterine growth retardation. The incidence is higher in males (twice as frequent as in females) and in the smaller of twins if the birth weight discrepancy exceeds 25% and the weight of the affected infant is less than 2000 grams. Symptoms occur in 50% to 90% of hypoglycemic infants. Small-for-dates babies have diminished stores of hepatic glycogen and diminished capacity for gluconeogenesis. They also possess a relatively increased mass of glucose-consuming tissue because the brain is least affected by growth retardation and is closest to normal weight compared with other organs, especially the liver. In normally grown neonates the liver, which is the principal glucose supplier, weighs one third as much as the brain, which is an active glucose consumer. In malnourished infants the liver weighs only one seventh as much as the brain. The hepatic source of glucose is thus quite reduced in malnourished babies. Most glycogen-depleted hypoglycemic infants are below the tenth percentile on the Colorado growth charts. Other hypoglycemic infants are affected for unknown reasons, although many seem to be subjected to excessive metabolic demands resulting from some type of stress. In addition to glycogen depletion, these infants have considerably reduced fat deposits for the provision of free fatty acids as a fuel substitute for glucose.

Symptoms usually appear between 24 and 72 hours of age; occasionally they begin as early as 3 hours and as late as 7 days of age. Severely hypoxic, hypothermic small-for-dates infants are most likely to become hypoglycemic within 6 hours after birth.

Monitoring blood sugar is thus important in small-for-dates infants and in any other stressed baby. Infants who place below the tenth percentile should have blood sugar assessment at least twice during the first 24 hours and at least three times daily thereafter until 4 days of age. Screening for low values is feasible with Dextrostix. A laboratory determination for blood sugar should be requested if the Dextrostix color change indicates a level less than 45 mg/100 ml. The Dextrostix is exquisitely sensitive, and because it is such a simple procedure it is commonly performed inaccurately. The blood must remain on the reactive tip for precisely 1 minute. Shorter periods do not permit a complete reaction; longer periods allow too much reaction. The blood must be rinsed off by a forceful stream of water from a plastic squeeze bottle. Care must also be exercised in touching the strip to the capillary blood flowing from a heel prick because the delicate membrane that covers the tip is easily disrupted by contact with the skin. Treatment of hypoglycemia is discussed later in this chapter.

Infants of diabetic mothers. Before the introduction of insulin over 40 years ago, few diabetic women conceived, and among those who did, the outcome of pregnancy was often catastrophic. Pregnancy in diabetic women is now commonplace, and in recent years screening during pregnancy has also identified women whose gestational diabetic tendencies were unsuspected in the nonpregnant state. As a result of more effec-

Table 11-2. White's classification of diabetes in pregnancy

Class A	Highest probability of fetal survival No insulin, little dietary regulation Includes gestational diabetes and prediabetes
Class B	Onset at age 20 or more Duration less than 10 years before pregnancy No vascular disease
Class C	Onset between 10 and 19 years of age Duration between 10 and 19 years Minimal vascular disease (retinal arteriosclerosis, calcification of vessels in the legs only)
Class D	Onset before age 10 years Duration 20 years or more Moderately advanced vascular disease (diabetic retinopathy, transient albuminuria, and hypertension)
Class E	Characteristics of class D plus calcification of pelvic vessels
Class F	Characteristics of class D plus nephritis
Class R	Active retinitis

tive management of diabetes, particularly during gestation, the offspring of diabetic mothers are now numerous, constituting a significant problem and a major challenge to the caretakers of high-risk infants. One in 500 to 1000 pregnant women is diabetic. The incidence of gestational diabetes is considerably higher—one in 120 pregnancies. Perinatal infant mortality and morbidity rates are inordinately high among infants of diabetic mothers. There is general agreement that diabetic pregnancies should be interrupted between the thirty-sixth and thirty-seventh weeks because earlier deliveries are associated with a high rate of neonatal mortality, whereas later ones are associated with a higher incidence of stillbirth. Fetal monitoring in diabetic and other high-risk pregnancies is discussed in Chapter 1.

The classification of diabetes during pregnancy that was introduced by Dr. Priscilla White is a universal reference for grading the severity of the maternal disease (Table 11-2). It differentiates severity according to duration of diabetes before pregnancy, age at onset, and extent of vascular involvement. Class A is the most common type; it includes gestational diabetes. Gestational diabetes is characterized by an abnormal glucose tolerance curve in an asymptomatic mother, which reverts to normal within 6 weeks after delivery. Whereas mortality in babies born of class A mothers is higher than in those of nondiabetic mothers, it is the lowest of all the groups in White's classification. The most unfavorable neonatal outcomes occur in classes D through F. Toxemia of pregnancy is more likely to occur in women with vascular disease (classes D through F), and this is probably an additional contributory factor to poor pregnancy outcome. Class A and B mothers give birth to large-for-dates babies; mothers in class C and below deliver small-for-dates babies (Chapter 5).

There is no well-defined explanation for all the abnormalities in infants of diabetic mothers. The hypoglycemia that commonly occurs within hours after birth is associated with increased insulin activity in the blood. Furthermore, hyperplasia and increased insulin content of the pancreatic islet cells are demonstrated at necropsy in virtually all these infants. Current consensus holds that fetal hyperglycemia, which results from high maternal levels of blood sugar, provides a relentless stimulus to the islets for insulin production, as evidenced by their hyperplasia. Sustained fetal hyperinsulinism and hyperglycemia ultimately lead to excessive growth and deposition of fat. This may explain the high incidence of infants who are large for gestational age. When the generous supply of maternal glucose is eliminated after birth, continued islet cell hyperactivity leads to hyperinsulinism and depletion of blood glucose. Within 2 to 4 hours hypoglycemia occurs. Although this hypothesis is plausible, it does not explain the obesity of offspring from mothers who are prediabetic, that is, those who are genetically predisposed to diabetes but have none of the characteristic abnormalities; nor does it explain the multiplicity of other abnormalities in infants of diabetic mothers.

The disorders that befall infants of diabetic mothers include hypoglycemia, hypocalcemia, hyperbilirubinemia, hyaline membrane disease (as a function of prematurity), renal vein thrombosis, and a considerably higher incidence of congenital anomalies than in infants of nondiabetic mothers.

At birth, blood glucose concentration is 80% or more of the maternal level. Within an hour in normal infants, it falls to a mean of 40 to 50 mg/100 ml, but in infants of diabetic mothers, hyperinsulinism causes a greater decline. Levels below 20 and 30 mg/100 ml whole blood (25 and 35 mg/100 ml serum) usually occur from 2 to 4 hours after birth, sometimes sooner, occasionally later. This decline is followed by a spontaneous rise between 4 and 6 hours of age. Approximately half the infants of treated diabetic mothers (classes B through F) develop glucose levels below 30 mg/100 ml. Among infants of gestational diabetic mothers (class A) approximately 20% are affected. Occasionally hypoglycemia is protracted.

Rarely it appears as late as 12 to 24 hours of age.

Hypocalcemia (serum calcium below 7 mg/100 ml or 3.5 mEq/L) often occurs with or without hypoglycemia. Low serum calcium is often present soon after birth. It is thought to be caused by depressed fetal parathyroid function that persists in the neonate temporarily Symptoms are usually imperceptible; those that do appear are not specific for hypocalcemia and are also seen in normocalcemic infants. They include irritability, coarse tremors, twitches, and convulsions. Low serum calcium levels are also requently observed in stressed premature infants of nondiabetic mothers. The treatment of hypocalcemia is described later.

Hyperbilirubinemia is more frequent among infants of diabetic mothers than in babies of like gestational age who are born of nondiabetic mothers. The characteristics and treatment of this disorder are identical in all premature infants.

Renal vein thrombosis is a rare occurrence. It may be unilateral or bilateral and is sometimes associated with radiologic evidence of calcification. The involved kidney is palpably enlarged, and hematuria and proteinuria are the rule. The survival of affected infants is in grave doubt. Nephrectomy is indicated if involvement is unilateral.

The incidence of all types of congenital anomalies is two to three times greater than in the general population. The incidence of congenital heart disease is increased threefold compared with infants of nondiabetic mothers.

Whether or not they are overtly ill, infants of diabetic mothers must be managed in an intensive care facility. Approximately half of them have an indisturbed course, but careful observation is necessary nevertheless. The severity of the maternal diabetes should be known and recorded as early as the first prenatal visit. The nursery should be notified when a diabetic woman begins labor.

The schedule for blood glucose monitoring of infants of diabetic mothers is different from that of small-for-dates infants because the timing of hypoglycemia differs. Since the lowest blood glucose levels in infants of diabetic mothers occurs at 2 to 4 hours of age, blood glucose determinations should be done on cord blood at birth and at 1, 2, 4, and 6 hours of age. Distressed infants, and all infants of classes B through F mothers, should be given 10% dextrose intravenously immediately after birth at a rate of 65 to 70 ml/kg of body weight.

Hypoglycemia and erythroblastosis fetalis. For years the danger of hypoglycemia in erythroblastotic infants was obscured by a preoccupation with the dramatic hematologic, cardiopulmonary, and central nervous system aspects of the disease. Low blood glucose levels may occur in almost a third of moderately or severely affected infants and in 5% of all erythroblastotic infants, regardless of severity. When cord hemoglobin is less than 10 grams/100 ml, the incidence of hypoglycemia is comparable to that in small-for-dates infants. As in the latter group, symptoms are often absent. When present, they are identical to those of hypoglycemia from other causes. Blood sugar levels may fall transiently before or after exchange transfusion, most often during the first day of life but occasionally later. Islet cell hyperplasia and increased insulin content of the islets and blood are similar to those of infants or diabetic mothers. Their cause is unknown. Blood glucose levels should be monitored every 4 to 6 hours during the first day and

regularly for the ensuing 3 days. Therapy is the same as for all forms of hypoglycemia.

Hypoglycemia in very small premature infants. Low blood sugar levels are not uncommon in infants whose birth weight is less than 1250 grams. Hypoglycemia may occur during the hours after birth and during the days that follow. Intravenous 10% dextrose is given routinely after birth and for variable periods thereafter. Presumably liver glycogen stores are low in these very immature infants, and the increased metabolic demands imposed by extrauterine life deplete glycogen supplies rapidly. The process is accentuated by cold stress, asphyxia, and respiratory difficulty, all of which are frequent in these small infants. Blood sugar data should be followed every 4 to 8 hours for the first 2 days of life and periodically thereafter. Since pH and blood gas determinations are usually necessary at frequent intervals, it is advisable to obtain glucose determinations simultaneously.

Treatment of hypoglycemia. Hypoglycemia requires treatment with intravenous glucose, whether symptoms are present or not. The method for administering glucose is identical for the hyperinsulinemic (infants of diabetic mothers, erythroblastotic infants) and the glycogen-depletion types of hypoglycemia (small-for-dates infants, smaller of twins). If a low blood sugar level is found in the first sample, a second is collected for confirmation, and treatment is begun immediately. If the baby is symptomatic, a 25% glucose solution is given in a dose of 2 to 4 ml/kg of body weight, followed by a solution that delivers glucose at 7 to 8 mg/kg/min. A 15% dextrose solution at 80 ml/kg/24 hr will deliver glucose at a rate of 8 mg/kg/min. A 10% dextrose solution at 120ml/kg/

24 hr will deliver glucose at the same rate. It is preferable to calculate glucose administration, whether for ordinary daily maintenance or for therapy of hypoglycemia, in terms of quantity given per minute. If the normal neonate generates approximately 5 to 8 mg/kg/min, therapeutic glucose for hypoglycemia should be given in at least these quantities. Failure to restore normoglycemia in 15 minutes is an indication to increase the dose of glucose, which can be as high as 14 mg/kg/min if necessary. This quantity of glucose may be given in a 20% dextrose solution at 100 ml/kg/24 hr or in a 15% solution at 140 ml/kg/24 hr. One may very simply convert glucose prescribed per minute into fluid per kilogram of body weight per 24 hours as follows:

Given as 10% dextrose solution IV:

mg glucose/kg/min × 15 = ml fluid/kg/24 hr

Given as 15% dextrose solution IV:

mg glucose/kg/min × 10 = ml fluid/kg/24 hr

Given as 20% dextrose solution IV:

mg glucose/kg/min × 7 = ml fluid/kg/24 hr

EXAMPLES:

IV Solution	Glucose/ kg/min	Factor	Amount fluid to give
10% D/W	10 mg	× 15	150ml/kg/24 hr
10% D/W	8 mg	× 15	120 ml/kg/24 hr
15% D/W	12 mg	× 10	120 ml/kg/24 hr
15% D/W	8 mg	× 10	84 ml/kg/24 hr
20% D/W	12 mg	× 7	70 ml/kg/24 hr

A strong case must be made (by reiteration) for calculation of actual quantities of glucose, rather than random selection of percent solution. It is no more appropriate to arbitrarily raise or lower the concentration of a dextrose solution for de-

sired changes in quantities of glucose than it is to change oxygen concentrations by ordering a different flow rate in liters per minute. Both practices are anachronistic. First, the quantity of glucose needed for adequate therapy must be determined. Second, the appropriate daily amount of fluid for the infant in question must be decided on. Third, the strength of the dextrose solution that best answers fluid and glucose needs must be calculated. Arbitrary choice of solution strength that totally disregards the quantity of glucose thus delivered, is an unacceptable practice.

There are those who believe that treatment of hypoglycemia with initial "push" dosage of 25% dextrose is ill-advised because the resultant abrupt rise in serum osmolality may cause intraventricular hemorrhage. There is indeed some evidence to indicate that hyperglycemia may have such an effect. However, the use of a continuous drip of 15% dextrose is associated with delayed restoration of normoglycemia in some babies—as much as 50 minutes. The long-term effects of this delay, though undocumented, are nevertheless a real concern. "Push" doses of 25% glucose should thus be given over at least a 10-minute interval so that abrupt elevations in osmolality are minimized or eliminated.

If the blood glucose level remains low after two subsequent determinations within 2 hours after onset of treatment, steroids should be added. Hydrocortisone, 5 mg every 6 to 12 hours, or 1 mg of prednisone every 6 to 12 hours, is generally used for this purpose. Oral milk feedings are started as soon as the infant tolerates them. Blood sugar level should stabilize at normal values for 24 to 48 hours before the dose of glucose is lowered. Except in the most protracted cases, steroids can usually be discontinued after 2 or 3 days.

Prognosis of neonatal hypoglycemia. Untreated symptomatic hypoglycemia in the neonate may cause death. Later in childhood the incidence of central nervous system dysfunction varies from 30% to 60% of untreated symptomatic small-for-dates infants. The incidence of later neurologic abnormality in asymptomatic infants may be considerably lower, but nevertheless significant. The destiny of asymptomatic small-for-dates babies with hypoglycemia is not known, since there are no well-controlled follow-up studies available. Clearly defined outcomes of well-treated hypoglycemic small-for-dates babies are also wanting. Data from a recent well-planned inquiry suggest that these infants still do not fare as well as normoglycemic controls, but many other unanswered questions have left the issue clouded. Outcome of the asymptomatic hypoglycemic infant has not been clarified. Until it is, the recommendation to treat such infants rapidly is virtually universal. The outcome for hypoglycemic infants of diabetic mothers has not been defined precisely. Some investigators have not found central nervous system abnormalities later in childhood; others have noted a low incidence of brain abnormalities, but no well-controlled, follow-up studies are available.

CALCIUM DISORDERS

The causes of neonatal hypocalcemia are multiple, and for the most part the mechanisms by which it is produced have not been unequivocally defined. Normal serum calcium levels vary from 8 to 10 mg/100 ml (4 to 5 mEq/L). Calcium levels below 7 mg/100 ml are considered abnormally depressed. The etiologic association of clinical signs with hypocalcemia, as with hypoglycemia, is difficult to establish because the symptoms occur in other unrelated disorders, and they are often nonexistent in hypocalcemic infants.

Two peaks of incidence occur, one during the first 48 hours and another between the fifth and tenth days of life. Typically, the infant with early hypocalcemia is premature, either AGA or SGA. Perinatal asphyxia increases the probability of hypocalcemia. The early type is thought to be related to temporary neonatal hypoparathyroidism. Serum calcium is low, phosphorus is high, and magnesium is sometimes diminished. Serum calcium is also related to gestational age: the shorter the gestation, the lower the calcium. Infants of diabetic mothers are often hypocalcemic. A history of abruptio placentae or placenta previa is not unusual. The symptoms of this early form of hypocalcemia, if any are discernible, often do not include neuromuscular involvement. Rather, they may be characterized by apnea, cyanotic episodes, edema, high-pitched cry, and abdominal distention; even these manifestations, however, have not been proved to be of hypocalcemic origin.

The form of hypocalcemia that begins during the fifth to tenth days is called *neonatal tetany*. It occurs in well-nourished infants who are fed evaporated milk formula that contains diminished concentrations of calcium in relation to phosphorus (increased Ca:P ratio), compared with concentrations in human milk. An increase in serum phosporus follows several days of feeding, and the resultant hyperphosphatemia depresses activity of the parathyroid gland. The effect of this suppression is to diminish serum calcium. Most proprietary brands of milk formula now contain a ratio of calcium to phosphorus closely simulating that of human milk. Neonatal tetany is rare in areas in which evaporated milk is not a prevalent formula. The signs of neonatal tetany are characterized by neuromuscular irritation—twitching, tremors, jitters, and focal or generalized convulsions. Convulsions frequently begin as the infant is taken up for a feeding. They vary in duration from a few seconds to as long as 10 minutes. Minor stimuli often provoke tremors or convulsive episodes, whereas in the undisturbed interim only restlessness may be apparent.

Maternal hyperparathyroidism is rare, but when it exists, the infant is quite likely to be hypocalcemic. A number of reports describe the diagnosis of maternal hyperparathyroidism only after identification of hypocalcemia in her newborn infant. Mothers of hypocalcemic infants should be investigated for this possibility. The pregnant woman with chronic hyperparathyroidism is hypercalcemic as a result of overactivity of that endocrine gland. Parathyroid hormone does not cross the placenta in either direction, but maternal calcium is actively taken up by the placenta; the fetus thus becomes hypercalcemic like the mother. Hypercalcemia depresses activity of the fetal parathyroid glands. At birth, with disappearance of the maternal oversupply of calcium, the neonate is left with a rapidly diminishing serum calcium level and with parathyroid glands that were depressed in utero. Parathyroid hormone is essential to calcium balance. It mobilizes calcium and increases serum levels. The neonate now has transient hypoparathyroidism and, as a result, is hypocalcemic.

Hypocalcemia is treated initially with intravenous injection of 10% calcium gluconate, 2 ml/kg of body weight (18 mg/kg of elemental calcium). The injection must be given slowly over a period of at least 10 minutes because sudden bradycardia frequently occurs during rapid administration. The heart rate should be monitored electronically or by auscultation. If it drops rapidly, the injection should be discontinued immediately. It may be resumed after a normal cardiac rate is maintained for approximately 30 minutes. Intramuscular administration of calcium gluconate is contraindicated because calcium precipitates rapidly; a calcemic mass and necrosis result. Caution is also required during intravenous infusion because accidental escape to extravascular tissue produces local calcification and sloughing. Calcium gluconate thus should not be administered through scalp veins. Orally administered calcium, added to formula, is begun as soon as feasible. Following the initial dosage, calcium gluconate should be added to intravenous fluids in a daily dose of 800 mg/kg (72 mg of elemental calcium). As normal serum levels are attained, the daily dose should be lowered gradually by half each day. Abrupt discontinuation may cause rebound hypocalcemia. If oral feedings are tolerated, calcium gluconate can be fed in amounts identical to those recommended parenterally, even after the initial "push" dose.

MAGNESIUM DISORDERS
Hypomagnesemia

Reports of tetany due to low magnesium levels have appeared with increasing frequency in the past few years. Normal serum magnesium concentration in the neonate is 1.2 to 1.8 mg/100 ml. Hypomagnesemia usually accompanies hypocalcemia. It occurs during or after exchange transfusions because magnesium becomes bound to the citrate in donor blood. For unknown reasons, it may also occur in infants of diabetic mothers. Serum magnesium determinations are essential for proper evaluation of babies with signs of neuromuscular excitability. They are especially important in hypocalcemic infants who do not respond to calcium therapy. If the signs are caused by magnesium deficiency, tetany and convulsions disappear promptly after appropriate therapy. An intramuscular dose of 50% magnesium sulfate (0.2 ml/kg of body weight) is given every 4 hours for the first day. The need for subsequent therapy is determined by serial serum magnesium determinations.

Hypermagnesemia

Magnesium sulfate is a preparation of choice for the treatment of preeclampsia. When it is administered by either the intramuscular or intravenous routes, serum magnesium levels in maternal and cord blood are higher than normal. The maternal normal range is 1.2 to 2.2 mEq/L; normal values in cord blood are 0.9 to 2.6 mEq/L. Most cases of neonatal hypermagnesemia reported to date have not been associated with clinical abnormalities, and there is some doubt that high magnesium levels are responsible for abnormal signs. However, there are several instances of severe neonatal illness associated with high serum magnesium concentrations. At high levels magnesium causes peripheral neuromuscular block (curare-like effect) and central nervous system depression as well. Clinical abnormalities in the neonate are believed by some authors to include hypotonia, weak or absent cry, and severe respiratory depression with apnea and cyanosis. The respiratory difficulty has necessitated mechanically assisted ventilation. Several investigators have used intravenous calcium in attempts to antagonize the depressive effects of excessive magnesium, but with little evidence of benefit. The consensus is that calcium therapy is not effective. However, a dramatic response to exchange transfusion has been well documented. Magnesium toxicity should be suspected in a symptomatic infant whose mother was treated vigorously with magnesium sulfate for preeclampsia.

REFERENCES

Adam, P. A. J., and Schwartz, R.: Diagnosis and treatment: should oral hypoglycemic agents be used in pediatric and pregnant patients? Pediatrics **42:**819, 1968.

Anderson, J. M., Milner, R. D. G., and Strich, S. J.: Pathological changes in the nervous system in severe neonatal hypoglycemia, Lancet **2:**372, 1966.

Avery, M.E., Oppenheimer, E. H., and Gordon, H. H.: Renal-vein thrombosis in newborn infants of diabetic mothers, N. Engl. J. Med. **265:**1134, 1957.

Ballard, F. J.: Carbohydrate metabolism and the regulation of blood glucose. In Stave, U., editor: Perinatal physiology, New York, 1978, Plenum Medical Book Co.

Barrett, C. T., and Oliver, T. K.: Hypoglycemia and hyperinsulinism in infants with erythroblastosis, N. Engl. J. Med **278:**1260, 1968.

Beard, A. G., et al.: Neonatal hypoglycemia: a discussion, J. Pediatr. **79:**314, 1971.

Brady, J. P., and Williams, H. C.: Magnesium intoxication in a premature infant, Pediatrics **40:**100, 1967.

Brazy, J. E., and Pupkin, M. J.: Effects of maternal isoxsuprine administration on preterm infants, J. Pediatr. **94:**444, 1979.

Clarke, P. C. N., and Carre, I. J.: Hypocalcemic, hypomagnesemic convulsions, J. Pediatr. **70:**806, 1967.

Cornblath, M., and Schwartz, R.: Disorders of carbohydrate metabolism in infancy, ed. 2, Philadelphia, 1976, W. B. Saunders Co.

Cottrill, C. M., McAllister, R. G., Jr., Gettes, L., and Noonan, J. A.: Propranolol therapy during pregnancy, labor, and delivery: evidence for transplacental drug transfer and impaired neonatal drug disposition, J. Pediatr. **91:**812, 1977.

Craig, W. S.: Clinical signs of neonatal tetany; with especial reference to their occurrence in newborn babies of diabetic mothers, Pediatrics **22**:297, 1958.

Craig, W. S., and Buchanan, M. F. G.: Hypocalcemic tetany developing within 36 hours of birth, Arch. Dis. Child. **33**:505, 1958.

Davis, J. A., Harvey, D. R., and Yu, J. S.: Neonatal fits associated with hypomagnesemia, Arch. Dis. Child. **40**:286, 1965.

Dorchy, H., and Loeb, H.: Correlation of Dextrostix values with true glucose in the range less than 50 mg/dl (editorial correspondence), J. Pediatr. **88**:692, 1976.

Epstein, M. F., Nicholls, E., and Stubblefield, P. G.: Neonatal hypoglycemia after beta-sympathomimetic tocolytic therapy, J. Pediatr. **94**:449, 1979.

Ertel, N. H., Reiss, J. S., and Spergel, G.: Hypomagnesemia in neonatal tetany associated with maternal hyperparathyroidism, N. Engl. J. Med. **280**:260, 1969.

Farquhar, J. W.: Prognosis for babies born to diabetic mothers in Edinburgh, Arch. Dis. Child. **44**:36, 1969.

Fischer, G. W., Vazquez, A. M., Buist, N. R. M., et al.: Neonatal islet cell adenoma: case report and literature review, Pediatrics **53**:753, 1974.

Fisher, D. A.: Insulin and carbohydrate metabolism. In Smith, C. A., and Nelson, N. M., editors: The physiology of the newborn infant, Springfield, Ill., 1976, Charles C Thomas, Publisher.

Fletcher, A. B.: Clinical and biochemical aspects of the infant of the diabetic mother. In Young, D. S., and Hicks, J. M., editors: The neonate: clinical biochemistry, physiology and pathology, New York, 1976, John Wiley & Sons, Inc.

Frantz, I. D., III, Medina, G., and Taeusch, H. W., Jr.: Correlation of Dextrostix values with true glucose in the range less than 50 mg/dl, J. Pediatr. **87**:417, 1975.

From, G. L. A., Driscoll, S. G., and Steinke, J.: Serum insulin in newborn infants with erythroblastosis fetalis, Pediatrics **44**:549, 1969.

Gentz, J., Persson, B., and Zetterstrom, R.: On the diagnosis of symptomatic neonatal hypoglycemia, Acta Paediatr. Scand. **58**:449, 1969.

Griffiths, A. D.: Association of hypoglycaemia with symptoms in the newborn, Arch. Dis. Child. **43**:688, 1968.

Gutberlet, R. L., and Cornblath, M.: Neonatal hypoglycemia revisited, 1975, Pediatr. **58**:10, 1976.

Habib, A., and McCarthy, J. S.: Effects on the neonate of propranolol administered during pregnancy, J. Pediatr. **91**:808, 1977.

Haworth, J. C.: Neonatal hypoglycemia: how much does it damage the brain? Pediatrics **54**:3, 1974.

Haworth, J. C., and McRae, K. N: The neurological and developmental effects of neonatal hypoglycemia: a follow-up of 22 cases, Can. Med. Assoc. J. **92**:861, 1965.

Jacobs, R. F., Nix, R. A., Paulus, T. E., et al.: Intravenous infusion of diazoxide in the treatment of chlorpropamide-induced hypoglycemia, J. Pediatr. **93**:801, 1978.

Keen, J. H.: Significance of hypocalcemia in neonatal convulsions, Arch. Dis. Child. **44**:356, 1969.

Lee, F. A., and Gwinn, J. L.: Roentgen patterns of extravasation of calcium gluconate in the tissues of the neonate, J. Pediatr. **86**:598, 1975.

Lilien, L. D., Grajwer, L. A., and Pildes, R. S.: Treatment of neonatal hypoglycemia with continuous intravenous glucose infusion, J. Pediatr. **91**:779, 1977.

Lipsitz, P. J.: The clinical and biochemical effects of excess magnesium in the newborn, Pediatrics **47**:501, 1971.

Lubchenco, L. O., and Bard, H.: Incidence of hypoglycemia in newborn infants classified by birth weight and gestational age, Pediatrics **47**:831, 1971.

Lucey, J. F., Randall, J. L., and Murray, J. J.: Is hypoglycemia an important complication in erythroblastosis fetalis? Am. J. Dis. Child. **114**:88, 1967.

Medovy, H.: Outlook for the infant of the diabetic mother, J. Pediatr. **76**:988, 1970.

Mizrach, A., London, R. D., and Gribetz, D.: Neonatal hypocalcemia: its causes and treatment, N. Engl. J. Med. **278**:1163, 1968.

Naeye, R. L.: Infants of diabetic mothers; a quantitative, morphologic study, Pediatrics **35**:980, 1965.

Neligan, G. A., Robson, E., and Watson, J.: Hypoglycemia in the newborn: a sequel of the intrauterine malnutrition, Lancet **1**:1282, 1963.

O'Sullivan, J. B.: Gestational diabetes: unsuspected, asymptomatic diabetes in pregnancy, N. Engl. J. Med. **264**:1082, 1961.

Pedersen, J.: The pregnant diabetic and her newborn, Baltimore, 1967, The Williams & Wilkins Co.

Pildes, R. S.: Metabolic and endocrine disorders: In Behrman, R. E., editor: Neonatal-perinatal medicine: diseases of the fetus and infant, ed. 2, St. Louis, 1977, The C. V. Mosby Co.

Pildes, R. S., Forbes, A., and Cornblath, M.: Studies of carbohydrate metabolism in the newborn infant. IX. Blood glucose levels and hypoglycemia in twins, Pediatrics **40**:69, 1967.

Pildes, R. S., Cornblath, M., Warren, I., et al.: A prospective controlled study of neonatal hypoglycemia, Pediarics **54**:5, 1974.

Raivio, K. O.: Neonatal hypoglycemia. II. A clinical study of 44 idiopathic cases with special reference to corticosteroid treatment, Acta Paediatr. Scand. **57**:540, 1968.

Raivio, K. O., and Osterlund, K.: Hypoglycemia and hyperinsulinemia associated with erythroblastosis fetalis, J. Pediatr. **43**:217, 1969.

Reisner, S. H., Forbes, A. E., and Cornblath, M.: The smaller of twins and hypoglycemia, Lancet **1**:524, 1965.

Robert, M. F., Neff, R. K., Hubbell, J. P., et al.: Association between maternal diabetes and the respiratory-distress syndrome in the newborn, N. Engl. J. Med. **294**:357, 1976.

Saville, P. D., and Kretchmer, N.: Neonatal tetany; a report of 125 cases and review of the literature, Biol. Neonate **2**:1, 1960.

Tsang, R. C., and Oh, W.: Neonatal hypocalcemia in low birth weight infants, Pediatrics **45**:773, 1970.

Tsang, R. C., Chen, I., Hayes, W., et al.: Neonatal hypocalcemia in infants with birth asphyxia, J. Pediatr. **84**:428. 1974.

Tsang, R. C., Chen, I-W., Friedman, M. A., et al.: Parathyroid function in infants of diabetic mothers, J. Pediatr. **86**:399, 1975.

Tsang, R. C., Kleinman, L. I., Sutherland, J. M., and Light, I. J.: Hypocalcemia in infants of diabetic mothers, J. Pediatr. **80**:384, 1972.

Tsang, R. C., Light, I. J., Sutherland, J. M., and Kleinman, L. I.: Possible pathogenetic factors in neonatal hypocalcemia of prematurity, J. Pediatr. **82**:423, 1973.

Wald, M. K.: Problems in metabolic adaptation; glucose, calcium, and magnesium. In Klaus, M. H., and Fanaroff, A. A., editors: Care of the high-risk neonate, Philadelphia, 1979, W. B. Saunders Co.

Yeung, C. Y., Lee, V. W. Y., and Yeung, C. M.: Glucose disappearance rate in neonatal infection, J. Pediatr. **82**:486, 1973.

Zucker, P., and Simon, G.: Prolonged symptomatic neonatal hypoglycemia associated with maternal chlorpropamide therapy, Pediatrics **42**:824, 1968.

Perinatal infection

Although of diverse etiology, perinatal infections have many attributes in common that distinguish them from infections in later life. Whether of bacterial, viral, or protozoan causation, the tissue damage wrought by these infections and the patterns of disease they produce are remarkably different from those observed in more advanced age groups. For instance, the bacteria generally implicated in fetal and neonatal disease are not ordinarily pathogenic in older children. Conversely, organisms that cause serious disease in mature patients, such as pneumococci, group A streptococci, and meningococci, are rarely encountered during the perinatal period. Diseases caused by rubella virus, cytomegalovirus, herpesvirus, and *Toxoplasma* are usually mild or asymptomatic in later life, but in the fetus and neonate these organisms produce extensive devastation of tissue, often resulting in death or dysfunctional survival.

In the pathogenesis of antepartal or intrapartal infection, maternal involvement, usually asymptomatic, always precedes fetal disease. The fetus may acquire disease from infected amniotic fluid, from the maternal bloodstream across the placenta, or by direct contact with infected maternal tissue in the birth canal. After birth the neonate must contend with the possibility of acquiring infection from other infants or from personnel or objects that surround him, particularly the equipment designed to save his life. The neonate's vulnerability to these hazards is determined by a number of variables, of which prematurity is clearly the most significant.

Another distinctive feature of perinatal infection is the immunologic response it stimulates. Special procedures are necessary to differentiate antibodies generated by the fetus and neonate from those received through the placenta from the mother. Serologic techniques that diagnose infections in older children are of little value in the newborn infant.

Physical signs of infectious disease, if any are indeed perceptible, are unique in their subtlety and their lack of specificity. Early in the course of infection one may not be aware of any disturbance, yet the disorder soon becomes rapidly fulminant and uncontrollable. Thus a severely septicemic premature infant may merely be hypoactive and refuse feeding. Furthermore, fever, the hallmark of infectious disease later in life, is often absent in the infected newborn. Coughing, which is almost universal in older children with pneumonia, is rare.

The choice of therapeutic antibiotics must usually be made before results of cultures are known. Such choices must be influenced by knowledge of the bacterial organisms most likely to cause disease. Their incidence is unique to the neonate. Equally important in the choice of therapy is an understanding of the immature pharmacologic response of the newborn infant. During the first 2 or 3 weeks of life, the absorption, metabolism, and excretion of drugs vary considerably from those observed in older patients, and the uninformed use of some drugs may have serious results. The disastrous consequences of ne-

glecting these differences were exemplified years ago by the widespread use of sulfisoxazole (Gantrisin) and chloramphenicol, which were administered in complete ignorance of the special hazards they imposed on the neonate. Sulfisoxazole caused an unexpectedly high incidence of kernicterus, and chloramphenicol caused numerous deaths.

This chapter discusses the salient aspects of perinatal infection, the fundamental reasons for its uniqueness, and the characteristics of its most important clinical entities.

ETIOLOGY
Bacterial agents

Most bacterial infections are caused by organisms comprising the flora of the mother's genital and intestinal tracts; beyond early infancy these agents are rarely pathogenic. Although varying lengthy lists of etiologic agents have emerged from numerous studies; a rather uniform pattern is apparent for the three major clinical entities: pneumonia, septicemia, and meningitis. Before the emergence of group B streptococci in the early 1970s as the most frequent etiologic agent, gram-negative rods produced 75% to 85% of these bacterial infections; *Escherichia coli* was predominant among them. *Pseudomonas aeruginosa* was the next most common agent. It is usually acquired postnatally; nursery equipment is a major source of its propagation. Staphylococci cause septicemia and pneumonia. Staphytococcal infection is virtually always acquired postnatally in the nursery, rarely from the mother during birth. Staphylococci are infrequently implicated in meningitis. During the worldwide nursery epidemics of the late 1950s and early 1960s, they were a prominent cause of pneumonia, and although still an

Table 12-1. Vertically transmitted viruses implicated in fetal and neonatal infection*

Virus	Fetal/neonatal disorders
Rubella virus	Microcephaly, meningoencephalitis (chronic), cataracts, microphthalmia, glaucoma, deafness, hepatitis, jaundice, hepatosplenomegaly, pneumonitis, cardiovascular anomalies, myocardial necrosis, thrombocytopenia, anemia, purpura, inguinal hernia
Cytomegalovirus	Microcephaly, cerebral calcification, hydrocephalus, encephalitis, chorioretinitis, hepatitis, jaundice, hepatosplenomegaly, pneumonitis, cardiac anomalies, thrombocytopenia, purpura, anemia, inguinal hernia
Herpesvirus hominis	Meningoencephalitis, microcephaly, cerebral calcification, herpetic rash, hepatitis, jaundice, pneumonitis, thrombocytopenia, anemia, coagulopathy, keratoconjunctivitis, chorioretinitis
Coxsackievirus group B	Meningoencephalitis, myocarditis, hepatitis, jaundice, thrombocytopenia
Varicella-zoster	Chickenpox rash, pneumonitis, hepatitis
Variola poxvirus	Smallpox rash, pneumonitis, hepatitis, meningoencephalitis
Vaccinia virus	Vaccinia rash, pneumonitis, hepatitis, stillbirth
Poliomyelitis	Spinal or bulbar polio similar to adult, myocarditis, pneumonitis, stillbirth, abortion
Rubeola	Measles as in later life (usually benign), stillbirth, abortion
Western equine encephalomyelitis	Meningoencephalitis
Myxovirus (mumps)	Congenital parotitis, ? congenital malformations
Hepatitis virus B	Neonatal hepatitis

*Modified from Sever, J. L., and White, L. R.: Annual Rev. Med. **19**:471, 1968.

important factor, they are now encountered with less frequency (see later). *Listeria monocytogenes* is a maternally derived gram-positive rod that also causes septicemia and meningitis. Most pediatric infections from this organism occur during the newborn period.

Viral agents

Viral diseases in the fetus and neonate are far less frequent than bacterial diseases, but they comprise an important cause of morbidity and mortality. They are generally transmitted from the mother but may also be acquired postnatally. Data on postnatally acquired viral disease are relatively meager, but considerable interest has been focused on infections acquired in utero. Thirteen viral agents are known to be vertically transmitted (from mother to fetus). These are listed in Table 12-1, accompanied by the prominent clinical findings for each. The importance of these perinatal viral diseases lies not only in the mortality they produce but in the more numerous infants who survive them with varying degrees of central nervous system damage.

Protozoan agent

Toxoplasma gondii is the most important protozoan agent involved in perinatal infection. Toxoplasmosis is discussed in detail later in this chapter.

PATHOGENESIS
Bacterial infections

Bacterial infections are acquired in utero, during descent through the birth canal, and after birth in the delivery room or nursery.

Intrauterine bacterial infection acquired by the ascending route. With few exceptions, bacterial infections are acquired prenatally by the ascending route; that is, organisms from the perineum and vagina gain entry into the uterine cavity through the cervix. Amniotic fluid is infected after passage of bacteria through a ruptured amniotic membrane, but sometimes the organisms permeate an intact one. They then gain entry into the fetus through the oral cavity and move to the lungs, gastrointestinal tract, and middle ear. Occasionally they enter the bloodstream from these sites.

The presence of organisms in amniotic fluid triggers an inflammatory response in the membranes consisting of infiltrates of polymorphonuclear leukocytes, which ultimately enter the amniotic fluid. Interestingly, the reaction begins in the maternal tissue and then spreads to the amniotic membrane, which is a fetal structure. The resultant lesion is known as chorioamnionitis. Benirschke and Driscoll have aptly pointed out that this is a unique example of response by one organism (maternal) to infection in another (fetal). The presence of bacteria in amniotic fluid thus produces chorioamnionitis and an outpouring of leukocytes into amniotic fluid. Chorioamnionitis and infected amniotic fluid do not always cause fetal disease. They merely expose the fetus to intrauterine infection. Based on the development of chorioamnionitis, several diagnostic procedures have been devised to identify exposure to intrauterine bacterial infection.

Identification of fetal infection. At birth three procedures are of possible value in identifying the risk imposed by exposure to infection, even though *most exposures do not produce active disease*. These procedures are applicable to premature infants, but results are equivocal and few nurseries utilize them. At neonatal facilities that do use them, antibotics are given to premature infants so identified even though they are asymptomatic. One procedure involves examination of gastric contents for the presence of neutrophils and bacteria. A second test employs microscopic examination of frozen sections of the umbilical cord immediately after birth. Infiltration of the cord by polymorphonuclear leukocytes is part of the overall response that characterizes chorioamnionitis. A third test utilizes microscopic examination of a section of amniotic membrane for the presence of infiltrate. It must be emphasized that *positive results from these procedures do not prove fetal disease*. For newborn infants in whom infection is later documented, however, these tests are positive with few exceptions.

Rupture of membranes and prolonged labor. There is general agreement that early rupture of amniotic membranes predisposes to chorioamnionitis and umbilical vasculitis (inflammation of the cord and its vessels) and that the possibility of fetal infection is thus enhanced. Most investigators consider that membrane rupture is early if it occurs at least 24 hours before delivery. Beyond this time the risk of infection increases as the interval between rupture of membranes and birth is prolonged. However, for reasons as yet unknown, numerous infections occur even when membranes rupture closer to delivery than 24 hours. Length of labor is not as clearly correlated with the incidence of infection. There is little doubt that the hazard is most serious when early membrane rupture and prolonged labor are combined. For the nurse, this type of information is valuable in anticipating and detecting the signs of infection. When an infant with a history of exposure to infection in utero is admitted to the nursery, cultures should be taken. The best sites for specimen collection are the throat, axillae, inguinal folds, and external auditory canals. If these cultures are taken within 1 or 2 hours after birth, the results reveal organisms to which the infant was exposed. If signs of illness appear subsequently, the results of cultures provide some basis for the selection of therapeutic antibiotics.

Gestational age and fetal infection. A strong positive association between short gestational age and increased incidence of chorioamnionitis, umbilical vasculitis, and neonatal infection has been cited universally. The shorter the gestational age, the higher their incidence. The incidence of septicemia, meningitis, and pneumonia is considerably higher among premature than among term infants.

Intrauterine bacterial infection acquired transplacentally. Syphilis and occasionally *Listeria monocytogenes* are transmitted across the placenta. Fetal tuberculosis is a rare infection, but when it occurs, it too is acquired through the placenta. Fetal infection from transplacentally derived pneumococcus, streptococcus, staphylococcus, and *Salmonella* is also rare. Before antibiotics were available, maternal septicemia due to these organisms was more frequent, and fetal infection by the placental route was an occasional sequel.

Bacterial infection acquired postnatally. Nursery personnel, infant cohorts, fixtures, and equipment utilized for care of the neonate comprise important sources of postnatal infection. In this respect the lessons learned from the worldwide scourge of staphylococcal epidemics are important to recall. Causative strains of staphylococci were repeatedly cultured from attendants, from other infants, and from articles in the environment such as airborne particles, linen, diapers, and blankets. An exchange between infants and environmental components was postulated by numerous investigators, and indeed the general pattern that emerged from most studies indicated as much. However, disagreement arose about the relative importance of each of these factors, and more fundamentally, about the original source of organisms. The bitter experience with staphylococcal epidemics over a period of several years led to a multiplicity of stringent hygienic measures and isolation techniques, some of which have been relaxed considerably because epidemiologic strains of staphylococci seemed to disappear from the nursery. The influence exerted by these stringent nursery practices is impossible to estimate. It is possible that a phase in the long-term natural life cycle of staphylococci has passed, largely unrelated to our feverish efforts to eliminate them. Infection control practices in the nursery are discussed later in this chapter.

Commensurate with the decline of staphylococcal disease, there was a rise in the incidence of postnatally acquired gram-negative rod infections. The increased use of mechanical equipment for the care of high-risk neonates has certainly been a factor in the upsurge of these infections. Epidemics caused by organisms such as *Pseudomonas aeruginosa, Serratia marcescens, Klebsiella, Aerobacter, Proteus, Achromobacter, Flavobacterium,* and *Alcaligenes faecalis* have been traced to a variety of unsuspected sources in the environment. Most of these organisms proliferate and thrive in water alone, and for this reason Wheeler has aptly dubbed them "water bugs." Epidemics of septicemia, meningitis, pneumonia, and conjunctivitis due to these organisms have arisen from one or more of the following sources:

Suction machines
Face masks
Resuscitation apparatus
Humidifying systems in incubators
Plastic sleeves on incubator portholes
Aerators on sink faucets
Dripping sink taps
Submerged water supply inlets in sinks
Cross connections between water inlets and
 waste lines
Dirty soap dispensers and soap trays
Bathing pans
Solutions used for eye irrigation
Benzalkonium (Zephiran) and other solutions
 used for cold sterilization

The lesson from the experience in recent years is clear: Vigilance in maintaining cleanliness of the physical environment is indispensable to the survival of all neonates.

Viral and protozoan infections

Fetal viral disease and toxoplasmosis are transmitted from the mother across the placenta. The only known exceptions are herpesvirus and cytomegalovirus infections, which are often acquired by the ascending route. Cytomegalovirus is also acquired transplacentally. The viruses listed in Table 12-1 have a presumed or proved capacity to permeate the placenta and enter the fetal bloodstream. Fetal infections may occur at any time during pregnancy. Rubella begins during the first trimester, occasionally slightly later. Cytomegalovirus infection may begin at any time during pregnancy, and in most cases herpesvirus disease is acquired in the third trimester.

Host defenses (immune response)

The mechanisms that comprise the host's defense against invasion by infectious agents are interdependent and multiple. Nonspecific factors include surface protection provided by the skin and mucous membranes, activity of phagocytic cells, and the inflammatory response. Specific factors involve the production of antibodies. They are specific in that they conteract a single organism and are effective against none other; in contrast the skin barrier, phagocytosis, and inflammation are active against any organism that encounters them.

Antibodies. The definitions of antibody and antigen are mutually dependent. An antibody is a protein synthesized by specific types of cells in response to antigenic stimulation; an antigen is a substance of any kind that stimulates the production of antibodies. One type of antibody is bound to cells, and another circulates in plasma (humoral antibodies); the latter are the immunoglobulins.

Most of the available data on the perinatal immune response concern the immunoglobulins. They are secreted into body fluids by lymphocytes and plasma cells, which are specialized cells in tissues. There are several varieties of immunoglobulins, the three major ones being IgG, IgM, and IgA (or gamma-G, gamma-M, gamma-A).

IgG. The IgG fraction contains antibodies to the majority of bacterial and viral organisms previously encountered by the mother. Of the three major immunoglobulins, only IgG crosses the placenta from the maternal to the fetal circulation. Maternally derived IgG first appears in the fetus during the third gestational month, accumulating progressively thereafter. Placental transfer is markedly increased during the last trimester. Length of gestation is thus a significant determinant of the IgG level at birth, which is lower in premature infants than in term infants. At 32 weeks, for example, a premature infant's cord blood contains only 400 mg/100 ml of IgG. In term infants the IgG concentration is at least equal to maternal levels, approximately 1000 mg/100 ml. Since most of the mother's circulating antibodies to bacterial and viral agents are in the IgG fraction, the fetus receives an ample supply of them from her. These antibodies are in effect an imprint of her own lifetime experience with infections. The uninfected neonate has virtually no other IgG at birth.

After birth, maternal IgG antibodies are catabolized, with resultant depletion over the first 3 months of life. The infant's synthesis of IgG increases gradually during the same period, and at approximately 3 months of age it is sufficient to supplant the loss of maternal IgG. The premature infant's IgG level reaches its lowest point much sooner because there was a low concentration at birth. There is thus a longer period of lower IgG levels until such time as the infant can generate significant amounts of the immunoglobulin. The fact that levels of protection are lower over a longer period may be a significant cause of the premature infant's greater susceptibility to infections and the high incidence of rehospitalization they require during the early months of

the first year. Total IgG concentration in term babies thus falls from about 1000 mg/100 ml at birth to 400 mg/100 ml at 3 months, at which time a gradual increase begins as a result of the infant's accelerated synthesis. The mother's protection against infection is thus bestowed on her baby, and these protective effects are extended well beyond intrauterine life. IgG contains specific antibodies against most of the common infectious agents, including gram-positive cocci (pneumococcus, streptococcus), meningococcus, and *Haemophilus influenzae,* the viruses, and the toxins of diphtheria and tetanus bacilli. This extended protection may explain partially, at least, the low incidence of these infections during the neonatal period, since most mothers possess antibodies to them. It should be noted in this connection that IgG does not contain antibodies against the enteric gram-negative rods; thus the infant is not protected against these infections by maternal antibody.

IgM. The fetus can produce significant amounts of IgM at about the twentieth gestational week. Since IgM does not cross the placenta, concentrations detected in the neonate clearly represent his own synthesis of it. At birth the normal serum IgM concentration is below 20 mg/100 ml. Normal adult levels are 75 to 150 mg/100 ml. Intrauterine infections of all sorts may produce an immunologic response in the fetus that often results in higher levels. Measurement of IgM has therefore been used to establish the presence of infection. However, IgM determinations are nonspecific indicators; they are no more specific for a particular type of infection than the erythrocyte sedimentation rate in older individuals. Identification of infection by elevated IgM levels is also limited by the time of appearance of such elevations as related to the onset of clinical disease. Elevations of IgM are not usually demonstrable for 5 to 10 days following the appearance of clinical disease. Our IgM determinations are performed twice weekly for at least 2 weeks following the onset of suspected infection. If within that interval IgM has not risen, we consider that an infectious process was unlikely. The onset time of clinical disease and the time of IgM elevation in a baby with congenital pneumonia is illustrated in Fig. 12-1. Abnormal signs were identified on the day of birth, yet an elevation was not evident until the fourth day of life. The stippled area represents the limits of normal IgM levels in our laboratory. In Fig. 12-2, a baby with postnatally acquired pneumonia became ill on the fifth day of life, yet an IgM level a day later was still normal. However, another determination on the ninth day was considerably above normal. Thus, although IgM

determinations are useful for confirmation of suspected infection, *they are useless as a primary screening procedure for the early identification of bacterial infection because the appearance of elevations is so delayed.* In the mother, IgM contains antibodies against gram-negative bacteria and a scattered variety of other antigens. In the neonate, IgM production is stimulated during the initial immunologic response to virtually all infectious agents.

IgA. IgA does not cross the placenta and is not detectable in most normal infants at birth. The fetus and neonate are slower to generate IgA than IgM, and it is thus found less regularly in serum of infected infants at birth. Normal adult levels are 200 to 400 mg/100 ml. IgA is also found over surfaces of intestinal and respiratory mucosa, as well as over renal epithelial surfaces in a form called "secretory IgA." At these sites it is notably active as an antibody. Its role in the intestine is best

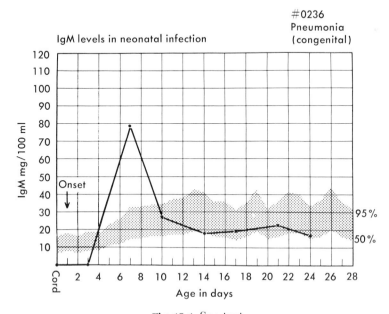

Fig. 12-1. See text.

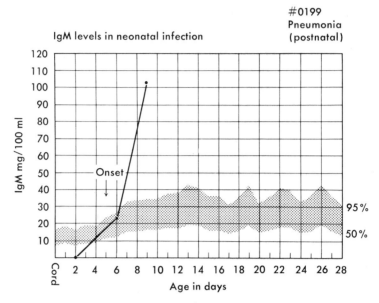

Fig. 12-2. See text.

known. Secretory IgA is present in breast milk in significant concentrations. Unlike serum IgA, IgM, and IgG, secretory IgA resists enzymatic digestion of gastric and intestinal juices. It therefore imparts immunity to mucosal surfaces of the intestine. For example, oral polio vaccine depends, for its effectiveness, on multiplication in the intestinal tract. The vaccine fails to immunize babies on breast milk from mothers with high antibody titers to poliovirus because vaccine virus is inactivated in the gut by secretory IgA from breast milk.

SPECIFIC BACTERIAL INFECTIONS
Pneumonia

Pneumonia is the most common of the serious neonatal infections. It has been cited as a cause of death in 10% to 20% of autopsies. Its peak incidence occurs during the second and third days of life. Pneumonia may be acquired in utero (congenital pneumonia) or from the nursery environment.

Congenital pneumonia is often, but not always, associated with obstetric abnormalities such as early rupture of membranes, prolonged duration of labor, maternal infection, and uncomplicated premature delivery. The bacteria most frequently involved are *Escherichia coli* and other enteric organisms and group B streptococcoi. Symptoms are evident at birth or within 48 hours thereafter. When affected infants are in distress at birth, they are flaccid, pale, or cyanotic. Resuscitation is often necessary. Once respirations are established, they are rapid and shallow. Slight retractions may be present, but they may not be as striking as those of hyaline membrane disease. If the infection is severe, repeated apneic episodes occur. Crepitant rales are sometimes audible. Temperature elevation is more likely in full-sized infants. Premature infants often have subnormal body temperature.

Postnatally acquired pneumonia is generally caused by *Pseudomonas aeru-*

ginosa, penicillin-resistant staphylococci, and enteric organisms. Clinical signs usually appear after 48 hours of life. A substantial number of infants are hypoxic at birth for reasons unrelated to infection. The most common presenting signs are rapid respiration, poor feeding, or aspiration during feeding. Vomiting and aspiration sometimes occur during feeding because previously unsuspected pneumonia is already present. The chest film in such instances reveals densities that cannot be attributed with certainty to effects of aspirated formula or to preexisting pneumonia. Recovery from postnatal pneumonia is more frequent than from congenital pneumonia.

Antibiotic therapy for pneumonia and other bacterial infections is discussed on p. 329.

Septicemia

Septicemia is a generalized infection characterized by the proliferation of bacteria in the bloodstream. The incidence of septicemia has not diminished since the introduction of antibiotics, but the etioloigic agents have changed and survival has increased. Before the antibiotic era, group A streptococci were predominant. Currently, coliform organisms and group B streptococci are the most frequent etiologic agents. The use of antibiotics has diminished mortality from 90% to a range of 13% to 45%, depending on the reporting investigator. Premature infants are most commonly involved; males are affected twice as often as females.

The early symptoms are vague and nonspecific. One expects chills, fever, and prostration in older infants, but the neonate may merely lose vigor, refuse feedings or lose weight. The nurse may simply note that he is "doing poorly." Other abnormal signs are less subtle and

as wide ranging as the bloodstream itself. Vomiting and diarrhea occur in approximately 30% of patients. Abdominal distention may be prominent. Abnormal respiration (apnea, tachypnea, and cyanosis) occurs in 20% to 30% of affected infants. Jaundice is a frequent finding. Hyperbilirubinemia may involve a high concentration of conjugated (direct) bilirubin, mostly in infants over 1 week of age. Hypoglycemia is not uncommon, being associated with gram-negative rod infection almost exclusively. It responds to increased concentrations of intravenous glucose, as described on p. 309. We have found that *hyperglycemia* is at least as frequently associated with septicemia as hypoglycemia. In sick babies who are not receiving excessive quantities of intravenous glucose, hyperglycemia has been a surprisingly strong indication of bacterial infection—usually septicemia. A wide variety of skin lesions occur. Pustules, furuncles, and subcutaneous abscesses are most often associated with streptococcal and staphylococcal infections, and less often with *Escherichia coli* and *Pseudomonas aeruginosa.* The latter organism also produces localized purplish cellulitis that breaks down into a black, gangrenous ulcer. Petechiae and ecchymoses are not common.

Meningitis occurs in a third of septicemic infants, although clinical signs are evident in only half the infants with this complication. The symptoms include convulsions, altered state of consciousness, irritability, spasticity, and fullness of the anterior fontanelle (see later).

The diagnosis of septicemia can be unequivocally documented only by recovery of organisms from blood culture, which requires at least 24 hours for growth. Since organisms are also present in the spinal fluid and urine, lumbar taps and suprapubic aspiration of the bladder are essential components of the diagnostic approach. By applying Gram's stain to centrifuged spinal fluid and urine, the morphologic identity of the bacteria may be established, thus affording a rational basis for immediate choice of antibiotics. Cultures of blood, spinal fluid, and urine must be taken before treatment is begun. If there is nothing to suggest the identity of the offending organism, kanamycin (Kantrex) or gentamicin (Garamycin) plus ampicillin are given immediately (p. 330).

Multiple exchange transfusions, one every 12 hours, are reportedly effective for septicemia with sclerema. We have sometimes seen dramatic disappearance of sclerema and obvious overall improvement. Four to six transfusions are often required.

The total leukocyte count alone is of little value in assessing the likelihood of bacterial infection. Instead, three other characteristics of the white blood cells are important: (1) the total *neutrophile* count, (2) the percent of the total neutrophiles that are immature forms (bands), and (3) the presence of toxic granulations in neutrophiles. A recently published study has demonstrated that among infants with documented bacterial infections, at least one of these three factors was abnormal. Furthermore, if all three were normal, the presence of bacterial disease was very unlikely. In the first week of life, neutropenia is primarily caused by septicemia (or other bacterial disease). It is also associated with maternal hypertension, severe asphyxia, and periventricular hemorrhage even in babies who are not infected. In the absence of the latter disorders, septicemia is a very likely diagnosis in the presence of a low total neutrophile count. By 72 hours, the minimum total neutrophile count is 1750/cu mm. Less than that number is

highly suggestive of infection in the absence of the other associated disorders mentioned above. Furthermore, infection is probable when the *percent of bands to total neutrophiles* exceeds 16% during the first 24 hours and approximately 12% thereafter. Thrombocytopenia (platelet count less than 150,000 cu mm) with or without associated evidence of disseminated intravascular coagulation (p. 281) is a common hematologic abnormality. IgM (p. 322) determination often reveals elevated levels (over 20 mg/100 ml in the first week of life). Usually the elevation is not evident for 3 to 7 days after onset of symptoms. High IgM levels generally confirm a diagnosis of bacterial infection days after the decision to treat with antibiotics has been made.

Meningitis

Almost half of all cases of meningitis in children occur during the first year of life, and the incidence is highest during the neonatal period. It is considerably more frequent in premature than in term infants and in males rather than in females. The causative organisms and the obstetric complications associated with meningitis are the same as those cited for septicemia.

Systemic symptoms cannot be differentiated from those of septicemia. Fullness of the anterior fontanelle is the most specific sign of meningitis. Stiffness of the neck, which is so frequent in older infants and children, is rare in the neonate. Opisthotonos occurs in one fourth of the infected infants; coma and convulsions occur in half of them.

The diagnosis must be confirmed by spinal fluid abnormalities and isolation of the organism from a cultured specimen. White cell content of spinal fluid may vary from 20 to several thousand per cubic millimeter. Polymorphonuclear leukocytes predominate. If the infection is due to *Listeria monocytogenes*, mononuclear cells are in the majority. Sugar content is usually low, and protein is elevated. Organisms are evident on Gram-stained smears of centrifuged spinal fluid. Blood cultures yield the etiologic agent in 75% of cases. Fatality rates vary from approximately 35% to 60%, and in approximately 30% to 35% of the survivors, central nervous sytem handicaps persist. In only 5% have these CNS handicaps required custodial care.

Treatment of meningitis utilizes the same antibiotics as that for septicemia. Therapy should continue for 2 weeks after the first sterile spinal fluid is obtained. The addition of intrathecal gentamicin by lumbar puncture to systemic administration was shown to be no more effective than systemic therapy alone. There was no less mortality or residual central nervous system abnormality among survivors.

Group B streptococcal disease

Special mention is made of group B streptococcal infection because of its startling increase in frequency during the last decade. The major diseases it produces are septicemia, meningitis, and pneumonia, but otitis media and conjunctivitis also occur.

Group B streptococcus was previously believed to be significant only as a cause of mastitis of cattle. It behaves in man, however, very much like the more familiar *Listeria monocytogenes*. Both organisms can be recovered from the cervices of asymptomatic pregnant women, and both are sometimes recovered from the urethras of asymptomatic male partners of such women. Maternal colonization during pregnancy may result in spontaneous abortion, severe neonatal septicemia, or a normal baby.

Two clearly defined syndromes occur, depending on their time of onset. The early-onset disease (so-called septicemic form), in which meningitis can nevertheless occur, is seen in the first few days after delivery. It is apparently acquired by the ascending route in utero or by contact with infected tissue during birth. It often progresses rapidly and relentlessly to cause death in 1 or 2 days. The lungs are heavily involved, and septicemia is almost the rule. In most instances meningitis is absent. The most frequent symptoms are respiratory distress, coma, shock, and jaundice. The organism can be cultured from any number of sites, including the nasopharynx, skin, external ear canal, meconium, and blood. Mortality ranges from 25% to 100%. The late-onset, or meningitic, form occurs several days to 3 months after discharge from the nursery. It almost invariably involves the meninges; its onset is not as abrupt as the early form, and its prognosis for survival is better. Mortality is approximately 20%.

From 4% to 6% of asymptomatic pregnant women have cervical cultures positive for group B streptococci. Cultures of the vulva and vagina have been positive more frequently, with up to 14% of vaginal cultures having been reported as positive. About 1% to 2% of all neonates are colonized with the organism, but colonization does not necessarily lead to disease. Approximately one in ten colonized babies becomes diseased. The organisms recovered from babies are usually identical to those grown from their mothers.

Group B infection departs from the usual pattern of perinatal infections in two ways: maternal complications are not necessarily increased (although in some uncontrolled series complications were said to be increased), and the term infant may be as vulnerable as the premature infant. In fact, in some series the incidence of the disease was higher in the term infants.

The organism is sensitive to penicillin and ampicillin. Group B disease has thus not been a problem in which the appropriate drug is not available. Most authors agree that the early form is an example of vertical transmission (mother to baby). The epidemiology of the late form is not yet clarified, but there are data suggestive of the role of nursery personnel in transmission of the late variety of the disease. Mother-to-infant transmission may also play a role, or the colonized infant may leave the hospital in health only to become ill later. This phenomenon is common in staphylococcal disease.

Diarrhea

Several bacterial agents can produce primary diarrhea. The most important is *enterotoxigenic* or *enteropathogenic Escherichia coli* (EEC). Salmonella, shigella, and staphylococci are infrequent causes. Serologic techniques have identified 140 groups of *E. coli;* somewhat over a dozen have been implicated in nursery epidemics of diarrhea.

Regardless of etiology, the early signs of infection consist of refusal to feed, weight loss, and hypoactivity. These may precede the diarrhea itself by a day or two. Blood and pus in the stool are rare, except in shigellosis, which itself is rare. As diarrhea continues, the infant becomes toxic, dehydrated, and acidotic (metabolic acidosis). These signs may appear abruptly during the early phase of explosive diarrhea. Dehydration is even more rapid if vomiting is also present. An ashen gray color, or pallor, is indicative of vasomotor collapse and impending

death. Rapid correction of metabolic acidosis and dehydration is therefore crucial. Milder forms of the disease are not unusual, being characterized by protracted diarrhea with fewer stools and a refusal to feed.

Institutional outbreaks are almost inevitable if an infected infant is in the nursery. The disease spreads from one bassinet to the next. Feces of infected babies contain an enormous quantity of organisms, and contamination occurs easily, mostly from unwashed hands of personnel and from gowns. Enteropathogenic *E. coli* has been cultured from the nasopharynx, thus suggesting that airborne spread occurs in some instances.

Diarrheal stools must be cultured as soon as they are evident. Most often a bacterial agent is not causative, and the microbiology laboratory will report that no pathogens are identifiable. When viral cultures are performed, they, too, are often negative. Enteropathogenic *E. coli* may cause explosive epidemics. For this reason oral neomycin or polymyxin, which constitutes effective therapy, is administered even before the results of cultures are returned. If these are positive, the infant should be removed from the nursery, and all other babies should be cultured and treated with the same antibiotics. An indication that diarrhea is of bacterial etiology may be gained from a smear of stool for polymorphonuclear leukocytes (pus cells). If the diarrhea is of bacterial etiology, pus cells are usually demonstrable. These cells are not present if diarrhea is caused by a virus or by any other agent.

Urinary tract infection

Neonatal urinary tract infections have been observed to occur as frequently as septicemia. For unknown reasons, renal infection in the neonate has received relatively scant attention. It is far more common in males than in females, the reverse of sex distribution in later childhood. Furthermore, its occurrence in a male does not strongly suggest underlying anomaly, as it does in older children.

Suspicion of infection should be aroused if more than 10% of body weight is lost during the first 5 days in an infant who is not especially ill. Fever is not unusual, particularly if the onset of symptoms is later than 5 days. A significant number of babies appear gray or cyanotic; abdominal distention and jaundice occur in relatively few. During the second week of life, however, jaundice with a high level of direct bilirubin is commonly associated with renal infection, almost always in males. Convulsions, in the absence of meningitis, occur in a small number of infants.

The organisms are gram-negative enteric rods with few exceptions. Blood cultures may be positive in up to 30% of affected babies. Two consecutive urine cultures, obtained by suprapubic aspiration, are diagnostic. Treatment is effective with appropriate antibiotics. Death occurs from complications of septicemia such as meningitis. Sometimes clinical symptoms, bacteriuria, and pyuria all disappear spontaneously, before treatment is begun.

Conjunctivitis

Infection of the conjunctivae may be acquired during the birth process or from the nursery environment. Bacterial conjunctivitis is usually due to staphylococcus, *Pseudomonas aeruginosa*, and enteric organisms. Clinical signs include swelling and redness of the conjunctiva, with varying amounts of purulent exudate. In its mildest form, conjunctivitis causes "sticky eyes," with little or no swelling.

Gonorrheal infection causes the most serious form of conjunctivitis. It is acquired during delivery by direct contact with infected maternal tissue. Initial symptoms are noted between the second and fifth days of life, sometimes later. Severe conjunctival redness, swelling of the eyelids, and copious pus are typically evident. Untreated, the infection may spread to the eyes, causing panophthalmitis and extensive destruction of ocular tissue. It also causes severe arthritis. Rapid diagnosis is possible from a Gram-stained smear of exudate from the eye, which reveals gram-negative cocci within pus cells.

Gonorrheal infection is treated with intramuscular penicillin. Conjunctivitis due to other organisms is effectively controlled by local instillation of an eye ointment containing polymyxin, bacitracin, and neomycin.

Omphalitis

Severe infection of the umbilical stump causes edema, redness, and purulent exudate in the region of the umbilicus. In milder infections there is no visible exudate, but redness and induration of the periumbilical skin are evident. Slight periumbilical erythema without induration is not pathologic. Inflammation of the umbilical stump may herald septicemia. Culture of the blood and the umbilicus is indicated, and treatment for septicemia should be started immediately.

ANTIMICROBIAL TREATMENT

The antibiotics of choice for neonatal infections are listed in Table 12-2. In most instances they must be chosen before results of cultures are available. It is

Table 12-2. Antibiotics of choice (1980)

Drug	Dose	Schedule	Route
Carbenicillin	200 to 300 mg/kg/24 hr	q. 8 hours (up to 7 days of age) q. 6 hours (7 days or older)	IM or IV
Kanamycin	15 mg/kg/24 hr	q. 12 hours (up to 7 days of age) q. 8 hours (7 days or older)	IM or IV
Gentamicin (Garamycin)	5 mg/kg/24 hr 7.5/mg/kg/24 hr	q. 12 hours (up to 7 days of age) q. 8 hours (7 days or older)	IM or IV
Penicillin G (aqueous crystalline)	100,000 U/kg/24 hr	q. 12 hours (up to 7 days of age) q. 6 hours (7 days or older)	IM or IV
Ampicillin	100 to 200 mg/kg/24 hr	Same as for penicillin	IM or IV
Methicillin (or oxacillin)	100 to 200 mg/kg/24 hr	Same as for penicillin	IM or IV
Nafcillin	50 mg/kg/24 hr	Same as for penicillin	IM or IV
Polymyxin B	3 to 4 mg/kg/24 hr 10 to 20 mg/kg/24 hr 1 mg (in 1 ml saline solution)	q. 12 hours q. 6 to 8 hours q. 24 hours	IM or IV Oral Intrathecal
Colistimethate sodium	8 mg/kg/24 hr	q. 12 hours	IM
Neomycin	50 to 100 mg/kg/24 hr	q. 6 hours	Oral

thus essential that they be effective against most of the organisms likely to infect the neonate. Major consideration must be given to the bacterial infections acquired in utero and during birth; they are derived from normal maternal intestinal flora (coliforms, group B streptococci). Penicillin-resistant staphylococci and *Pseudomonas aeruginosa* are more likely to be etiologic in postnatally acquired infections than in congenital ones. When onset of symptoms occurs after 48 to 72 hours, additional consideration must be given to these possibilities.

The overall effectiveness of some antibiotics has diminished through the years.

About three decades ago streptomycin was highly active against coliform infections, but it ultimately lost its effectiveness and was replaced by kanamycin (Kantrex). Now the activity of kanamycin against *E. coli* has begun to decline significantly. In the years immediately following its introduction, kanamycin was active against 90% to 95% of *E. coli* strains; currently it eliminates approximately 60% or less in some hospitals. In the early phases of their use both streptomycin and kanamycin were also effective against staphylococci, and this effectiveness, too, was soon lost. Diminished activity of these drugs is related to their widespread use. At present, gentamicin is a satisfactory alternative to kanamycin, but its effectiveness is also declining, while disuse of kanamycin in recent years is now associated with a return to its initial effectiveness. Gentamicin is also effective against *Pseudomonas aeruginosa*, thus offering a decided advantage in the treatment of bacterial infection.

For over two decades penicillin has remained useful against most strains of staphylococci that are not hospital acquired, streptococci, syphilis, *Listeria monocytogenes*, and gonorrheal organisms. However, ampicillin has largely replaced penicillin because it is active against the same organisms and a majority of *E. coli* strains as well. The staphylococci that are resistant to penicillin must be treated with nafcillin or a similar type of drug specifically active against penicillin-resistant strains.

Infections manifest during the first 48 hours are best treated with kanamycin or gentamicin plus ampicillin because they are probably congenitally acquired. Onset at a later age implies that hospital-acquired organisms may be etiologic. For these infections carbenicillin with gentamicin plus nafcillin may be used.

SPECIFIC VIRAL INFECTIONS

The viruses implicated in perinatal infections are listed in Table 12-1. They are transmitted across the placenta from mother to fetus, except for herpesvirus, which is usually acquired by the ascending route, and cytomegalovirus, which is sometimes acquired similarly. Maternal transmission may occur early in pregnancy, causing chronic intrauterine infections such as rubella or cytomegalovirus, or closer to delivery, causing postnatal onset of infections such as herpesvirus, Coxsackievirus, varicella, and smallpox. One of several consequences may befall the fetus or neonate as a result of maternal infection: (1) death may occur in utero or after birth as a result of fetal disease, (2) intrauterine death may follow severe maternal toxicity, (3) survival may occur despite infection but with congenital malformations or destruction of tissue (brain and liver), or often with no apparent aftermath, or (4) the virus may not be transmitted to the fetus.

The intrauterine infections of primary importance are rubella, cytomegalovirus infection, and herpesvirus infection.

Rubella

The congenital rubella syndrome is a chronic virus infection of the fetus and neonate that begins during the first trimester of pregnancy and usually persists for months after birth. The virus has been recovered from abortuses, placentas, and amniotic fluid. At autopsy it has been grown from virtually every organ of the body. In life it has been cultured from the throat, urine, meconium, conjunctival secretion, and spinal fluid, from surgically removed segments of the ductus arteriosus, from cataractous lenses, and from liver specimens. The majority of infants may harbor virus as long as 3 months. In some infants the virus persists for several months or years longer. Virus has been recovered from the lens of a 3-year-old child. Persistently infected infants may be a source of contagion; small epidemics among hospital personnel have been traced to them. Pregnant women are thus at risk when exposed to these infants.

Approximately 10% to 20% of gravid women are susceptible to rubella. Estimates of the risk of fetal disease after maternal infection have varied through the years from one epidemic to the next. In general, maternal infection during the first gestational month causes disease in 33% to 50% of exposed fetuses; during the second month 25% are affected, and during the third month 9% are affected. There is a distinct but smaller risk during the fourth month of pregnancy; 4% of exposed fetuses may be affected, primarily by lifelong hearing impairment.

Whether positive or negative, a history of infection is unreliable because at least half the infected older children and adults are asymptomatic. Furthermore, the clinical signs of rubella are difficult to interpret during nonepidemic periods, since they mimic several other virus infections. During the extensive epidemic of 1964, half the mothers of diseased infants were unaware of infection during pregnancy. Fetal disease is no less severe in the asymptomatic mother than in the symptomatic one.

The cardinal clinical signs are intrauterine growth retardation, congenital heart disease, and cataracts. The organs of growth-retarded infants are hypoplastic because rubella virus impairs the proliferative (mitotic) phase of growth (p. 116). Several types of cardiac malformation have been noted; the most common are patent ductus arteriosus and stenosis of the peripheral pulmonary arteries. Severe myocardial degeneration also occurs in a few infants. Cataracts may be bilateral or unilateral; they are usually present at birth, but occasionally they develop days or weeks later. Other eye abnormalities include microphthalmia, glaucoma, and a pigmented retinopathy. Thrombocytopenia and petechiae are present in 40% to 80% of infected neonates. Enlargement of the liver and spleen is common, and unconjugated hyperbilirubinemia, largely due to hemolysis, is also frequent. When hepatitis occurs, it further contributes to the retention of unconjugated bilirubin, but it also causes elevations of direct bilirubin as well (obstructive jaundice). Occasionally rubella hepatitis progresses to cirrhosis. Interstitial pneumonia is not uncommon, the virus having been recovered from affected lungs. Neurologic abnormalities are present in a minority of neonates; they usually appear later in infancy. Microcephaly, for instance, ordinarily develops after the newborn period. Spinal fluid abnormalities consist of elevated protein concentration and increased white cells, usually lymphocytes. In the neonate they are more frequent than clinical neurologic abnormalities.

The diagnosis of congenital rubella is strongly suggested by the combined presence of cataracts and congenital heart disease. Elevated IgM levels are usually detectable at birth. Serologic documentation is possible by demonstrating rubella antibody in serum IgM. Other serologic tests are not helpful because they measure maternal IgG antibody, which may be present as a result of an infection that preceded pregnancy by many years.

The immune status among nursery personnel of childbearing age should be determined at the onset of employment. If serologic tests indicate susceptibility, attenuated rubella virus vaccine should be administered. Infected infants are contagious; susceptible personnel who are exposed while unknowingly pregnant are at risk of having an infected fetus.

Cytomegalovirus (CMV) infection

The cytomegaloviruses are ubiquitous agents that cause infections in populations of all ages throughout the world. Perinatal infections are acquired transplacentally from asymptomatic mothers. In the presence of primary acute maternal infection, 50% of fetuses are affected. The acutely infected mother is more likely to transmit the disease early in pregnancy than later. Early gestational transmission also seems to be associated with greater severity of fetal disease. Beyond the neonatal period, acquired cytomegalovirus infections are usually asymptomatic; the excretion of virus in urine (viruria) is thus required for the identification of infected individuals. Maternal viruria at the time of delivery has been noted in 3% to 4% of apparently normal women. Postive cultures from the cervix at the time of delivery have been demonstrated in 4.5% of women in Pittsburgh and as many as 28% in Japan. Similar studies have identified viruria in 1% of randomly selected newborns, most of them apparently normal, in whom viruria often persists through the first year of life. Cytomegalovirus has been recovered from an abortus as early as the twelfth gestational week. The fate of apparently healthy viruric neonates has not been documented, but estimates of later central nervous system damage range from 10% to 25%. The only report of postnatal acquisition of the disease in the nursery concerns two premature infants who may have become infected from blood transfusions.

The results of congenital infection range from widespread tissue damage that is incompatible with life, to survival associated with extensive brain damage, and to complete absence of signs during the neonatal period. Diseased infants are often small-for-dates and hypoplastic. The principal target organs are the blood, brain, and liver, although virtually every organ of the body can be affected. Hemolysis causes anemia and unconjugated hyperbilirubinemia. Thrombocytopenia with petechiae and ecchymoses in the skin is quite frequent. Obstructive jaundice (direct hyperbilirubinemia) is a consequence of liver damage. Enlargement of the liver and spleen are common. Cytomegalovirus also produces encephalitis; the resultant clinical signs vary from lethargy and hypoactivity to convulsions. Microcephaly may be present at birth, or it may develop over the ensuing few months. Skull x-ray examinations may reveal calcification in the brain, which is also present in infants with toxoplasmosis. Chorioretinitis is discernible in 10% to 20% of symptomatic infants; this lesion, too, is similar to the eye findings in infants with toxoplasmosis. Pneumonia occurs occasionally.

The diagnosis is best established in babies with typical clinical signs by recovery of virus from urine. There is considerable diagnostic value in the demonstration of elevated IgM levels, but these are not specific for CMV. Specific identification of cytomegalovirus antibodies within the IgM fraction is the most accurate serologic method. Although several antiviral drugs have been utilized for treatment, their efficacy has not been clearly established.

Herpesvirus infection

Herpesvirus is classified into type 1 and type 2 varieties, each with distinctive serologic attributes and clinical implications. Type 1 causes the common, and often recurrent, lesions in the lips of older children and adults. It also produces gingivostomatitis and skin lesions above the waist. Type 2 causes the vast majority of lesions in the cervix, vagina, and external genitalia. Most neonatal infections are due to type 2 virus. The fetus acquires herpesvirus by the ascending route from infected genitalia or by direct contact with these tissues during the birth process. Neonatal herpesvirus is thus a venereal disease acquired by the infant in a manner similar to gonorrhea. Transplacental acquisition probably occurs, but it is apparently rare, having been reported in only a few suggestive cases. Delivery by cesarean section has been recommended for infants whose mothers are known to have genital herpes. The value of this prophylactic approach is not established, but most authorities recommend it nevertheless. If membranes rupture 6 hours or more before section is performed, ascent of virus may infect the fetus. A number of instances have been reported in which herpes infection followed delivery by cesarean section.

Like most other infectious agents that affect the neonate, herpesvirus produces a broad spectrum of clinical signs. The neonatal disease exists in disseminated and nondisseminated forms. The disseminated variety is fatal to 96% of affected infants. Although microscopic lesions may be found in every organ of the body, the most extensive involvement occurs in the adrenals, liver, brain, blood, and lung. Initial symptoms may be present at birth, or they may not appear until 3 or 4 weeks of age. Fever is detectable in approximately one third of infected infants. Other common signs include hepatosplenomegaly, hepatitis with jaundice (associated with direct hyperbilirubinemia), bleeding diathesis, and neurologic abnormalities. These neurologic signs are described later. Vesicular skin lesions are almost pathognomonic, but unfortunately they occur in only one third of the patients. They are usually sparsely distributed over the entire body; occasionally they appear in clusters. Sudden bleeding from the gastrointestinal tract, needle punctures, and circumcision sites portends death within 48 hours. Most infants

so affected have been shown to have disseminated intravascular coagulation.

Several nondisseminated forms are composed of central nervous system, skin, and eye abnormalities, which occur singly or in combination. In none of them is there visceral involvement. These varieties of the disease cause death in 25% of the infants, but over half the survivors have residual damage to the brain and eyes. Neurologic abnormalities are the most frequent. They include convulsions (focal or generalized), abnormal muscle tone, opisthotonos, bulging fontanelle, and lethargy or coma. The spinal fluid contains an elevated protein concentration and increased leukocytes (predominantly lymphocytes). The eye signs include cloudy corneas (keratitis), conjunctivitis, and chorioretinitis. In a substantial proportion of infants with nondisseminated infection, skin involvement is the sole manifestation. As a rule they survive, but psychomotor damage is residual in some. New skin lesions continue to appear for several days; occasionally they recur sporadically up to 2 years of age. These recurrences may be associated with routine immunizations, unrelated febrile disease, or trauma. Most often the lesions appear for no known reason.

The most seriously disabling sequelae among surviving infants are neurologic. They consist of microcephaly or hydrocephalus and varying degrees of psychomotor retardation. Ocular residua may cause total or partial blindness as a result of scars in the cornea (from keratitis) and retina (from chorioretinitis).

In the absence of skin lesions, the diagnosis is elusive because the symptoms are otherwise nonspecific, most often being confused with septicemia. Cultures of virus from skin vesicles and the throat or identification by electron microscopy are the most reliable diagnostic procedures. Positive culture results are observable within 24 to 48 hours.

Antiviral drugs have been used as therapy for neonatal herpesvirus infection, but their efficacy has not been determined. They include iododeoxyuridine (IDU), cytosine arabinoside (ara-C), and adenine arabinoside (ara-A). They are toxic, particularly to the hemotopoietic system, and all of them are immunosuppressive. Ara-A appears to be least toxic of the three drugs. A controlled trial of these drugs is now in progress among twenty centers in the United States.

PROTOZOAN INFECTION
Toxoplasmosis

Toxoplasmosis, caused by the protozoan *Toxoplasma gondii*, is usually an asymptomatic infection in older individuals. It is widespread to varying degrees among different populations over the world. In the United States it occurs in 1 to 4 per 1000 live births—approximately 3000 infected infants annually. It is an important perinatal infection, being transmitted across the placenta from an apparently healthy, but infected, mother. The acutely infected mother is more likely to transmit the organism to her fetus in late rather than early pregnancy. Fetal infection from maternal illness is 17%, 24%, and 62% in the first, second, and third trimesters, respectively. The reasons for this phenomenon are unknown. Symptoms appear in the infant at birth or soon thereafter, but many infants are asymptomatic for the first several weeks of life. The organism has been found in every cell type in the body except the red blood cell, and the resultant clinical signs are thus variable. An array of neurologic abnormalities includes convulsions, coma, severe generalized hypotonia, microcephaly, or hydrocephalus. Skull films may reveal diffuse, comma-shaped intracranial calcifications. Chorioretinitis occurs in most symptomatic infants; microphthalmia is also common. Other signs include hepatosplenomegaly, jaundice (direct and indirect hyperbilirubinemia), petechiae and ecchymoses of the skin (thrombocytopenia), and pallor (anemia). The fatality rate among diseased neonates is 12%. Neurologic deficits are extremely common in survivors.

Serologic diagnosis is feasible immediately after birth by demonstration of specific toxoplasma IgM antibodies. Other serologic procedures, if they reveal sufficiently high titers, also establish the diagnosis (hemagglutination inhibition).

CONTROL OF NURSERY INFECTION

Because of continuous presence in the nursery and involvement with hour-by-hour care, the nurse is the baby's most supportive caretaker. However, a lack of concern for hygienic practices can become a serious threat to the infant's survival. The prenatal acquisition of bacterial infection is in large measure unpreventable, but with few exceptions postnatally acquired infectious disease can indeed be avoided. Quite aside from the strict sterility that is obviously required during administration of parenteral fluids and medications or during performance of invasive procedures, the practices of nursery personnel need only be predicated on a few simple rules of hygiene. Realistically there is nothing aseptic about these practices; rather, they are clean to the utmost. The provision of a continuously germ-free environment is impossible, even in most sophisticated nurseries; nor does it seem desirable when one considers that animals maintained in such environments experience a significant delay in their capacity to produce antibodies because of the absence of antigenic stimuli.

Traditionally the practices advocated for prevention of infections have also tended to make the nursery a forbidding place to enter. Such an atmosphere is particularly inadvisable for neonatal intensive care units because the infants in them require greater attention from more people than any other type of patient in the hospital. Surgeons, cardiologists, neurologists, hematologists, anesthesiologists, x-ray technicians, laboratory technologists—all these individuals, besides the nursery staff itself, must regularly converge on sick infants. The resultant traffic is often something to behold. This type of care requires unimpeded access to the nursery, but careful hygienic demeanor is mandatory for all concerned. The simpler and more rigid the rules, the more consistently they are followed. A number of studies have provided a scientific basis for discarding needless and obstructive so-called aseptic techniques. The nurse's role in all this is pivotal. Daily practices must protect patients from exposure to infection, and, in addition, the nurse should be the most effective and vociferous promulgator of established rules of hygienic technique.

Infections are propagated by people and by things. In addition to a predisposition to infection because of illness, the sick neonate is also at great risk because a large cohort of personnel must use a multiplicity of objects in giving care. Furthermore, the nature of a special care nursery is such that it attracts referrals from other institutions. As a consequence, a relatively large number of profoundly ill infants are housed in one facility for extended periods, thus increasing the hazard of cross-contamination. The practices to be described are applicable to any nursery—routine or special care. The risks they are designed to minimize are greater in special care facilities.

Propagation of infection by personnel

Personnel carriers of various organisms have been studied extensively, and their role in epidemics has been conjectural. There is some evidence that they may spread infection by the airborne route, but the current consensus is that direct contact by contaminated hands is the principal modality.

Most published studies concern the spread of staphylococci and their colonization among infant cohorts. Colonization of staphylococci occurs when organisms settle on the skin, in the nose, and in the throat without producing disease. The colonized infant is at considerably higher risk of subsequent disease than the noncolonized one. For instance, staphylococcal skin infection has been noted in 20% of infants who become colonized in the first 2 days of life, whereas only 1.4% of noncolonized infants are similarly afflicted. Colonization has been noted in as many as 100% of infants in a single nursery during epidemic years, but high rates also occur during nonepidemic periods. The significance of staphylococcal colonization is not restricted to the diseases that may subsequently appear during the nursery stay; discharged infants often become ill at home. They may also spread the organism to cause household epidemics, even though they remain healthy.

It thus follows that the effects of various procedures for minimizing nursery infections can be gauged from colonization rates and the incidence of overt disease. A number of excellent studies have in fact utilized this approach, and they are in general agreement on the validity of some of these procedures. In each instance the investigators caution that the conclusions reached are directly applicable to conditions in their respective facilities and that universal adoption of their practices may or may not be valid.

Failure to wash hands properly between handling of different infants is undoubtedly the principal mode of spread of infection by any organism. Nothing is more fundamental to proper nursery hygiene than handwashing. On first entering the nursery, personnel should wash to a level above the elbows for at least 2 minutes. Between patients, washing for 15 seconds should be adequate. Currently the use of any type of soap or an iodinated detergent is recommended. The iodinated preparations are preferable, at least for the initial 2-minute scrub, because they are active against gram-positive cocci and gram-negative rods as well, but they sometimes cause skin sensitivity.

In December, 1972, statements from the Food and Drug Administration and the American Academy of Pediatrics recommended that routine total body bathing of infants, utilizing hexachlorophene-containing detergents, be discontinued. Although clinical signs of toxicity in human infants had not been documented, diffuse cystic lesions were observed in the brains of monkeys who were bathed daily for 90 days with a detergent containing hexachlorophene. Furthermore, blood levels of hexachlorophene in human newborns had been demonstrated, presumably absorbed from the skin. Several weeks after these statements were issued, the Center for Disease Control (Atlanta) reported approximately sixty nursery outbreaks of staphylococcal disease throughout the nation. Whether or not these outbreaks were related to the discontinuation of hexachlorophene

bathing is still conjectural. The temporal relationship between the two events suggests as much, although documentation is lacking. The original statements of the Food and Drug Administration and the American Academy of Pediatrics were subsequently modified to recommend that hexachlorophene bathing may be utilized in the presence of a staphylococcal outbreak, but it is unlikely to halt the spread of infection. The modified statements also emphasized the fundamental importance of handwashing and the necessity to investigate all nursery practices to determine the sources of staphylococcal colonization and disease. The preferred method of skin care is now "dry skin care" (see Skin Care of Newborns, Statement, Fetus and Newborn Committee, American Academy of Pediatrics).

Nursery personnel should wear short-sleeved scrub dresses to accommodate washing to the elbows. At some facilities the use of gowns by physicians and other personnel has been discontinued if infants are not removed from incubators. However, long-sleeved gowns should be worn and changed between handling infants if they are taken from an incubator or bassinet, whether to feed or to perform a procedure (individual gown technique). Caps, masks, and hairnets are no longer recommended.

Isolation and suspect nurseries are not considered essential, but infants with diarrhea and draining infections must be removed from the nursery. Infants with bacterial meningitis, septicemia, and pneumonia need not be isolated, nor is there a need to remove infants if amniotic membranes have ruptured early (even if the fluid is purulent), if there is a history of antepartum or postpartum maternal fever, or if the baby was born anywhere outside the delivery room.

Several studies have revealed that colonization rates and the incidence of infectious disease are not increased when parents are permitted in the nursery. This development is particularly important in light of the recent realization that a profound impact is exerted on the mother by protracted separation from her sick newborn; it may significantly alter her attitude for some time afterward (Chapter 14). The precautions regarding handwashing and gowning for personnel are similarly applicable to parents.

Details of nursery techniques and measures for the management of nursery epidemics are fully presented in a recent revision of *Standards and Recommendations for Hospital Care of Newborn Infants* (1977), published by the American Academy of Pediatrics. A copy of this publication should be available at every facility that cares for newborn infants.

Infection from equipment and fixtures

The widespread use of indwelling catheters, at the umbilical site and in peripheral veins, has added another potential source of serious infection. The risk of infection involved in umbilical vessel catheters is well known. It is not generally appreciated, however, that catheters in peripheral veins cause a considerably higher incidence of bacteremia and local infections. These catheters must be placed with meticulously aseptic technique. They should be managed in the same fashion as the deep vein catheters that are used for total parenteral alimentation.

A group of gram-negative organisms, aptly dubbed by Wheeler as "water bugs," has been identified as an important cause of individual and epidemic infection. These organisms are spread primarily from contaminated equipment. Infants are infected by an enormous in-

oculum of bacteria capable of proliferating in clear water. Illness usually begins several days after birth or some time later if the nursery stay is protracted.

Pseudomonas is the most prevalent of these organisms. Other frequent offenders are *Aerobacter, Alcaligenes, Achromobacter, Flavobacterium, Serratia,* and *Erwinia* (implicated in contaminated caps on bottles of intravenous fluids). The epidemics caused by these bacteria may be widespread in the nursery during a short period, or the infections may occur sequentially in one or a few infants over a protracted interval. They emanate from any piece of equipment, particularly those associated with high humidity or moisture of any kind. Plumbing fixtures are also important sources of contamination. A list of these objects is presented on p. 321.

Regularly obtained cultures from most of these articles are an essential component of bacteriologic surveillance. Furthermore, autoclaving or gas sterilization is indicated for all items that lend themselves to these processes. Water in the reservoirs of incubators has been discontinued in many nurseries. Oxygen humidifiers are changed daily, and the water within them is changed every 8 hours. Disposable plastic tubes from oxygen outlets are discarded every 24 hours. Mist generators that provide clouded moisture in incubators for infants in respiratory distress are avoided because such treatement is useless, and it increases the incidence of "water bug" infections. Sterile distilled water from previously unopened bottles that is used in ultrasonic nebulizers is changed every 8 hours. Cotton balls are not stored in solutions of benzalkonium chloride (Zephiran) because in these circumstances *Pseudomonas* has been repeatedly recovered from the disinfectant. It is disconcerting to realize that bacteriologists use compounds related to benzalkonium chloride in their media to encourage the growth of *Pseudomonas* by impairing proliferation of other organisms.

The sources of infection in the nursery have multiplied commensurate with recent advances in the care of sick infants. It is essential for the nurse supervisor to execute a program of bacteriologic surveillance and sterilization of equipment. The staff nurse must be certain that the equipment she is using has been cleaned or sterilized in accordance with this program. These programs must be planned in conjunction with the physician in charge of the nursery, an infectious disease expert, an epidemiologist, and a representative from the hospital bacteriology laboratory.

The spread of organisms from people and from things must be eliminated, or at least minimized, by applying sensible techniques of proved value. As in so many other aspects of newborn care, the nurse can assure or destroy the success of infection control procedures better than any other staff member. Close and continuous contact with the babies qualifies the nurse as a perceptive monitor of the incidence of infection, and repeated contacts with physicians and other personnel provide the opportunity to appraise and regulate their demeanor in regard to infection control.

REFERENCES

Ablow, R. C., et al.: A comparison of early-onset group B streptococcal neonatal infection and the respiratory distress syndrome of the newborn, N. Engl. J. Med. **294**:65, 1976.

Alford, C. A., Neva, F. A., and Weller, T. H.: Virologic and serologic studies on human products of conception after maternal rubella, N. Engl. J. Med. **271**:1275, 1964.

Alford, C. A., et al.: A correlative immunologic, microbiologic and clinical approach to the diagnosis of acute and chronic infections in the newborn infant, N Engl. J. Med. **277**:437, 1967.

Anderson, G. S., et al.: Congenital bacterial pneumonia, Lancet **2**:585, 1962.

Baker, C. J., Barrett, F. F., Gordon, R. C., and Yow, M. D.: Suppurative meningitis due to streptococci of Lancefield group B: a study of 33 infants, J. Pediatr. **82**:724, 1973.

Barrie, D.: Incubator-borne *Pseudomonas* pyocyanea infection in a newborn nursery, Arch. Dis. Child. **40**:555, 1965.

Barton, L. L., Feigin, R. D., and Lins, R.: Group B beta-hemolytic streptococcal meningitis in infants, J. Pediatr. **82**:719, 1973.

Benirschke, K.: Routes and types of infection in the fetus and the newborn, Am. J. Dis. Child. **99**:714, 1960.

Benirschke, K., and Driscoll, S. G.: The pathology of the human placenta, New York, 1967, Springer-Verlag New York, Inc.

Bergstrom, R., Larson, H., Lincoln, K., and Winberg, J.: Studies of urinary tract infections in infancy and childhood. XII. Eighty consecutive patients with neonatal infection, J. Pediatr. **80**:858, 1972.

Blanc, W. A.: Pathways of fetal and early neonatal infection, viral placentitis, bacterial and fungal chorioamnionitis, J. Pediatr. **59**:473, 1961.

Cabrera, H. A., and Davis, G. H.: Epidemic meningitis of the newborn caused by flavobacteria. I. Epidemiology and bacteriology, Am. J. Dis. Child. **101**:289, 1961.

Davies, P. A., and Aherne, W.: Congenital pneumonia, Arch. Dis. Child. **37**:598, 1962.

Davis, L. E., et al.: Cytomegalovirus mononucleosis in a first trimester pregnant female with transmission to the fetus, Pediatrics **48**:200, 1971.

Desmond, M. M., et al.: Congenital rubella encephalitis, J. Pediatr. **71**:311, 1967.

Eichenwald, H. F.: Congenital toxoplasmosis: a study of 150 cases, Am. J. Dis. Child. **94**:411, 1957.

Eickhoff, T. C., Klein, J. O., Daly, A. K., et al.: Neonatal sepsis and other infections due to group B beta-hemolytic streptococci, N. Engl. J. Med. **271**:1221, 1964.

Ermocilla, R., Cassady, G., and Ceballos, R.: Otitis media in the pathogenesis of neonatal meningitis with group B beta-hemolytic streptococcus, Pediatrics **54**:643, 1972.

Evans, H. E., Akpata, S. O., and Baki, A.: Bacteriologic and clinical evaluation of gowning in a premature nursery, J. Pediatr. **78**:883, 1971.

Foley, J. F., et al.: *Achromobacter* septicemia—fatalities in prematures, Am. J. Dis. Child. **101**:279, 1961.

Franciosi, R. A., Knostman, J. D., and Zimmerman, R. A.: Group B streptococcal neonatal and infant infections, J. Pediatr. **82**:707, 1973.

Gehibach, S. H., Gutman, L. T., Wilfert, C. M., et al.: Recurrence of skin disease in a nursery: ineffectuality of hexachlorophene bathing, Pediatrics **55**:422, 1975.

Gitlin, D., Kumate, J., Urrusti, J., et al.: The selectivity of the human placenta in the transfer of plasma proteins from mother to fetus, J. Clin. Invest. **43**:1938, 1964.

Gluck, L., and Wood, H. F.: Staphylococcal colonization in newborn infants with and without antiseptic skin care; a consideration of epidemiologic routes, N. Engl. J. Med. **268**:1265, 1963.

Hanshaw, J. B., and Dudgeon, J. A.: Hepatitis viruses. In Viral diseases of the fetus and newborn, Philadelphia, 1978, W. B. Saunders Co.

Hardyment, A. F., et al.: Observations on the bacteriology and epidemiology of nursery infections. I. Staphylococcal skin infections, Pediatrics **25**:907, 1960.

Hildebrandt, R. J., et al.: Cytomegalovirus in the normal pregnant woman, Am. J. Obstet. Gynecol. **98**:1125, 1967.

Hoffman, M. A., and Finberg, L.: *Pseudomonas* infections in infants associated with high humidity environments, J. Pediatr. **46**:626, 1955.

Horn, K. A., Zimmerman, R. A., Knostman, J. D., and Meyer, W. T.: Neurological sequelae of group B streptococcal neonatal infection, Pediatrics **53**:501, 1974.

James, L. S.: Hexachlorophene, Pediatrics **49**:492, 1972.

Kohen, D. P.: Neonatal gonococcal arthritis: three cases and review of the literature, Pediatrics **53**:436, 1974.

Kopelman, A. E.: Cutaneous absorption of hexachlorophene in low-birth-weight infants, J. Pediatr. **82**:972, 1973.

Korones, S. B., Ainger, L. E., Monif, G. R., et al.: Congenital rubella syndrome: new clinical aspects with recovery of virus from affected infants, J. Pediatr. **67**:166, 1965.

Korones, S. B., Roane, J. A., Gilkeson, M. R., et al.: Neonatal IgM response to acute infection, J. Pediatr. **75**:1261, 1969.

Korones, S. B., Todaro, J., Roane, J. A., et al.: Maternal virus infection after the first trimester of pregnancy and status of offspring to 4 years of age in a predominantly Negro population, J. Pediatr. **77**:245, 1970.

Kresky, B.: Control of gram-negative bacilli in a hospital nursery, Am. J. Dis. Child. **107**:363, 1964.

Light, I. J., and Linnemann, C. C., Jr.: Neonatal herpes simplex infection following delivery by cesarean section, Obstet. Gynecol. **44**:496, 1974.

Light, I. J., Brackvogel, V., Walton, R. L., and Sutherland, J. M.: An epidemic of bullous impetigo arising from a central admission-observation nursery, Pediatrics **49**:15, 1972.

Lockhart, J. D.: How toxic is hexachlorophene? Pediatrics **50**:229, 1972.

Manroe, B. L., Weinberg, A. G., Rosenfeld, C. R., and Browne, R.: The neonatal blood count in health and disease. I. Reference values for neutrophilic cells, J. Pediatr. **95**:89, 1979.

McCracken, G. H.: Changing pattern of the antimicrobial susceptibilities of *Escherichia coli* in neonatal infections, J. Pediatr. **78**:942, 1971.

McCracken, G. H., Jr., and Nelson, J. D.: Antimicrobial therapy for newborns: practical application of pharmacology to clinical usage, New York, 1977, Grune & Stratton, Inc.

McCracken, G. H., Hardy, J. B., Chen, T. C., et al.: Serum immunoglobulin levels in newborn infants. II. Survey of cord and follow-up sera from 123 infants with congenital rubella, J. Pediatr. **74**:383, 1969.

Miller, D. R., Hanshaw, J. B., O'Leary, D. S., and Hnilicka, J. V.: Fatal disseminated herpes simplex virus infection and hemorrhage in the neonate: coagulation studies in a case and a review, J. Pediatr. **76**:409, 1970.

Monif, G. R. G., Avery, G. B., Korones, S. B., et al.: Postmortem isolation of rubella virus from three children with rubella-syndrome defects, Lancet **1**:723, 1965.

Monif, G. R. G., Egan, E. A., Held, B., and Eitzman, D. V.: The correlation of maternal cytomegalovirus infection during varying stages in gestation with neonatal involvement, J. Pediatr. **80**:17, 1972.

Nahmias, A. J., Alford, C. A., and Korones, S. B.: Infection of the newborn with herpesvirus hominis, Adv. Pediatr. **17**:185, 1970.

Olding, L.: Bacterial infection in cases of perinatal death, a morphological and bacteriological study based on 264 autopsies, Acta Paediatr. Scand. **171**(supp.):1, 1966.

Overall, J. C., Jr.: Neonatal bacterial meningitis: analysis of predisposing factors and outcome compared with matched control subjects, J. Pediatr. **76**:499, 1970.

Overbach, A. M., Daniel, S. J., and Cassady, G.: The value of umbilical cord histology in the management of potential perinatal infection, J. Pediatr. **76**:22, 1970.

Peter, G., Lloyd-Still, J. D., and Lovejoy, F. H., Jr.: Local infection and bacteremia from scalp vein needles and polyethylene catheters in children, J. Pediatr. **80:**78, 1972.

Powell, H., Swarner, O., Gluck, L., and Lampert, P.: Hexachlorophene myelinopathy in premature infants, J. Pediatr. **82:**976, 1973.

Prod-hom, L. S., Choffat, J. M., Frenck, N., et al.: Care of the seriously ill neonate with hyaline membrane disease and with sepsis (sclerema neonatorum), Pediatrics **53:**170, 1974.

Rosen, F. S.: Immunity in the fetus and newborn. In Gluck, L., editor: Modern perinatal medicine, Chicago, 1974, Year Book Medical Publishers, Inc.

Sever, J. L.: Possible role of humidifying equipment in spread of infections from the newborn nursery, Pediatrics **24:**50, 1959.

Sever, J. L.: Perinatal infections affecting the fetus and newborn, Proceedings of a Conference on Mental Retardation Through Control of Infectious Diseases, June 9-11, 1966, Public Health Service Publication no. 1962, Washington, D.C., 1966, Government Printing Office.

Sherman, J. D., et al.: Alcaligenes faecalis infection in the newborn, Am. J. Dis. Child. **100:**212, 1960.

Shuman, R. M., Leech, R. W., and Alvord, E. C., Jr.: Neurotoxicity of hexachlorophene in humans. II. A clinicopathological study of 46 premature infants, Arch. Neurol. **32:**320, 1975.

Silverman, W. A., and Homan, W. E.: Sepsis of obscure origin in the newborn, Pediatrics **3:**157, 1949.

Silverman, W. A., and Sinclair, J. C.: Evaluation of precautions before entering a neonatal unit, Pediatrics **40:**900, 1967.

Snowe, R. J., and Wilfert, C. M.: Epidemic reappearance of gonococcal ophthalmia neonatorum, Pediatrics **51:**110, 1973.

South, M. A.: Enteropathogenic *Escherichia coli* disease: new developments and perspectives, J. Pediatr. **79:**1, 1971.

Sprunt, K., Redman, W., and Leidy, G.: Antibacterial effectiveness of routine hand washing, Pediatrics **52:**264, 1973.

Starr, J. G., and Gold, E.: Screening of newborn infants for cytomegalovirus infection, J. Pediatr. **73:**820, 1968.

Stern, H., and Tucker, S. M.: Prospective study of cytomegalovirus infection in pregnancy, Br. Med. J. **2:**268, 1973.

Swartzberg, J. E., and Remington, J. S.: Transmission of toxoplasma, Am. J. Dis. Child. **129:**777, 1975.

Watson, D. G.: Purulent neonatal meningitis: a study of forty-five cases, J. Pediatr. **50:**352, 1957.

Weller, T.: The cytomegaloviruses: ubiquitous agents with protean clinical manifestations, I and II, N. Engl. J. Med. **285:**203, 1971.

Wheeler, W. E.: Water bugs in the bassinet, Am. J. Dis. Child. **101:**273, 1961.

Wilson, M. G., et al.: New source of *Pseudomonas aeruginosa* in a nursery, J.A.M.A. **175:**1146, 1961.

Yeung, C. Y.: Hypoglycemia in neonatal sepsis, J. Pediatr. **77:**812, 1970.

Zuckerman, A. J.: The problem and control of hepatitis B infection in the fetus and the newborn. In Krugman, S., and Gershon, A. A., editors: Infections of the fetus and the newborn infant, New York, 1975, Alan R. Liss, Inc.

CHAPTER 13

Central nervous system disorders of perinatal origin

Concern for survival of sick neonates is surpassed only by an anxiety to avoid residual brain damage. Although the incidence of residual neurologic impairment has diminished considerably since the advent of fetal medicine and neonatal intensive care, there remains an unacceptable number of infants whose lives are destined to be of limited quality and longevity. Our success in avoiding these tragic sequelae is substantial but partial, and the implications of our failures are diffuse. The lives of the immediate family of the affected infant are disrupted. Also, those who are responsible for management of these sick infants are beset with ethical considerations that usually remain unresolved, largely as a function of our inability to predict long-term effects. There is also a concern about the potential number of handicapped survivors and the resulting fiscal liabilities.

This chapter is devoted to a discussion of the principal forms of noninfectious brain damage that are incurred during the perinatal period, their etiologies insofar as these are known, the possibilities of prevention, and the available modes of therapy. Discussion will focus on those central nervous disorders that are largely attributable to asphyxia; those due to birth trauma are discussed in Chapter 2.

THE CENTRAL NERVOUS SYSTEM SEQUELAE OF PRENATAL AND POSTNATAL ASPHYXIA AND ISCHEMIA OF THE BRAIN

The occurrence of damage to a previously normal brain during the antepartum and intrapartum periods is most often the result of oxygen deprivation. This may occur either as a result of diminished blood oxygen content in the presence of normal perfusion or as a result of diminished perfusion (ischemia) even if oxygen content is normal. The prenatal causes of hypoxia-ischemia are usually a consequence of the chronic fetal distress that is associated with maternal toxemia, other causes of placental insufficiency, severe postmaturity, and occasionally maternal diabetes. The other causes of protracted fetal distress are listed in Table 2-1. Acute hypoxia is more likely to occur during labor and delivery. The causes of these acute episodes, such as abruptio placentae, placenta previa, and prolapsed cord, are also listed in the same table. Hypoxia-ischemia that occurs postnatally is generally due to severe cardiorespiratory distress and vascular collapse (hypotension) from severe infection.

Other causes of damage to the brain include infections acquired prenatally and postnatally, maternal drug habits and drug therapy, postnatal metabolic disorders such as hypoglycemia, and congenital malformations.

We are concerned here with the aftermath of hypoxic-ischemic episodes, whether these occur before or after birth. Ninety percent of them occur prenatally. A variety of lesions may be produced, depending on the severity of the insult and the gestational age. In term infants, the most common consequence of hypoxia-ischemia is *cerebral necrosis*. In the premature infant, *periventricular necrosis (periventricular leukomalacia) and intraventricular hemorrhage* are most frequent. Another hemorrhagic consequence of hypoxia (and sometimes of trauma) is *primary subarachnoid hemorrhage* in both premature and term infants.

Cerebral (neuronal) necrosis

Cerebral (neuronal) necrosis is restricted to the term infant. The damage is incurred as the result of hypoxemia or the diminished cerebral perfusion that accompanies systemic hypotension. Usually, both of these factors are operative. Varying degrees of cellular necrosis occur in selected areas of the cerebral cortex, basal ganglia, brain stem, and cerebellum. Often, the initial insult is followed very shortly by edema of the brain. These changes occur to a varying extent, according to the severity of the hypoxic-ischemic episode. If the infant survives, cerebral atrophy is demonstrable by computerized tomographic (CT) scan several months later. The long-term sequelae of major concern include seizures, motor deficits, choreoathetosis and ataxia, and mental retardation. This combination of clinical signs is often referred to as "cerebral palsy." It should be understood, however, that cerebral palsy does not necessarily include mental retardation.

Clinical course. The clinical course of affected term infants has been followed by a number of investigators whose findings have been presented in terms of time intervals following birth. The major abnormalities involve the sensorium, muscle tone, seizure activity, and abnormal eye findings. As a rule, the fewer the symptoms or the more rapid the recovery from those that are present, the better the long-term outcome.

In light of present knowledge, *it is inadvisable to predict the quality of life based on a particular clinical course.* Persistence of abnormalities is usually associated with long-term neurologic impairment, but the precise extent of this impairment is generally unpredictable. The earlier the disappearance of an abnormal sign, the better the outlook. The description of abnormalities that follows is applicable only to term infants.

Sensorium. Alertness is diminished to the point of lethargy, or in the extreme, to stupor. Some improvement usually occurs within 12 to 24 hours, even in severely affected babies. Those who are mildly affected may progress to alertness within a shorter period. Following the period of improvement, the more severely affected infants relapse into stupor or coma between 24 and 72 hours after birth. In most infants, alertness may be regained in a few days, but stupor persists for weeks in the most severely affected babies.

Eyes. During the first 12 to 24 hours the pupils are reactive to light. Frequently, coordinated (conjugate) roving eye movements occur. Abnormal extraocular movements appear some time between 24 and 72 hours after birth in moderately and severely affected infants. Thus, "bobbing" eye movements may be in evidence. They are characterized by conjugate, but random, vertical motion. Skew deviation may also occur. Vertical position of the eyes is disparate; one eye is lower than the other.

Muscle tone. During the first 12 to 24 hours most infants are flaccid; their spontaneous movements are absent or markedly diminished. During the next 12 to 24 hours, muscle tone improves along with consciousness and spontaneous movement appears. Between 24 and 72 hours, severely affected infants become markedly hypotonic again; their spontaneous movements disappear. Beyond 72 hours they remain hypotonic for protracted periods.

Seizures. Some form of seizure activity is identifiable in approximately 50% of affected infants. The seizure activity is not often discernible before 6 hours of age. Early manifestations include sustained horizontal conjugate eye deviation; repeated blinking of the lids; sucking, smacking, and tongue thrusting movements; and swimming motions of the limbs. Apneic episodes are frequent. Tonic and clonic convulsive movements are multifocal. It is a peculiarity of the neonate that the tonic and clonic movements occur at random, not in the ordered sequence so characteristic of older children and adults. These blatant convulsive movements sometimes accompany the very early subtle signs of convulsions, but more frequently they follow them within hours. Within 6 to 24 hours, seizure activity may worsen. Tonic and clonic movements are predominant. These convulsions are difficult to control pharmacologically. Apneic episodes become more frequent and protracted. The most profoundly injured infants have status epilepticus. Severe seizure activity may continue for 48 to 72 hours and then disappear. In some infants, convulsions recur sporadically over the next few weeks. Sometimes jitteriness occurs between convulsive episodes when these are sporadic. Jitteriness is not always a benign sign, even if it occurs in the absence of convulsions.

Anterior fontanelle. Since the response to hypoxia often involves swelling of brain cells, water content is increased and intracranial pressure is elevated. Often, between 24 and 48 hours after birth, tight bulging of the anterior fontanelle and separation of the sutures of the skull first appear. These findings may persist for several days, and they are usually associated with the *syndrome of inappropriate secretion of antidiuretic hormone* (Chapter 7).

In the extreme, infants who are most profoundly damaged remain lethargic or stuporous and are unable to feed, thus requiring nasogastric feedings. Feeding difficulty generally improves over a few days or occasionally over a period of several weeks. Beyond the first 72 to 96 hours after birth, many infants who will have long-term effects remain hypotonic and cannot take feedings.

Treatment. Since cerebral edema is such a common manifestation of this type of brain injury, fluids are restricted in infants who are thought to have experienced intrauterine asphyxia. Thus, we administer approximately 50 ml/kg/24 hr to affected babies. The treatment of seizures is described later in this chapter.

A number of attempts are under way to evaluate several agents for the alleviation of cerebral edema. The use of hyperosmotic agents such as mannitol and glycerol is under study. Diuretics such as furosamide are also being investigated. Corticosteroids have been advocated on a trial basis because of their salutary effect in older patients, particularly those with cerebral edema following trauma. The protracted type of cerebral edema that follows hypoxic-ischemic injury apparently does not respond similarly. The status of corticosteroid therapy is thus far undetermined.

Periventricular leukomalacia

Periventricular leukomalacia occurs in premature infants. It is largely the result of diminished blood flow and is thus an area of infarction. The affected regions of the brain are adjacent to the lateral ventricles. Most often, the lesion does not include a hemorrhagic component. Many affected infants are not symptomatic during the neonatal period, but they may be simply lethargic and hypotonic. The motor fibers that descend from the cortex to the extremities run through the infarcted area of brain. Thus, injury to these fibers results in the long-term abnormality known as *spastic diplegia*, which does not necessarily include mental retardation. Spastic diplegia is grouped with the other abnormalities that constitute "ce-

rebral palsy." It is a permanent abnormality that is unique to premature infants. Although all four limbs may be affected by spastic paralysis, the lower limbs are characteristically more involved. A remarkable diminution in the incidence of spastic diplegia has been observed in numerous centers since the advent of neonatal intensive care.

Intraventricular (periventricular) hemorrhage

Intraventricular hemorrhage is a common consequence of hypoxia-ischemia that is peculiar to premature infants. It has been reported in a few term infants, but as a rule, the shorter the gestational age, the higher the incidence of hemorrhage. The term *intraventricular* implies that the hemorrhage bursts into the cerebral spinal fluid to circulate within the ventricular system. This does in fact occur in 85% of the cases, but the hemorrhage occurs first in the tissue immediately adjacent to the ventricular wall and it may occasionally remain there, never to burst into the cerebral spinal fluid in the ventricles.

The incidence of intraventricular hemorrhage is difficult to estimate. Just a few years past, the only methodology available for the diagnosis of these lesions was examination of cerebral spinal fluid extracted by lumbar puncture. The lumbar puncture was performed only after the appearance of clinical neurologic abnormalities. With the use of CT scanning, new clinical correlations with the appearance of intraventricular hemorrhage have come to light. Thus in a recent survey of 46 infants who weighed less than 1500 grams, 20 of them (43%) had evidence of intraventricular hemorrhage as demonstrated by the CT scan. Among the infants with hemorrhage who survived, seven were identified by the scanning technique *even though they were apparently asymptomatic*. Furthermore, although this study involved a relatively small number of infants, it was possible to grade the severity of the lesions according to the CT scan appearance. We have entered an era in which the relationship of perinatal clinical events to long-term outcome will be identified and etiologic factors that are applicable to prevention will be demonstrated. In the study previously mentioned, the frequency of intraventricular hemorrhage among infants who weighed less than 1500 grams (43%) is astonishing. Previous studies have demonstrated at *autopsy* that intraventricular (periventricular) hemorrhage was identifiable in 50% to 70% of infants *who died*. In another recent study, a follow-up of fifteen infants who survived intraventricular hemorrhage demonstrated that six (40%) were normal between 12 and 36 months of age. Moderate or severe neurologic handicaps were identifiable in only three of the fifteen babies (20%). In the remaining six (40%), neurologic handicaps were of minor significance. We are thus coming to the realization that this lesion is far more frequent than previously suspected, and that intact survival, or survival with minor impairment, is quite common. The contemporary difference in this new outlook is the result of an ability to detect these hemorrhages by surveillance techniques that do not depend on the appearance of clinical signs. At present, with only preliminary information, it appears that the incidence of survival, and its quality, approximates that which has been reported for neonatal bacterial meningitis. Furthermore, based on CT scan appearance, the extent (severity) of these lesions can be graded. Thus far, grade I (the mildest) through grade IV (the most severe) seem to correlate with the severity of residual handicap and with the appearance of hydrocephalus.

Clinical signs. Clinical signs are variable. At one extreme, these lesions occur in infants who are asymptomatic, while on the other, a catastrophic sequence of events results in death within minutes or hours. The catastrophic course is characterized by worsening of existing respiratory difficulty (apnea, hypercapnia, hypoxemia) in spite of previously adequate mechanical ventilatory support. The blood pressure drops precipitously. Normal body temperature is difficult or impossible to maintain. Cyanosis persists in spite of vigorous attempts to provide optimal respiratory support. Hypotonia is severe. Within a few hours the anterior fontanelle is tight and bulging. Seizures occur soon after the onset or within several hours. Opisthotonic posture, coma, and fixed, dilated pupils are frequent. The hematocrit falls at least 20% from its previous level, often by as much as 50% or 60%. Metabolic acidosis is severe and persistent, presumably as a result of vascular instability and poor general perfusion. The cerebral spinal fluid is bloody, but this is usually difficult to distinguish from the bloody fluid of a traumatic lumbar puncture. However, if the infant survives at least 24 hours, lumbar puncture later yields dark red-brown fluid that represents old blood. To us, this has been a most reliable sign of intraventricular hemorrhage. Some investigators have assigned great significance to abnormalities in thespinal fluid, others find only an irregular association between abnormal findings and outcome.

A less severe clinical course is probably most frequent. These signs are usually milder or evanescent. In some instances, they are virtually undetectable, while biochemical data is highly suggestive. Thus, a number of infants may manifest jaundice that is otherwise unexplained, while abnormal neurologic signs are barely discernible. Persistent metabolic acidosis or the sudden appearance of hyperglycemia or hypoglycemia may similarly suggest an intraventricular hemorrhage in which clinical signs are difficult to detect. More often, such infants become lethargic and hypotonic; they may also have intermittent opisthotonos. Focal seizures may occur and often disappear quite rapidly. In other instances subtle clinical signs, the significance of which cannot be determined, may be followed in 1 to 2 weeks by enlargement of the head, tightness of the anterior fontanelle, and separation of sutures. The use of the CT scan has revealed numerous instances of ventricular dilatation that has preceded enlargement of head circumference by a considerable period. The symptoms of intraventricular hemorrhage may appear, disappear, and reappear intermittently prior to ultimate cessation, or they may persist for several days and then disappear only to be followed by enlargement of the head. Of all the mild clinical signs, lethargy and hypotonia are most frequently encountered.

Pathogenesis. Intraventricular hemorrhage occurs in an area of the brain called the *germinal matrix*. The germinal matrix is located adjacent to the walls of the ventricles; its capillary blood supply is copious. The germinal matrix is an early developmental structure that is not present in the term infant. Therefore, hemorrhage in this area is unique to the premature infant. The capillaries in the germinal matrix are extremely fragile; they are almost devoid of supportive connective tissue. They are thus vulnerable to

rupture with relative ease. Furthermore, the capillaries become particularly vulnerable to disruption because hypoxic-ischemic events damage their walls. In most instances of hemorrhage into the germinal matrix, blood breaks through the ependymal wall into the ventricles and circulates in the cerebral spinal fluid. Obstruction to the flow of cerebral spinal fluid often occurs as a result, and the ventricles dilate in response to accumulating pressure. *This ventricular dilatation progresses for at least 1 to 2 weeks before enlargement of the head is clinically perceptible.* Hydrocephalus was previously thought to occur in approximately 80% of infants with intraventricular hemorrhage. More recently the incidence of hydrocephalus is cited in 44% of such affected infants.

Treatment. Supportive treatment to remedy hypoxemia, acidosis, and hypotension is the highest priority. Following stabilization of the baby, the most promising regimen involves daily lumbar punctures to relieve the pressure within the ventricular system. Removal of spinal fluid also serves to remove the blood therein and probably diminishes the possibility of obstruction to flow. From preliminary data, it appears that this regimen may diminish the incidence of hydrocephalus. Hyperosmotic agents such as glycerol have been used in an attempt to minimize the accumulation of fluid within the ventricles, but they are not conclusive.

Primary subarachnoid hemorrhage

Hemorrhage into the subarachnoid space may be primary or it may occur secondarily as an extension of bleeding that originated elsewhere (intraventricular hemorrhage or subdural hematoma). *Primary subarachnoid hemorrhage* involves bleeding into the subarachnoid space that does not involve other areas. The most common cause of such hemorrhage is hypoxia; birth trauma is a less frequent etiologic factor. Three fourths of the affected infants are premature.

In most instances, symptoms of primary subarachnoid hemorrhage are absent or mild. In a substantial number of infants, however, seizure activity occurs—particularly in term infants. These seizures characteristically appear on the second day of life; they are sporadic and persist for several days. This disorder is unique in that infants who convulse repeatedly seem to be well in the interim. In premature infants, primary subarachnoid hemorrhage is an infrequent cause of recurrent apnea in the absence of seizures.

Sequelae of this lesion are rare. Hydrocephalus may result from obstructed flow or impaired absorption of cerebral spinal fluid over the convex surfaces of the cerebral hemispheres. Massive subarachnoid hemorrhage is even more infrequent. It is usually associated with severe hypoxia or trauma and rarely culminates in death.

NEONATAL SEIZURES

Neonatal seizures may be subtle and barely discernible or blatant and lifethreatening. They are nonspecific symptoms that are caused by a variety of serious disorders. Recognition of their significance and identification of their causes are prerequisite to effective therapy.

The signs of seizure activity are frequently subtle and are most likely to escape the attention of inexperienced observers. These signs include sustained horizontal deviations of the eyes, paroxysms of horizontal or vertical nystagmus, blinking, chewing, sucking or vigorous tongue thrusting, transient abrupt loss of muscle tone, and vasomotor instability that is manifested by evanescent mottling or blotching. A number of less subtle signs are more likely to attract attention, including rowing motions of the upper extremities and bicycle movements of the lower ones, sudden assumption of a rigid posture, and fist clenching so forceful that it blanches the hand. Apnea has also been identified as a component of seizure activity, but rarely by itself. More frequently, apnea occurs in association with one or several of the more subtle manifestations.

The progressive tonic-clonic seizure that occurs in older infants is not observed in the neonate. Rather, convulsive episodes are usually one or the other, tonic or clonic. Tonic convulsions may involve the entire body. The infant stiffens; the back may arch. The lower extremities are in rigid extension; the toes point upward. The upper extremities are also stiff as they extend outward or forward. Occasionally, tonic postures are restricted to one or more of the extremities. Clonic activity consists of repetitive jerks at a rate of one to three per second. It is multifocal, migrating from one extremity to another in a disorganized fashion. In addition, facial twitches may be quite prominent. In a minority of instances, clonic seizures are focal; that is, they are restricted to one extremity, while unaccompanied by an altered state of consciousness. The distribution of localized tonic or clonic seizure activity bears no relationship to the location of lesions in the brain. Localized seizures are usually the result of diffuse cerebral disturbance.

Myoclonic seizures, rare in the neonate, are characterized by discrete gross jerks of one or more extremities. They are sometimes associated with abnormal eye movements and blinking.

Jitteriness is a rather frequent occurrence that must be differentiated from true seizures. Jitteriness is often benign and is most commonly associated with hyperactive and agitated states that are precipitated by hunger, thirst, or discomfort. If the infant's neurologic status is otherwise normal, jitteriness is not indicative of neurologic abnormality. However, jitters may be a sign of serious disorders such as hypocalcemia, hypoglycemia, drug withdrawal, and hypoxic-ischemic encephalopathy. Jitteriness is characterized by rapid alternating movements of equal amplitude in both directions. In contrast, clonic movements during true seizures have a fast and slow component and are not usually so rapid. Jitteriness can be stimulated by a disturbance of any kind, and it can be eliminated by gently touching or flexing an involved extremity. Seizures are rarely initiated by disturbances. Furthermore jitteriness is not associated with any of the subtle signs of seizure activity such as blinking or abnormal ocular motion.

Once the infant's abnormal movements are identified as seizures, the need to demonstrate etiologic factors becomes urgent. The clinical entities that produce seizures are numerous, but they can be grouped into five categories:

Perinatal difficulties (asphyxia, trauma)
Metabolic disorders
Infectious diseases
Drug withdrawal
Congenital malformations of the brain

Perinatal difficulties, primarily those that occur during labor and delivery, are the most frequent causes of neonatal seizures. Intrauterine asphyxia is responsible for most cases of hypoxic-ischemic encephalopathy. In most instances prenatal asphyxia is caused by maternal difficulties and/or placental abnormalities. In a minority, traumatic labor and delivery is causative, such as occurs from pro-longed labor with transverse arrest, high forceps extraction, breech presentation, or difficult manual extraction. Low Apgar scores of infants who have experienced intrauterine asphyxia reflect a continuation of the misadventure that began in utero. Trauma generally causes cerebral contusion, which is most frequent in term infants. Subarachnoid hemorrhage and skull fractures occur less frequently; subdural hematoma is now rare. Intraventricular hemorrhage is virtually always a disorder of premature infants. It is a sequel to asphyxia, and seizures appear approximately 6 hours after the hemorrhage (Chapter 2).

Hypoglycemia and hypocalemia are the principal metabolic disorders that produce seizures. Others that occur less frequently are the aminoacidurias, bilirubin encephalopathy (kernicterus), hypernatremia or hyponatremia; and drug withdrawal (narcotics and alcohol). Hypoglycemia is usually defined as a blood glucose level less than 20 mg/100 ml in premature babies and less than 30 mg/100 ml in term infants. However, most hospital laboratories perform glucose determinations in serum rather than whole blood, and hypoglycemic levels in serum are higher. Hypoglycemia occurs at serum levels of 25 mg/100 ml in premature infants and at 35 mg/100 ml in term infants. The longer the duration of hypoglycemia, the more likely is seizure activity. Most hypoglycemic infants are asymptomatic. Among symptomatic babies, approximately 20% manifest some type of seizure activity. Immediate diagnosis by Dextrostix is the method of choice, but laboratory determination of glucose levels must be performed to verify the results of the Dextrostix.

Hypocalcemia is defined by a serum calcium less than 7 mg/100 ml. The incidence of hypocalcemia clusters around the first 2 or 3 days and again at 6 to 10 days of age.

The latter group of infants are usually born at term and are given milk preparations that contain an inappropriate calcium-phosphorus ratio. In recent years, late onset hypocalcemia has become infrequent because of widespread use of proprietary formulas that contain a higher calcium-phosphorus ratio. Early onset hypocalcemia occurs in infants who have experienced perinatal stress. In them, low serum calcium concentrations are associated with other factors such as asphyxia, trauma, and hypotension. In such circumstances, the role of hypocalcemia in the causation of seizures can be established only if seizures disappear within minutes following intravenous administration of calcium solution. Such is rarely the case in early onset hypocalcemia.

The infectious diseases that produce neonatal seizures (Chapter 12) are those that include meningitis and encephalitis. Bacterial infections predominate and among them *E. Coli* and group B streptococcal septicemia with meningitis are the most common. Both these organisms are usually acquired by the fetus from the mother during the birth process. Thus, clinical signs of disease usually appear within 5 days of age. However, bacterial meningitis may begin at any time during the nursery stay if the infant is inoculated from the environment or by personnel carriers. Other etiologic agents of infectious disease include the nonbacterial group (toxoplasma, rubella virus, cytomegalovirus, and coxsackievirus). Seizures occur in affected babies by virtue of the encephalitis produced by these agents.

The two underlying disorders that most urgently require specific diagnosis are hypoglycemia and bacterial infection. Dextrostix for blood sugar will adequately determine the presence of the former; immediate examination of spinal fluid for cells and organisms will demonstrate the latter. Hypoglycemic levels demonstrated by Dextrostix should be verified by laboratory determination of calcium, sodium, potassium, and magnesium. Variations in the infant's history and physical findings may indicate additional determinations or delete others.

Management of the convulsing infant is comprised of specific therapy for metabolic disorders (hypoglycemia, hypocalcemia, hypomagnesemia) and for bacterial infection. It is also comprised of anticonvulsant medication and supportive therapy for adequate respiratory function, hydration, electrolyte balance, and body temperature. When seizures first appear, we determine the presence of hypoglycemia by Dextrostix and draw blood for glucose, calcium, phosphorus, and magnesium. If the Dextrostix indicates normoglycemia, we administer phenobarbital as described below.

For hypoglycemia we infuse 2 to 4 ml of 25% glucose intravenously over a period of approximately 5 minutes. This is followed by continuous administration of a solution that provides 0.5 gm to 0.8 gm/kg of glucose per hour, depending on the results of repeated Dextrostix and laboratory determinations of glucose levels. Anticonvulsant medication is not indicated for treatment of hypoglycemia.

Specific therapy for hypocalcemia is instituted only after serum calcium levels are known. We administer 150 mg to 200 mg/kg of calcium gluconate intravenously (3 to 4 ml/kg of a 5% solution) over a period of approximately 10 minutes. Heart rate is monitored by a cardiotachometer during the infusion of calcium. A sudden fall in heart rate requires that calcium administration be halted. If seizures are severe and continuous, we use phenobarbital when calcium administration cannot be continued. Late onset hypocalcemia is frequently associated with hypomagnesemia which, if untreated, will cause persistence of the convulsive state in spite of calcium therapy. Magnesium sulfate is given intramuscularly in a dose of 0.2 ml/kg/24 hr as a 50% solution. Overdoses of magnesium may produce severe muscle paralysis by virtue of the curare-like effect that the magnesium ion produces.

Phenobarbital is the anticonvulsant drug of choice. In the absence of hypoglycemia or hypocalcemia, we give an initial intravenous dose of 10 mg/kg. If seizures have not subsided in 30 minutes, the same dose is repeated. In most instances, the seizures subside. Thereafter, phenobarbital is maintained at 5 mg/kg/24 hr in divided doses every 12 hours. Convulsions caused by perinatal asphyxia are notoriously difficult to control; maintenance doses of phenobarbital up to 10 mg/kg may be required.

We do not use diazepam to control seizures because phenobarbital is quite effective, the effect of diazepam is relatively transient, and diazepam may cause vascular collapse particularly when used with phenobarbital. Furthermore, the vehicle in which the drug is administered contains sodium benzoate, which displaces bilirubin from its albumin-binding sites. The result is a vulnerability to kernicterus because of the increased quantity of free bilirubin that has become unbound from albumin.

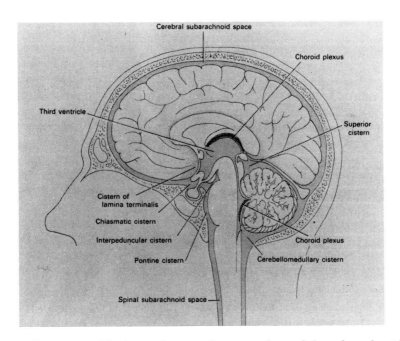

Fig. 13-1. Midline view of the brain showing the ventricles and the subarachnoid space in the shaded area. The two choroid plexuses are in the third (uppermost) and fourth ventricles. Spinal fluid flows from the choroid plexus into the ventricles within the brain to the subarachnoid space that envelops its external surfaces. (From Carpenter, M. B.: Human neuroanatomy, Baltimore, 1976, The Williams & Wilkins Co.)

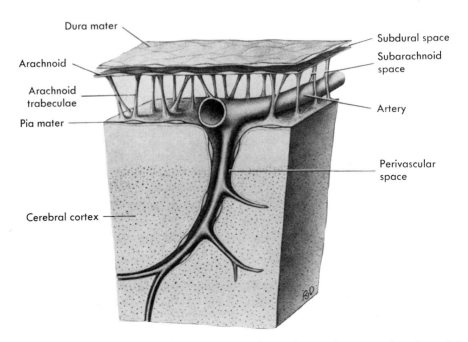

Dura mater

Arachnoid

Arachnoid trabeculae

Pia mater

Cerebral cortex

Subdural space

Subarachnoid space

Artery

Perivascular space

Fig. 13-2. The subarachnoid space is shown in relationship to the external surface of the brain, the blood vessels, and the meninges. (From Carpenter, M.B.: Human neuroanatomy, Baltimore, 1976, The Williams & Wilkins Co.)

HYDROCEPHALUS

Hydrocephalus is an abnormal physical finding that is produced by a number of underlying disorders. It is characterized by the accumulation of cerebral spinal fluid (CSF) within the ventricular system secondary to an obstruction of normal flow. Intraventricular pressure rises; the ventricles become distended. Ultimately, distension of the ventricles progresses and within days or weeks enlargement of the head is obvious. At this point, the anterior fontanelle is tight and bulging; the skull sutures are widened.

Cerebral spinal fluid is generated by the choroid plexus and by the brain substance as well. It is produced at an average rate of 0.4 ml/min, ranging from 0.26 to 0.65 ml/min. Normally, fluid flows from the lateral ventricles into the third ventricle after passing through the fora-

men of Monro. From the third ventricle it enters the aqueduct and proceeds to the fourth ventricle, from which it leaves the ventricular system by passing through the foramina of Luschka and Magendie. Fluid next flows over the convex surfaces of the cerebral hemispheres within the subarachnoid space and is returned to the sagittal sinus to reenter the blood stream (Figs. 13-1 and 13-2).

Obstruction to the flow of spinal fluid may occur anywhere along the pathway just described. The obstruction may be due to tumor, blood clot, adhesions, or congenital malformations, and it may be located within the ventricles or outside them. In the neonate, hydrocephalus occurs most frequently as a sequel to intraventricular hemorrhage and bacterial meningitis. In both instances, the obstruction is a result of residual adhesions from the initial disease process.

Hydrocephalus produces only one early clinical sign—enlargement of the head. If other neurologic abnormalities are evident, they are the result of the underlying disorder that caused the hydrocephalus. Head enlargement is also produced by a number of other entities such as subdural hematoma, porencephaly, hydranencephaly, and achondroplasia. The spurt in growth that occurs following adequate feeding of a malnourished infant is often characterized by transient rapid enlargement of the head.

The most reliable diagnostic procedure is the CT scan. Ultrasound scans at the bedside will in the future provide a more convenient and rapid method for demonstration of ventricular enlargement. If the remaining cerebral cortex is thin, transillumination of the skull (p. 165) can demonstrate the accumulated fluid.

The treatment of hydrocephalus is generally unsatisfactory. Pharmacologic therapy, whether aimed at diminishing the production of cerebral spinal fluid or withdrawing it from the ventricular system into the bloodstream, has not been successful. Surgical treatment is currently the most acceptable approach, despite its difficulties. It consists of the placement of a shunt from the ventricles into the peritoneal space or the heart. This provides an ongoing run-off for excessive intraventricular fluid. Shunts in small infants must generally be revised later as their growth proceeds. The shunting catheters frequently become obstructed, and they also may become infected at either the intracranial or distal end. In spite of these complications, there is unfortunately no better method available for the management of hydrocephalus.

REFERENCES

Fitzhardinge, P. M.: Complications of asphyxia and their therapy. In Gluck, L., editor: Intrauterine asphyxia and developing fetal brain, Chicago, 1977, Year Book Medical Publishers, Inc.

Freeman, J. M., and Brann, A. W.: Central nervous system disturbances. In Behrman, R. E., editor: Neonatal-perinatal medicine: diseases of the fetus and infant, ed. 2, St. Louis, 1977, The C. V. Mosby Co.

Horwitz, S. J., and Amiel-Tison, C.: Neurologic problems. In Klaus, M. H., and Fanaroff, A. A., editors: Care of the high risk neonate, Philadelphia, 1979, W. B. Saunders Co.

Krishnamoorthy, K. S., Shannon, D. C., DeLong, G. R., et al.: Neurologic sequelae in the survivors of neonatal intraventricular hemorrhage, Pediatrics **64:**233, 1979.

Mitchell, W., and O'Tuama, L.: Cerebral intraventricular hemorrhages in infants: a widening age spectrum, Pediatrics **65:**35, 1980.

Palma, P. A., Miner, M. E., Morriss, F. H., et al.: Intraventricular hemorrhage in the neonate born at term, Am. J. Dis. Child. **133:**941, 1979.

Papile, L.-A., Burstein, J., Burstein, R., and Koffler, H.: Incidence and evolution of subependymal and intraventricular hemorrhage: a study of infants with birth weights less than 1500 gm, J. Pediatr. **92:**529, 1978.

Seay, A. R., and Bray, P. F.: Significance of seizures in infants weighing less than 2500 grams, Arch. Neurol. **34:**381, 1977.

Volpe, J. J.: Perinatal hypoxic-ischemic brain injury, Pediatr. Clin. North Am. **23:**383, 1976.

Volpe, J. J.: Observing the infant in the early hours after asphyxia. In Gluck, L., editor: Intrauterine asphyxia and the developing fetal brain, Chicago, 1977, Year Book Medical Publishers, Inc.

Volpe, J. J.: Neonatal intracranial hemorrhage: pathophysiology, neuropathology, and clinical features, Clin. Perinatol. **4:**77, 1977.

Volpe, J. J.: Neonatal periventricular hemorrhage: past, present, and future, J. Pediatr. **92:**693, 1978.

CHAPTER 14

Impact of intensive care on the parent-infant relationship

Jean Lancaster

The development of an affectionate, nurturing, and reciprocal relationship between infant and parent is essential for a healthy psychologic outcome. Recent studies have increased our understanding of the early development of parent-infant relationships; however, the precise process of attachment is unknown. Attachment refers to the quality of affectional ties between mother and infant that begin to develop early in pregnancy, appear to increase when fetal movement is felt, and are intensified with seeing, touching, and caring for the infant after birth.

EARLY SEPARATION: EFFECTS ON ATTACHMENT

Several studies suggest that these bonds of affection can be disrupted when the newborn infant experiences minor or major illness that necessitates separation from the mother. Animal studies suggest that early separation is detrimental to the developing mother-child relationship. When newborn goats were separated from their mothers immediately after birth and reunited several hours later, the mothers were either unable or unwilling to accept their offspring. Some dams fed the kids indiscriminately; others butted them away. Among rats and mice, total rejection of the young did not occur, but maternal behavior was lessened when early separation had occurred. In contrast, when lambs were kept with their mothers for 4 days, then separated and later reunited, the mothers always returned to their own lambs and exhibited normal maternal behavior. It seems that for many animal species physical contact with the young in the immediate postnatal period is essential for the development of normal mothering behavior. Whether a similar critical period exists for humans is conjectural, but two studies suggest such a possibility. In one of them, groups of mothers were allowed differing amounts of physical contact with their infants during the newborn period. Follow-up observations at discharge and at 1 month indicated that mothers who had the earliest and most frequent contact with their babies showed more en face and fondling behavior and were more soothing during a physical examination. In a related study, primiparous mothers who had early contact with their premature infants showed more confidence in their caretaking abilities than those denied early contact.

For both animals and humans, touch seems to play an important role in the establishment of the relationship. The human mother first uses touch to become acquainted with her baby, and later uses it to express love. She explores the infant's body with her fingertips, gradually using more of her hands and finally enfolding him in her arms, holding him close to her body. Mothers of term infants will often complete this process within 10 minutes. Mothers who have been separated from their premature infants often express difficulty in believing that they have a child. Yet when these mothers have contact with their babies, they use the same touching behaviors as mothers of term infants but proceed at a slower pace.

Eye-to-eye contact between human mothers and their children is a powerful elicitor of maternal affection. Similarly, the performance of caretaking activities and the derivation of satisfaction from the child both seem to be necessary preludes to the development of maternal love. Prolonged separation of mother and child may hinder the natural evolution of these phenomena.

It is quite apparent that the moments after birth are exquisitely sensitive for the *initiation* of attachment. In recent years the long- and short-term benefits of this encounter between mother and child have acquired a mystic aura of indispensability. Even more than that, there is a pervasive persuasion among the laity and professionals that absence of this early contact inflicts irrevocable maternal disaffection, which in turn ultimately influences the attitude of the child. It is unfortunate that a simple, understandable, and natural desire to experience the sheer joy of first contact after birth has become complicated by the idea that nothing will ever be right if for any reason these moments are missed. They are indeed missed when the neonate requires resuscitation and when separation of mother and infant is unavoidable because intensive care must be instituted. Now, the unrealistic fear of future disaffection is added to the guilt and grief of giving birth to a troubled baby. We have observed this phenomenon repeatedly, particularly in well-educated mothers. However desirable this early contact may be, we should advise parents that its absence does not preclude a normal relationship in the future. The attachment of mother and child is ongoing and dynamic. In normal circumstances it is highly resistant to permanent disruption.

Besides physical separation, there is evidence that a mother suffers emotional estrangement from her high-risk infant. The causes of these feelings are varied and complex. She has lost the normal child she anticipated during pregnancy, and the realization that her baby is less than perfect initiates a grief reaction.

To therapeutically assist parents in working through this grief process, health professionals must understand it and must be able to identify and interpret behavior patterns that parents should anticipate.

GRIEF

Grief is a normal and characteristic response to the loss of, or separation from, a significant person. It creates emotional and physical pain. Uncomplicated grief seems to run a predictable course; it is influenced by the abruptness of the loss, preparation for the loss, and the relationship between the survivor and the lost object. Grief includes an initial period of shock that is usually followed by either denial or panic. Essentially, the same sequence of events occurs during grief caused by death, premature birth or birth of a severely handicapped infant.

Denial is a defense mechanism that cushions the impact of loss and has been called a "human shock-absorber" to tragedy. Emotions are temporarily defused; the sense of time is suspended in an attempt to delay the impact of loss. This allows a bereaved individual some time to organize inner resources and to search for an appropriate response to the devastating event. Yet the expression of denial is often inconsistent. To the physician, for example, the parents may exhibit vehement denial when told their infant is critically ill. Thus, after being informed, the mother may say: "My baby will be ready to go home with me when I am discharged from the hospital." On the other hand, she may talk openly with the social worker. Apparently, grieving parents often find it inappropriate to share their hurt with the physician (or perhaps the nurse as well) who must care for their child; they fear that their own pessimism will influence the treatment that is provided. They feel safer divulging their deep feelings with staff members who are not directly involved in medical care.

In response to their loss, some parents panic. When stability is disrupted by the loss of a significant relationship, emotional expressions often have no limit. Panic is manifested by intense anxiety, excitement, and/or paranoid ideas. Panic can usually be minimized if calm and authoritative management is provided by a responsible professional—nurse, physician, or social worker. A person in panic is desperately seeking resources to restore order to inner chaos.

As shock and denial are replaced by awareness of reality, strong feelings of anger, guilt, shame, and helplessness emerge. Crying, sleep disturbances, loss of interest in daily activities, and somatic symptoms of distress and pain are commonly experienced. If these feelings are not openly expressed, perhaps because of strong inhibitions for any number of reasons, anger is sealed within, guilt evolves, and release from shock is experienced as severe depression. Depression is a response to loss; it is a device for coping. Depression often signals a need to verbalize suppressed fear and anxiety. Recovery is impeded when we do not interpret such behavior accurately. An environment must be provided to allow verbalization of feelings. Short-term depression is a normal response to loss. Its absence indicates an abnormal coping behavior. The grieving parents must externalize their feelings of anger, guilt, and disappointment.

Parents' attempts to make sense of their loss are often manifested in such questions as: "Why me? What did I do wrong? Why did God let my baby die?" Behind these questions are anxiety, poor self-image, and a desperate desire for someone who cares enough to listen to their real fears. We must be open and honest; we should encourage verbalization, rather than restrain it.

Finally, the grieving person enters the phase of acceptance and recovery when grief continues, but the trauma of loss is gradually overcome and a state of equilibrium is once again established. This period of grief is very trying for parents, particularly those whose infants have major abnormalities or do not survive. Many parents feel that the grief has been resolved, only to find themselves depressed and their daily routines hampered by exhaustion. Family and friends fail to recognize that grief takes months to resolve. They often unknowingly abandon the grieving family after the initial crisis. Many parents express the fear that the revitalization of their feelings indicates that they have lost control or that they will never be able to resolve the loss. This is a time when parents need to communicate openly with each other and with close friends. Group meetings, such as Parents Experiencing Perinatal Death (Memphis, Tennessee) or groups for parents of infants with specific anomalies, are extremely helpful. At such meetings, communication with parents in similar situations provides effective support. Such communication also demonstrates that the behavior they fear in themselves is actually pervasive and normal and that in time the impact of their loss will diminish.

Although grieving is painful, it is necessary for a healthy outcome. In the extreme, failure to mourn a significant loss is associated with long-term depression, psychosomatic illness, and other pathologic consequences.

PREMATURE BIRTH

The long-awaited physical contact with a newborn, the anticipated interaction, and the provision of nurturing care to their offspring, are all fantasies of parents-to-be and are all abruptly terminated by the birth of a sick, premature infant.

Fears for the survival and intactness of the child are paramount. The parents experience the loss of the perfect child of their dreams, as well as blow to their self-esteem because the child they have created is imperfect. Their grief is different from that of parents whose infant has died. They must surrender the baby of their dreams to form a relationship with their real child, who may be normal or handicapped. If the baby's survival is in doubt, the parents may be reluctant to invest in a relationship. Anticipatory grief is evident at this time. Study and experience have documented the pervasiveness of anticipatory grieving by parents of infants transferred to a regional neonatal center. Parents prepare themselves for the death of their infant, while at the same time continuing to hope that their baby will live. In our experience, the most common manifestation of anticipatory grief is delayed naming of the baby until survival is assured. In the presence of electronic monitors, catheters, and other forbidding equipment, it is understandably difficult for parents to focus on their baby; their attention is fixed on the equipment and the threatened loss that it symbolizes.

The work of anticipatory grief can be accelerated by frequent visiting and providing specific caretaking activities for the parents. Yet in many instances, initiation of a close relationship with the baby is unlikely until the parents are convinced that a favorable outcome is certain.

Working with parents of premature infants

The ultimate goal of our work with parents of premature infants is to foster the development of an attachment to their baby. Since the birth of a premature infant creates a sense of loss, attachment cannot be achieved totally until the parents have resolved their grief. To facilitate the grieving process and to enhance the reality of the living child, parents must be allowed to see their infant at the earliest opportunity. They must discuss the condition of their infant with identifiable members of the health care team. Parents need compassionate and knowledgeable personnel with whom they can share their fears and concerns without fear of being judged.

Prior to their first visit, the nurse must prepare the parents for the baby's appearance and for the equipment in use. At the bedside, the function of each item and its role in promoting recovery should be explained. Comments about the baby's individuality are particularly helpful, and statements such as "He likes to hold my finger while I feed him" or "She is very active" will help the parents see their baby beyond the equipment. Phototherapy should always be temporarily discontinued and eye patches should be removed to permit eye-to-eye contact between parents' and child, except when the baby is so ill that he cannot open his eyes. The nurse must be present with the parents at the beginning of the visit. Later, parents should be left alone with their baby. Constant supervision and hovering by personnel tends to inhibit mothering responses such as touch and eye-to-eye contact. Some mothers can tolerate only brief visits in the beginning. When they indicate a need to leave, they should be reassured that their reactions are normal and that they are welcome to return at will.

For the mother who has been hospitalized elsewhere, we have found it helpful to send a picture of the baby. The picture provides some visual contact that is otherwise impossible. Typically, the mother's fantasy is worse than reality. She is encouraged to call the nursery at any time to talk with the nurse who cares for her baby. Night hours are extremely stressful for parents; we receive many telephone calls between 10 PM and 1 AM.

In our center, parents are encouraged to visit their babies and touch and fondle them while they are still in incubators. Observations at several centers have not demonstrated an increased risk of infection if parents are allowed to visit the nursery. In fact, one investigator noted that mothers observed isolation precautions more carefully than medical personnel. In the case of a premature infant, the nurse must prepare parents for the generalized startle reaction to touch, instead of the expected localized physical response. They must also be informed about the lack of response of a depressed infant, regardless of maturity. For example, when the premature infant who is touched by his mother simply exhibits a Moro reflex and cries, the mother may perceive the response as displeasure. She should not be allowed to believe that she is unwanted by her baby, that her attention has been repelled. She should be told of this expected response to spare her the agony of a misinformed reaction.

Mothers who wish to breast feed should be encouraged to do so. Although the premature infant may be unable to nurse at the breast, mothers can be taught to express the milk, freeze it, and bring it to the center. Breast feeding offers the mother of the hospitalized premature infant an opportunity to provide something that no one else can.

As soon as it is appropriate, our mothers are asked to perform selective caretaking activities for their infants. These activities should elicit positive reinforcement of the mother's endeavors. She must be protected from feelings of incompetence lest she withdraw further from her baby. All mothers are encouraged to feed and bathe their babies repeatedly before discharge. Since a mother may interpret poor feeding, sleeping during feeds, or regurgitation as indications of her own ineptness, she should be forewarned of the normal nature of these occurrences. The nurse should not immediately take the infant who feeds poorly from the mother and then feed the baby successfully in her presence. The resultant feelings of inadequacy and resentment are thus cruelly imposed on her already existing emotional difficulties. Rather, the nurse should help by demonstrating techniques such as gentle rotation of the nipple or stroking of the infant's cheek to initiate a sucking reflex.

Diminishing the impact of psychologic separation is somewhat more difficult. Some understanding of the parents' feelings is prerequisite to any attempt to alleviate them. The physician, nurse, and social worker must assist parents in their attempts to deal with grief and accept the infant so they can become involved in his care. Consistency in communication is necessary to prevent parental misunderstanding. Communication failures often lead to a less than optimal adjustment to the crisis. Effective intervention and communication with parents requires observation of behavior and identification of the stage of grieving. Parents should know that their feelings are common. As previously stated, the mother (and father as well) usually progresses through shock, a developing awareness of reality, and finally an acceptance of reality. During the period of shock, she cannot comprehend what is said to her. She fre-quently claims that everything is unreal or dreamlike. She may deny the reality of her predicament. Although the neonatal nurse rarely encounters the mother at this stage of her grief process, she can, in collaboration with social workers and nurses on the maternity floor, keep the mother continuously informed about the baby's status. However, it is important to realize that a mother in this phase of grief can ill afford to be overwhelmed with too much information. An honest, simple explanation is all that is needed; it is certainly all she can understand for the time being. Problems at hand should be discussed; predicting problems such as jaundice, preumothorax, retardation, or possible death must be avoided in an attempt to prevent completion of the grief process. Once the grief process is completed, parents must reestablish a relationship with a baby who is perceived as dead and buried; frequently, the reestablishment of this relationship is never accomplished.

Active intervention into the grief process by describing reality and by encouraging the mother to express her feelings will assist her progress. She must not be pushed into discussing her feelings. With a developing awareness of reality, the mother has moved into the second stage of grief. Now she may be overcome with feelings of anger, guilt, and shame. She may lash out at those who come to her aid; she may berate herself or her spouse for dreadful failure. Transfer of parental guilt and anger to medical and nursing staff is common. It is a great temptation for the staff to categorize such a mother as "difficult." As a result of this categorization, personnel withdraw from the mother in question; in fact, complete abandonment is not uncommon. Yet the patient has merely grasped at anger and hostility as an immediately available mode of coping with her catastrophy. No greater harm can be inflicted at that moment than abandonment by the only individuals who could be supportive and who could thereby avert a potentially long-term attitudinal difficulty. The mother must be encouraged to express these negative emotions; they indicate attempts to cope with a stressful situation. Only as she externalizes them can she begin to move toward acceptance of reality, and only then can she begin to establish the bonds of relationship with her baby.

One indication of progress is the development of an interest in the infant and his care. However, when she asks the same questions over and over again in her struggle to grasp the situation, those who work with her should be genuinely concerned and patient. It is during this time that she can first be taught to care for her baby and thus relate to him. Impatience with frequent questions turns her away and impedes ultimate acceptance of her baby. Several studies have shown that mothers who fail to visit or call about their baby, who exhibit little anxiety in relation to the child's prematurity or illness, who seek little information about their baby, and who are unable or unwilling to share their own fears and concerns are destined for a difficult, if not pathologic, relationship with their child. Identification of such behavior urgently requires parental counseling by others besides the nurse. A significant correlation between lack of interest and a paucity of telephone calls and visits has been observed. Furthermore, the incidence of children who are destined for parental battering increases in the face of these signs of detachment or neglect.

If survival of the infant is in doubt, parents may emotionally prepare for death while simultaneously maintaining hope for survival. They may physically withdraw from their infant during such a crisis; yet they usually maintain contact by phone. They must begin to accept the reality of an uncertain prognosis. It is important for both parents to be accurately informed about the baby's condition. Cautious optimism must be utilized in counseling parents about their infant's condition. Informing them that death is a certainty or that mental retardation is a likelihood will be detrimental to the establishment of an acceptable relationship should the baby survive. Parents must not be allowed to develop unrealistic optimism, but close contact should nevertheless be encouraged. Close early contact with an infant who later dies does not cause a dangerous increase in grief among mothers with no history of emotional difficulty. The last stage of the grief process, acceptance of reality, may take several months and indeed may never be accomplished, particularly if the infant is handicapped.

Mothers need frequent praise and reassurance as they learn to care for their babies. The nurse should guide a mother who has difficulty with a caretaking activity, rather than supplant her. The impressive competence of the nurse may well discourage the mother from trying to learn.

Nurses can evaluate a mother's emotional state by being alert to signs of tension, such as rapid breathing, muscle tension, perspiration, and rapid or stilted conversation. When the mother is participating in care of her baby, her approach to touching and holding him often reveals a great deal about her emotional state. During the learning period, if she is unsure of herself, she will handle the baby rather stiffly and awkwardly, tend-ing to hold him away from her body. At first she prefers only to touch him with her fingertips rather than enfold him in her arms. A distant sort of handling and holding is often manifest during feeding. The mother who is at ease with her baby holds him closely, with his head resting in the crook of her elbow in proximity to, or touching, her breast. She usually holds him turned toward her, and she seeks repeated eye contact with him. Both baby and mother are relaxed in a comfortable position. In contrast, the mother who is uneasy and anxious usually assumes an awkward, uncomfortable position. Her arm is stiff and it tires easily. In her insecurity she is preoccupied with the mechanics of the feeding process and thus makes no attempt to establish eye contact with her infant. She seeks reassurance from the nurse repeatedly and must receive positive responses from her baby, such as consuming all of the offered formula or sleeping postprandially. She is visibly upset if the baby fails to take all of the milk or if he regurgitates. This behavior reinforces feelings of incompetence and is often perceived as rejection. Eventually, with support from an adept nurse, this mother will develop a comfortable relationship with her baby.

An occasional mother, for one reason or another, fails to establish a firm attachment to her baby. She holds him on her knee with his head on her forearm but at a distance from her breast. The baby will likely be on his back or perhaps turned away from her. Instead of making eye contact, she gazes around the room, apathetic and disinterested. Because she pays little attention to the baby, the bottle is tilted incorrectly, so that the nipple is filled with air rather than milk. This mother needs counseling if she is ever to form a healthy relationship with her

baby. Identifying such a mother in the early phase of her relationship with the baby and referring her for help may prevent multiple problems in the future. It should be noted that most mothers transiently exhibit some signs of discomfort with their babies; it is the predominant and persistent behavior patterns that are important.

As mother and baby become acquainted, she seeks some indication that she is successfully meeting his needs. Relaxation and sleep are the most common early signs of such success. Unfortunately, because of their biologic difficulties, high-risk babies are often at first unable to respond favorably to the mother's ministrations. Mothers should be taught that this lack of response is not a reflection of poor mothering, so that the baby's inability to respond does not further jeopardize the relationship.

DEATH OF A NEWBORN

Until recently, few health professionals appreciated the depth of grief that is experienced by parents whose newborn infant dies. Studies indicate that parents' grief from loss of a neonate is little different from that which is associated with the loss of an older child or adult.

The mourning response may begin immediately after death, it may be delayed, or it may be entirely absent if strong denial mechanisms exist. One long-term study demonstrated that one third of the mothers who experienced perinatal death developed severe psychiatric problems. Our personal experience suggests that mothers who do not see or touch their infant before death seem to have more difficulty in completing the grief process than those who did. The health professional's role must thus continue after death of the infant. The principal tasks are to facilitate the parents' acknowledgment of the death as a reality, to assure that grieving progresses to acceptance, and to be available to the parents during the resolution process. Several meetings with parents are usually required to accomplish these ends.

Parents should be informed of their infant's death in a quiet and private place. Privacy allows expression of emotions without inhibitions or fears of judgment by others. The events surrounding the death should be discussed in appropriate detail; parents' questions must be answered. They should be offered the opportunity to see and hold their infant after death because loss of the infant and resolution of the grief process seems to be enhanced thereby. Observations of 25 mothers who had touched, but never held, their infants have demonstrated the same behavior pattern after death that one sees when the baby is alive—poking the extremities, rubbing the extremities, trunk, and head, and finally embracing the infant. All these mothers, except one, embraced the infant, kissed the infant, and made very personal remarks expressing both love and sadness. At the end of the holding period, every mother remarked, "You can have him now," or "She is yours now." Apparently, as mothers hold their dead infants, their need to caress and identify is satisfied, denial is eliminated, and death becomes a reality.

Contact with parents should recur 2 to 3 weeks after the baby's death. The purpose of this visit is to answer questions concerning the death, review autopsy findings, evaluate their reaction to the loss, and help them understand their feelings and behavior. Many parents are concerned about losing control of their emotions and having feelings of impending insanity. Mere verbalization of these

fears often brings relief. The importance of encouraging ongoing communication between spouses and with their living children cannot be overemphasized. It is not unusual for husbands and wives to find themselves at different stages of grief. Marital difficulties are virtually unavoiable when husband and wife communicate poorly following the death of their baby. Parent groups are extremely helpful during the long grieving period.

The third scheduled contact with parents should occur some 2 to 3 months after the infant's death. The primary purpose of this contact is to make sure that the grieving process is moving towards acceptance. At this time, parents usually express feelings of depression, anger, and isolation. Depression indicates that death has become a reality. During this time, parents are beset with introspection regarding the meaning of life, death, religion, and the baby's care before death. Feelings of isolation are often magnified. Relatives and friends often incorrectly view parental return to routine activity as a sign of the termination of grief. The health professional who is aware of the length of the grieving process and that such is not the case can be helpful to parents at this time.

In some parents, pathologic grief reactions may be identifed at this time. Symptoms include total denial of the loss, inappropriate hostility or cheerfulness, severe depression, psychosomatic disorders, and inability to cope. Recognition of the symptoms and referral for psychiatric assistance is indispensable.

In time, parents who have successfully worked through their anger and depression in response to their infant's loss will reach a stage of acceptance in which they are neither angry nor depressed. They simply accept the fact that the infant is dead. Periods of sadness are recurrent, particularly on special occasions such as birthdays and family holidays.

CONGENITAL MALFORMATION

The birth of an infant with congenital malformations precipitates a major family crisis. The idealized, healthy infant has not materialized. Parental reactions are greatly influenced by the type of malformation, visibility of the malformation, social and personal values, and previous relationships with family and friends. Attitudes of health professionals toward the infant's defect also contribute to the parental response.

Mourning the loss of the "perfect" infant requires time; the process requires parents to gradually relinquish the dreams of their wished-for child and to adapt to the handicapped baby who was born. Parents have little time to grieve their loss before demands are made to invest in a relationship with the imperfect child. Grief is complicated by preoccupation with demands of the child's physical care.

Parents of children with congenital anomalies need continuing support from a variety of professionals to deal with their shock and disappointment and to facilitate their long-term attachment. They should be gently informed of the infant's problems as soon as possible. Allowing parents to see the infant helps to overcome denial and alleviate exaggerated and grotesque fantasies by providing the opportunity to discuss the normal characteristics of the infant. Images of the unseen are invariably worse than the actual problem. Early and frequent contact allows parents to become acquainted with the infant's features; usually the contact supports positive maternal feelings. This identification and initiation of a relationship is a major step in reducing the emotional turmoil associated with the birth of a handicapped child. Parental self-esteem is increased as they become involved in the care of their infant and as responses from the infant are appreciated.

Parents need to know the purpose of care rendered, what to expect from their infant, and community services that are available. Protracted counselling with parents is essential and is best accomplished by perinatal social workers. It is only by learning parents' fears and concerns that one can assess their stage of adaptation. Dealing with reality decreases the tendency of parents to deny their problems. Persistent denial should be avoided because it prolongs grief.

Mourning the birth of a handicapped child is an exhausting experience that cannot be hurried or denied. Parents need the opportunity to discuss all aspects of the child's condition and treatment. They should discuss their feelings in an uninhibiting environment; their role in caring for the infant must be active. With support, most parents identify many positive aspects of their infant, and they eventually provide the love and nurture that are fundamental to parent-infant attachment.

REFERENCES

Averill, J. R.: Grief, its nature and significance, Psychol. Bull. **70:**721, 1968.

Barnard, M. U.: Supportive nursing care for the mother and newborn who are separated from each other, Am. J. Nurs. **1:**107, 1976.

Barnett, C. R., Leiderman, P., Grobstein, R., and Klaus, M.: Neonatal separation: the maternal side of interactional deprivation, Pediatrics **45:**197, 1970.

Beckwith, L., Cohen, S. E., Kopp, C. B., et al.: Caregiver-infant interaction and early cognitive development in preterm infants, Child. Dev. **47:**579, 1976.

Benfield, D. G., Leib, S. A., and Reuter, J.: Grief response of parents after referral of the critically ill newborn to a regional center, N. Engl. J. Med. **294:**975, 1976.

Bibring, G. L.: Some considerations of the psychological processes in pregnancy, Psychoanal. Study Child **14:**113, 1959.

Blau, A., Slaff, B., Easton, K., et al.: The psychogenic etiology of premature births, Psychiat. Med. **25:**201, 1963.

Bowlby, J.: Processes of mourning, Int. J. Psychoanal. **42:**22, 1961.

Brazelton, T., Scholl, M., and Robey, J.: Visual responses in the newborn, Pediatrics, **37:**284, 1966.

Campbell, S. B. G., and Taylor, P. M.: Bonding and attachment: theoretical issues, Semin. Perinatol. **3:**3, 1979.

Clark, A. L., and Affonso, D. D.: Maternal-child relationships, Am. J. Nurs. **1:**94, 1976.

Cohen, R. L.: Some maladaptive syndromes of pregnancy and the puerperium, Obstet. Gynecol. **27:**562, 1966.

Cullberg, J.: Mental reactions of women to perinatal death. In Morris, N., editor: Psychosomatic medicine in obstetrics and gynecology, New York, 1972, S. Karger.

Davidson, G. W.: Death of the wished-for child: a case study, Death Educ. **1:**265, 1977.

Davidson, G. W.: Living and dying, religion and medicine series, Minneapolis, 1975, Augsburg Publishing House.

De Chateau, P.: Effects of hospital practice on synchrony in the development of the infant-parent relationship, Semin. Perinatol. **3:**45, 1979.

De Chateau, P., and Wiberg, B.: Long-term effect on mother-infant behavior of extra contact during the first hour post partum. I. First observations at 36 hours, Acta. Paediatr. Scand. **66:**137, 1977.

De Chateau, P., and Wiberg, B.: Long-term effect on mother-infant behavior of extra contact during the first hour post partum. II. Follow-up at three months. Acta. Paediatr. Scand. **66:**145, 1977.

Deutsch, H.: The psychology of women: a psychoanalytic interpretation. II. Motherhood, New York, 1945, Grune & Stratton, Inc.

Drotor, D., Bashiewicz, A., Irvin, N., et al.: The adaptation of parents to the birth of an infant with a congenital malformation: a hypothetical model, Pediatrics **56:**710, 1975.

Dubois, D. R.: Indications of an unhealthy relationship between parents and premature infant, J. Obstet. Gynecol. Nurs. **4:**21, 1975.

Elliott, B. A.: Neonatal death: reflections for physicians, Pediatrics **62:**96, 1978.

Engle, G. L.: Is grief a disease? Psychosom. Med. **23:**18, 1961.

Fanaroff, A. A., Kennell, J. H., and Klaus, M.: Follow-up of low birth weight infants: the predictive value of maternal visiting patterns, Pediatrics **49:**287, 1972.

Friedman, S. B., Chodoff, P., Mason, J. W., et al.: Behavioral observations on parents anticipating the death of a child, Pediatrics **32:**610, 1963.

Funke, J., and Irby, M. I.: An instrument to assess the quality of maternal behavior, J. Obstet. Gynecol. Nurs. **7:**19, 1978.

Furman, E. P.: The death of a newborn: care of parents, Birth and Fam. J. **5:**214, 1978.

Gibson, J. J.: Observation of active touch, Psychol. Rev. **69:**477, 1962.

Giles, P. F. H.: Reactions of women to a perinatal death, Aust. N.Z.J. Obstet. Gynaecol. **10:**207, 1970.

Green, M., and Solnit, A. J.: Reactions to the threatened loss of a child: a vulnerable child syndrome. III. Pediatric management of the dying child, Pediatrics **34:**58, 1964.

Greenberg, M., and Morris, N.: Engrossment: the newborn's impact upon the father, Am. J. Orthopsychiatry **44:**520, 1974.

Hersher, L., Richmond, J., and Moore, A.: Maternal behavior in sheep and goats. In Rheingold, H., editor: Maternal behavior in mammals, New York, 1963, John Wiley & Sons, Inc.

Johnson, S. H., and Grubbs, J. P.: The premature infant's reflex behaviors: effect on the maternal-child relationship, J. Obstet. Gynecol. Nurs. **4:**15, 1975.

Kahn, E., Wayburne, S., and Fouche, M.: The Baragwanath Premature Baby Unit: an analysis of the case records of 1,000 consecutive admissions, S. Afr. Med. J. **28:**453, 1954.

Kaplan, D., and Mason, E.: Maternal reactions to premature birth viewed as an acute emotional disorder, Am. J. Orthopsychiatry **30:**539, 1960.

Kennedy, J. C.: The high-risk maternal-infant acquaintance process, Nurs. Clin. North Am. **8:**549, 1973.

Kennell, J. H., and Klaus, M. H.: Care of the mother of the high-risk infant, Clin. Obstet. Gynecol. **14:**926, 1971.

Kennell, J. H., and Rolnick, A. R.: Discussing problems in newborn babies with their parents, Pediatrics **26:**832, 1960.

Klaus, M. H., and Kennell, J. H.: Mothers separated from their newborn infants, Pediatr. Clin. North Am. **17:**1015, 1970.

Klaus, M. H., Jerauld, R., Kreger, N. C., et al.: Maternal attachment: importance of the first postpartum days, N. Engl. J. Med. **286:**460, 1972.

Klaus, M. H., Kennell, J. H., Plumb, N., and Zuehike, S.: Human maternal behavior at the first contact with her young, Pediatrics **46:**187, 1970.

Klopfer, P. H.: Mother love: what turns it on? Am. Sci. **59:**404, 1971.

Leifer, A. D., Leiderman. P. H., Barnett, C. R., and Williams, J. A.: Effects of mother-infant separation on maternal attachment behavior, Child Dev. **43:**1203, 1972.

Lindemann, E.: Symptomatology and management of acute grief, Am. J. Psychiatry **101:**141, 1944.

Mandelbaum. A.: The group process in helping parents of retarded infants, Children **14:**227, 1967.

Manguiten, H. H., Slade C., and Fitzsimons, D.: Parent-parent support in the care of high-risk newborns, J. Obstet. Gynecol. Nurs. **8:**275, 1979.

Mason, E. A.: A method of predicting crisis outcome for mothers of premature babies, Public Health Rep. **78:**1031, 1963.

Mercer, R. T.: Mother's response to their infants with defects, Nurs. Res. **23:**133, 1974.

Minde, K., Trehub, S., et al.: Mother-child relationships in the premature nursery: an observational study, Pediatrics **61:**373, 1978.

O'Connor, S., Vietze, P., Hopkins, J., et al.: Post partum extended maternal-infant contact: subsequent mothering and child health, Pediatr. Res. **11:**380, 1977.

Owens, C.: Parents' reactions to defective babies, Am. J. Nurs. **64:**83, 1964.

Parkes, C.: Bereavement and mental illness. Part I. A clinical study of the grief of bereaved psychiatric patients, Br. Med. J. Psychol. **38:**1, 1965.

Powell, L. F.: The effects of extra stimulation and maternal involvement on the development of low birth weight infants and maternal behavior, Child Dev. **45:**106, 1974.

Raphael, D.: The tender gift: breastfeeding, Englewood Cliffs, N.J. 1973, Prentice Hall, Inc.

Robson, K. S.: The role of eye-to-eye contact in maternal-infant attachment, J. Child Psychol. Psychiatry **8:**13, 1967.

Rose, I., Boggs, T. R., Jr., Adlerstein, A., et al.: The evidence for a syndrome of "mothering disability" consequent to threats to the survival of neonates: a design for hypothesis testing including prevention in a prospective study, Am. J. Dis. Child. **100:**776, 1960.

Rowe, J., Clyman, R., Green, C., et al.: Follow up of families who experience a perinatal death, Pediatrics **62:**166, 1978.

Rubenstein, J.: Maternal attentiveness and subsequent exploratory behavior in the infant, Child Dev. **38:**1089, 1967.

Rubin, R.: Basic maternal behavior, Nurs. Outlook **9:**683, 1961.

Rubin, R.: Maternal touch, Nurs. Outlook **11:**828, 1963.

Saylor, Rev. D. F.: Nursing response to mothers of stillborn infants, J. Obstet. Gynecol. Nurs. **6:**39, 1977.

Seigler, M.: Pascals' Wager and the hanging of crepe, New. Engl. J. Med. **293:**853, 1975.

Solnit, A., and Stark, M.: Mourning the birth of a defective child, Psychoanal. Study Child **16:**523, 1961.

Spitz, R. A.: Hospitalism, Psychoanal. Study Child **1:**53, 1945.

Taylor, P. M., and Hall, B. L.: Parent-infant bonding: problems and opportunities in a perinatal center, Semin. Perinatol. **3:**73, 1979.

Thaler, O. F.: Grief and depression, Nurs. Forum **5:**8, 1966.

Ujhely, G. B.: Grief and depression: implications for preventive and therapeutic nursing care, Nurs. Forum **5:**23, 1966.

CHAPTER 15

Organization and functions of a neonatal special care facility

Advanced diagnostic and therapeutic techniques during the past decade have resulted in the evolution of a new type of facility for the care of sick neonates. Prior to the 1960s, infants were admitted to a term or a premature nursery. Infected babies were admitted to a separate, irregularly staffed nursery that was reserved solely for contagious disease. Uninfected sick infants were managed in the premature or term nursery to which they were originally admitted. In many hospitals an observation nursery was set aside for infants with unproved but suspected infection. Postoperative neonates were treated in surgical areas along with children of all ages and, in many instances, with adults as well.

The contemporary special care facility arose in response to an awareness of the singular characteristics of perinatal disorders. A newly acquired understanding of pathophysiologic phenomena during this period of life, and the capacity to apply this knowledge clinically, required an appropriate setting in which the severely ill baby could be managed. These developments occurred simultaneously with advances in electronics and biochemistry. Practical methods for the evaluation of numerous crucial parameters of fetal and neonatal illness were thus made available. Continuous monitoring of cardiorespiratory function became a reality. The performance of multiple biochemical determinations on minute quantities of blood was facilitated by new microtechniques. Conservation of body heat became feasible with the availability of radiant heaters and servocontrolled incubators. With confidence in improved methods for the control of infection, a direct impetus was provided for housing all medically and surgically ill infants in a common area, whether they were premature or mature, infected or noninfected. This approach revolutionized requirements of nursery architecture, fixtures, and equipment, but more important, a need was created for specially trained personnel in several disciplines who must function cohesively if lives were to be saved. Today, optimal performance by all personnel requires a spirit of camaraderie in which traditional ideas of hierarchy are minimized in the nursery organization. Every worker in a special care unit is indispensable to its successful operation.

Although survival is an obvious end point by which to gauge the success of these vigorous efforts, *intact* survival is the overriding consideration. There is good reason to assume that diminished mortality and decreased incidence of central nervous system damage among survivors go hand-in-hand. The factors that contribute to perinatal mortality may, if present to a less severe degree, result in central nervous system dysfunction rather than death. By minimizing the effects of these deleterious factors, diminished mortality is probably associated with a decreased incidence of dysfunctional survival.

Do mortality rates decrease when intensive care is applied? There is excellent evidence that they do indeed. In the Province of Quebec, among hospitals with special care units or with access to them by transfer of sick infants, mortality during the first week of life was approximately half that of hospitals without such services. Similar benefits have been reported from Nova Scotia and from several large centers in the United States. In Arizona the mortality rate of babies with hyaline membrane disease who were *not* transported to an intensive care unit was 59% (1967 to 1970); among those who *were* transported the mortality rate was 32%. In the same state, in intensive care institutions themselves, the mortality rate of babies between 1000 and 2500 grams fell from 11.5% in 1964 to 5.9% in 1970. At Vanderbilt University Hospital,

the mortality rate of babies in the same weight bracket was 11.8% before intensive care; it was 6.5% afterward. At Mount Zion Hospital in San Francisco, the mortality rate of low birth weight infants was 21.8% before intensive care and 6.6% after it was introduced. At the Robert B. Green Hospital in San Antonio, Texas, in just 2 years (1969 to 1971), the mortality rate of infants who weighed 1500 to 2500 grams was reduced from 18% to 7.8%. There is little doubt that intensive care programs have indeed increased survival.

What has happened to the survivors? Follow-up studies have been encouraging. For infants below 1500 grams, studied outcomes reveal some sort of neurologic defect in 7% to 10% of infants. For the specific handicap called spastic diplegia, in which intellectual function is seldom impaired, the fall in incidence is dramatic. From Sweden, a decline of 50% is recorded. From Britain an incidence of 10.3% fell to zero. From other centers in that country and elsewhere, the incidence is 3.6% or less. There has been a reduction in *all* forms of cerebral palsy among children of very low birth weight reported from virtually all centers in which such data have been recorded. An improvement in IQ has been associated with the decline in physical handicaps among low birth weight babies. Although IQ is still below the norms for term infants at certain centers, 80% to 90% of survivors below 1500 grams had no serious residual handicaps.

During the first year of our own special care program at the University of Tennessee, there was decline of 28% in the mortality rate of low birth weight infants from the average of the preceding 8 years. We attribute this decline to the training of personnel; new equipment was not acquired until the last 5 or 6 months of that period. Although electronic monitors, mechanical respirators, and other such items are important, they are nevertheless a secondary consideration. *The care of sick babies cannot be intensive unless personnel perform with intensity.* Without this ingredient, complex equipment is useless. The heavy staffing requirements imposed by special care units should preclude indiscriminate establishment of these facilities by hospitals that merely seek to enhance or maintain their community images. The concept of regionalization of perinatal care offers the best means for an appropriate distribution of institutions that offer different levels of care.

REGIONALIZATION OF PERINATAL CARE

The professional advice and supervision that constitute perinatal care must be made available to every pregnant woman and her newborn child. Although the vast majority of the newly born are healthy, intact survival is jeopardized in a substantial number who require complex medical attention for severe illness. In many instances these severe neonatal illnesses can be anticipated, ameliorated or eliminated by special management of high risk mothers. In the extreme, this type medical attention entails the recruitment of a variety of professional personnel who are generally concentrated in densely populated communities. It is in these larger communities that the full spectrum of medical consultants, nurse specialists, laboratory capabilities and facilities with equipment are to be found. Yet the complex medical management of high risk mothers and infants must be qualitatively the same, regardless of the size of the community in which patients reside. That perinatal mortality and morbidity are significantly reduced by the application of our best contemporary technology has been plainly documented for several years. From this fact alone, there arises a sense of urgency to make such technology available to all mothers and infants, to eliminate any existing inaccessibility to complex care, and to assure a high quality of medical attention in every hospital that renders it regardless of the complexity of care or location of the hospital.

Optimal care is thus planned for a region as a whole. Available resources, primarily personnel and money, are allocated to avoid duplication of facilities and to assure proper utilization of services, both of which affect the ultimate quality of care. The needs of individual patients will be fulfilled by designating Perinatal Regions. All levels of care will be available within each region. Each level of care, no matter how uncomplicated or complex, must be of optimal quality. The sole determinants of where care will be administered within a region, and by what type of personnel, are the severity and complexity of the illness. Services should be available as close to home as possible, but the transfer of patients from one hospital to another is inevitable if all levels of care are to be delivered to the residents of a Perinatal Region.

A coordinated system within a region first requires the designation of certain hospitals for provision of care levels according to their capacity to provide them. Beyond the designation of care levels, activation of an effective pattern of communication for consultation, and for transport of patients, will provide functional continuity between diverse hospitals within a region. Fundamental to all these activities is a regional program for continuing education of personnel; without it the system will falter.

Although these guidelines are addressed to hospitals as institutional providers of perinatal care, the basic emphasis is on the role of physicians, nurses and other personnel who are the direct and personal providers of such care. The three (3) types

Table 15-1. Services provided by perinatal facilities*

Services	Level I	Level II	Level III
Complete prenatal care for maternity patient with no complications or with minor complications	X	X	X
Complete prenatal care for maternity patients with most complications		X	X
A special diagnostic and management clinic for high-risk prenatal patients			X
Risk identification scoring system	X	X	X
Management of uncomplicated labor and delivery of normal term fetus	X	X	X
Prompt management of unexpected complications occuring during labor and delivery, including anesthesia, cesarean section, and blood administration	X	X	X
Management of complicated labor and delivery		X	X
Intrapartum intensive care			X
In-house anesthesia service		X	X
Electronic fetal monitoring	±	X	X
Physically separated facilities for obstetrics	X	X	X
Capability for resuscitation of depressed neonate at every delivery	X	X	X
Care for the healthy newborn	X	X	X
Stabilization and risk assessment of all neonates	X	X	X
Intravenous fluid administration to neonates	X	X	X
Management of most neonates who have complications up to short-term assisted ventilation		X	X
Continuous neonatal monitoring capability		X	X
Blood gases available on 24-hr basis		X	X
Neonatal intensive care including assisted ventilation and hyperalimentation			X
Neonatal surgical capability			X
Availability of pediatric subspecialists in cardiology, genetics, and hematology			X
Care of mothers with no complications postpartum	X	X	X
Management of unexpected postpartum complications including hemorrhage and sepsis	X	X	X
Management of most postpartum complications		X	X
Data collection on performance and outcome	X	X	X
Laboratory services for electrolytes, bilirubin, blood glucose, calcium on 24-hr basis	X	X	X
X-ray services with portable film capability on 24-hr basis	X	X	X
Laboratory services to assess fetal well-being and maturity		X	X
Diagnostic x-ray and ultrasound		X	X
Nutritional consultation		X	X
Social service		X	X
Respiratory therapy consultation		X	X
Sterilization and family planning services	X	X	X
Follow-up developmental assessment clinic			X

*From Graven, S. N.: The organization of perinatal health services. In Behrman, R. E., editor: Neonatal-perinatal medicine: diseases of the fetus and infant, ed. 2, St. Louis, 1977, The C. V. Mosby Co.

of hospital facilities herein are different from each other primarily in the services performed by their personnel, and only secondarily in the equipment they possess.*

A regionalized system should include three types of facilities within designated geographic perinatal care areas. They are designated by levels of care according to the *extent* of their respective capacities. *These designations do not indicate quality of available care; they refer only to the extent of care.* Table 15-1 lists the suggested functions of the three levels of care.

Level I facilities

The Level I facility has three principal functions: (1) the management of normal pregnancy, labor, and delivery, (2) the earliest possible identification of high-risk pregnancy and/or high-risk neonates after birth, and (3) the provision of competent emergency care in the event of unanticipated obstetric and/or newborn emergencies. These facilities are generally located in small communities within hospitals that are vital to the overall health care of the area. They are defined as primary (Level I) care centers only by virtue or their limited capacity to manage perinatal complications. There is little justification for hospitals in densely populated (urban) areas to offer the necessarily limited facilities that characterize Level I care. Level I facilities generally deliver approximately 500 livebirths annually. Since the occurrence of complications is an infrequent event, staffing and equipment requirements are not as demanding as for Level II and III care.

---

*Modified from the Introduction to guidelines for regionalization, hospital care levels, staffing and facilities, Nashville, 1978, Tennessee Perinatal Care System.

Level II facilities

These are larger perinatal services in hospitals that serve more densely populated areas, generally urban and suburban communities. The ideal Level II facility should be capable of managing 75% to 90% of maternal and neonatal complications. However, this must necessarily vary according to the capacity of an individual hospital. In any event, a Level II facility must manage a number of perinatal complications in addition to offering a full-range of maternity and newborn care in uncomplicated circumstances. As in the case of the previously described Level I unit, the activities of a Level II institution are assumed to be of the highest quality compatible with contemporary practice. The designation implies that a few functions are not within the capacity of a Level II unit, which must therefore be obtained at a Level III facility.

Level III facilities

Level III facilities, in addition to offering a complete spectrum of care for uncomplicated maternity and newborn patients, should have the capacity to manage the most complex of all perinatal disorders. Thus in the case of neonatal disorders, the Level III facility has at its disposal a complete roster of pediatric subspecialists, pediatric surgeons, pediatric radiologists, geneticists and hospital epidemiologists. This facility should deliver all the modalities of complex care that constitute sophisticated contemporary practice. In a densely populated region in which there is more than one Level III unit, only one of them should be designated as a *regional center*. The regional center has the responsibility for coordinating the perinatal activities of its geographically delineated perinatal region. It is also responsible for maintaining consultative services for obstetricians, pediatricians, and the respective nursing services. It is expected that at all Level III units, and at regional centers in particular, a staff of *perinatal social workers* will be available to manage the multiplicity of problems that arise among families whose infants receive intensive care. The regional center must conduct ongoing continuing education programs intramurally and in other hospitals of the region as well.

The Level III unit, whether or not it is a designated regional center, must have a full-time obstetrician who is a subspecialist in maternal-fetal medicine and a full-time pediatrician who is a subspecialist in neonatal-perinatal medicine. Clinical nurse specialists in obstetrics and in newborn care should direct their respective nursing services in coordination with the efforts of the physicians. Staff physicians in the neonatal intensive care unit should also be subspecialists in neonatal-perinatal medicine.

CLINICAL FUNCTIONS

The clinical functions performed in a special care unit include direct observation of patients by nursing personnel and physicians, physiologic monitoring with electronic equipment, biochemical monitoring by laboratory personnel, diagnostic and therapeutic procedures, and promotion of maternal-child contact to the fullest feasible extent. The success of the last-mentioned function is almost exclusively dependent on skillful nursing and counselling by social workers.

Direct observation of infants

The components of direct observation of sick infants have been described throughout this book. This phase of special care is reiterated to emphasize its fundamental importance. It is thus unwise to provide electronic equipment for remote observation of sick babies from centrally located consoles similar to those in adult intensive care units. Severe difficulty can be better detected in the earliest stages by an alert nurse who notes slight cyanosis, even though uninterrupted respirations and heart rate have not yet tripped the alarms of monitors. A monitor cannot signal the regurgitation of a feeding until the baby becomes apneic after aspiration of milk. Optimal outcomes are basically dependent on constant scrutiny of infants by personnel rather than by gadgets. The crucial factors listed here are direct observations that can be made only by well-trained nurses. *None of them is detectable by monitors:*

1. Acceptance of feedings; course of weight gain
2. Early detection of regurgitation to prevent aspiration of vomitus
3. Abdominal distention; frequency and character of stools
4. Changes in activity (lethargy, convulsive phenomena, hyperactivity)
5. Jaundice
6. Pallor and early cyanosis
7. Skin lesions that indicate infection
8. Deviations from prescribed volumes of intravenous infusions
9. Edema
10. Respiratory distress characterized by tachypnea, retractions, flaring of alae nasi, and grunting
11. Quality of breath sounds
12. Character and location of heart sounds

Physiologic monitoring and therapy: electronic and other types of equipment

Electronic monitoring has greatly facilitated the detection of cardiovascular and respiratory difficulties. *These instruments are intended for use by skillful personnel; they are not intended to re-*

place them. In addition to cardiorespiratory monitoring, the control of temperature and ambient oxygen concentrations is also feasible with appropriate instrumentation. Following are the general categories of equipment required for intensive neonatal care:

I. Monitors
   Respiration (apnea)
   B. Heart rate
   C. Blood pressure
   D. Temperature (rectal, ambient, or skin probes), with or without controller
   E. Electrocardiogram (oscilloscopes, writers)
   F. Oxygen analyzers (ambient)
   G. Transcutaneous sensors for P_{O_2}, P_{CO_2} and pH
II. Therapeutic equipment
   A. Incubators, with sevocontrolled temperature
   B. Infusion pumps for intravenous fluid administration
   C. Phototherapy lamps
   D. Radiant heaters
III. Oxygen administration
   A. Plastic head hoods
   B. Humidifier warmers, preferably with variable temperature control
   C. Repirators (positive pressure with pressure or volume limiters; negative pressure)
IV. Resuscitation equipment
   A. Insufflation bags with masks
   B. Endotracheal tubes and adapters
   C. Laryngoscopes with premature blades
   D. Defibrillator

Biochemical monitoring

The special care unit should have its own laboratory staffed by technologists who are aware of the clinical significance of their efforts. At the very least, blood gas and pH determinations should be available within minutes after they are ordered for infants in respiratory distress and for periodic monitoring of other conditions such as late metabolic acidosis of prematurity. Since large units are usually located in sprawling hospital complexes whose central laboratories are at some distance from the nursery, the special care unit's laboratory should provide as many biochemical parameters as possible. Reliability and immediate availability of results are best assured when laboratory personnel are involved with newborn medicine on a full-time basis and are thus familiar with the special problems of sick infants. Blood glucose, bilirubin, and electrolyte determinations are indispensable. Hemoglobin and hematocrit determinations, stained blood smears, and Gram stains are also important.

Radiologic diagnosis

Chest films are the most frequent radiologic need in the nursery. They are best procured with minimal disturbance to the infant and thus should be taken by portable x-ray equipment, with the infant in an incubator. Films of the skull, abdomen, and extremities also can be taken with portable equipment. Gastrointestinal series and intravenous pyelograms should be performed in an x-ray room within the special care unit. If such a room is not available, the infant should be transported to the hospital radiology department only if accompanied by a nurse or a physician. A transport incubator with its own battery to provide heat, and its own portable source of oxygen, must be available for this purpose.

STRUCTURAL COMPONENTS

The complete tertiary unit contains areas designed for intensive, intermediate, and minimal care. Infants are admitted directly to these areas, depending on their status, or they may be moved from one section to another according to changes in conditions. Thus an infant who was successfully treated for hyaline membrane disease, perhaps with ventilatory assistance, can be transferred with ease from the intensive care to the intermediate care area. Minimal care sections are generally devoted to convalescent growing infants.

Special care facilities should be as close as possible to the labor and delivery rooms. Currently, most new neonatal units are constructed by remodeling existing facilities, thus imposing severe limitations on optimal location, floor plan, and space. A number of notable units in the United States and in Canada are housed in children's hospitals rather than in general hospitals. These centers function solely as referral units, since they are usually at some distance from obstetric facilities.

The ideal center should accommodate infants who are distributed among the three graduated care areas. Complete units for fewer than fifteen to twenty infants who are similarly distributed may be too expensive to operate. They may also fail to provide sufficient clinical ma-

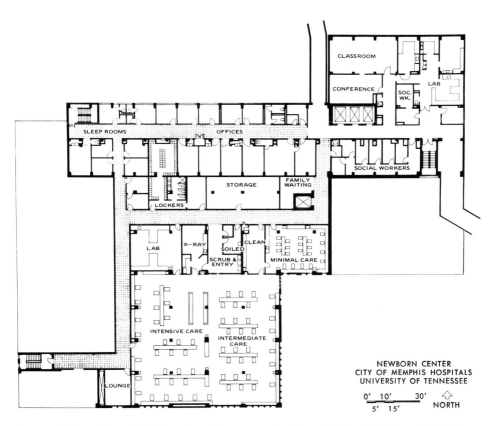

Fig. 15-1. Floor plan of the Newborn Center at the City of Memphis Hospital, University of Tennessee. (Courtesy of Yeates, Gaskill, and Rhodes, Architects, Memphis, Tennessee.)

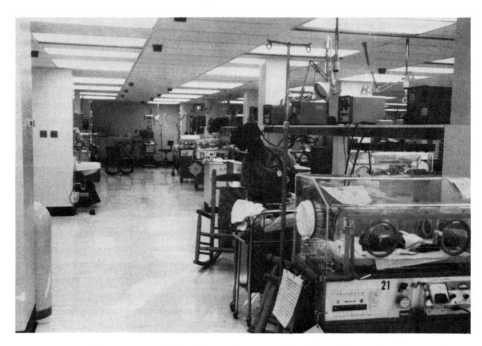

Fig. 15-2. Recently constructed Newborn Center at the City of Memphis Hospital, University of Tennessee. The facility houses a total of 80 infants in all three levels of care.

terial to maintain the interest and skill of personnel.

The number of bassinets and incubators within each of the three graduated care areas must be determined individually for each institution. These calculations depend on the population to be served. In some hospitals or communities the incidence of low birth weight is 7% of live births; in others, such as our own, it may be 15% to 17%. Since the principal source of infants requiring special care is the low birth weight group, the number of maximal care stations is largely determined by the incidence of small babies. The extent of referrals from the community is another important consideration in these calculations.

Current trends are toward housing all infants who need special care in a single large room, with sections organized administratively for the three levels of graduated care. Such an arrangement permits assignment of personnel according to their respective skills while providing ease of movement of patients and personnel from one area to another. An average of at least 80 square feet per infant should be allocated, 100 square feet is far more practical. More space is provided for each infant in the maximal care area than in the other sections.

The Newborn Center at the University of Tennessee Center for the Health Sciences (City of Memphis Hospital) will be briefly described because it is an example of a modern special care unit (Figs. 15-1 and 15-2). It is comprised of a single large room, 6000 square feet, for sixty maximal and intermediate care babies and a number of other rooms for ancillary functions. A smaller room, adjacent to the larger one, houses twenty minimal care babies in an area of 1000 square feet. The plan was developed to conserve nursing energy by minimizing walking distances entailed in use of the telephone, procurement of instruments and supplies, and recording of notes in charts that are otherwise stored at a central desk. The diagram of our floor plan (Fig. 15-1) shows the disposition of incubators or bassinets and the placement of wall cabinets and other cabinets throughout the room. Supplies are stored as close to the infant as possible, permitting the nurse to remain in the area to which she is assigned. Formula in individual bottles is stored in the cabinets. Extensive work surface adjacent to each infant is provided by the counter tops. Daily notes are made at the cribside. The area contains ten sinks operated by foot pedals for convenient handwashing. Telephone extensions are placed at several points in the room. At least ten electrical outlets are available for each care station. Two oxygen lines and a suction and two air outlets serve each incubator. In addition to copious illumination from lighing fixtures, an adjustable work light is suspended from the ceiling over each maximal care incubator. Infant stations in the intermediate care areas are provided with identical service receptacles as those in the maximal care area. Each incubator or open radiant-heated bed is placed 6 feet apart. A red light in the ceiling over each infant station is synchronized with the infant's monitor so that when the alarm sounds on the monitor, the appropriate red light flashes. These lights were installed to circumvent the frustrating lack of direction that is characteristic of the alarm sounds on most cardiorespiratory monitors.

Appropriate space for all supportive services is located on the same floor as the infant area. Thus there are six offices for each of the social workers, appropriate offices for supervising nurses, fellows, and physician faculty. The laboratory is immediately adjacent to the large infant area. An x-ray developing room is situated adjacent to the laboratory. All x-ray films are developed in the unit and remain at the infant's bedside until discharge. The radiologist reads all x-ray films in a designated area within the unit. A classroom that seats sixty individuals and a conference room that seats twenty to thirty are located on the same floor. Sleeping accommodations for physician staff and laboratory personnel are available for six individuals.

A baby-viewing area was not provided. Based on the concepts presented in Chapter 14, parents are encouraged to visit their infants in the nursery.

The delivery suite is located two floors below the special care unit. An express elevator transports infants from the delivery room directly to the nursery. The facility for normal term infants is one floor below the special care nursery.

STAFF

No problem is more vexing than the procurement of adequate numbers of qualified personnel. The heavy staffing requirement of these units invariably taxes hospital budgets. Administrative officials thus find it difficult to provide funds for the ideal staffing pattern.

A corps of registered nurses, practical nurses, and nurse assistants or technicians must be deployed to match training and skill with the level of care required for each infant. For every shift, optimal staffing should provide one nurse for two infants in the maximal care area and one nurse for three to six infants in the other sections. In calculating the total number of personnel required for 24 hours, the needs for each shift must be multiplied by a factor of 4.4 to allow for vacations, sickness, and days off. Ward secretaries, laboratory technologists, social workers, and housekeeping personnel are essential for complete staffing. In a large center the physician-in-charge must be a full-time neonatologist; in a smaller center a pediatrician may be employed part time. Large units are also staffed with residents who rotate through the nursery during their pediatric training and with fellows in neonatology. Nursing students and postgraduate nurse trainees are regularly present in units that are affiliated with schools of nursing and medicine.

EDUCATIONAL PROGRAMS

The tertiary care center that proposes to manage high-risk infants who are born in a large hospital, as well as those referred from the community, is committed to an extensive educational program of high quality. Training should be provided for the unit's nurses and for other nurses from hospitals throughout the region. In-service programs should begin with a series of lecture sessions devoted to the principles of perinatal medicine, combined with cribside instruction in the various sections of the unit. This initial phase of training requires at least 3 months. Ongoing education must thereafter include periodic sessions devoted to case presentations and to special subjects such as the basic principles of electricity and their application to the prevention of shock hazards, demonstration and practice of endotracheal intubation utilizing models specially made for this purpose, and discussions of important current literature. Training sessions are given primarily by the clinical nurse supervisors.

The unit must also participate in advanced degree programs sponsored by the school of nursing and in the instruction of student nurses according to the school's curriculum.

The education of other members of the nursing team (assistants, practical nurses) is also indispensable. This phase of the program should be administered primarily by the clinical nurse supervisor and staff.

We have been gratified by our weekly social work conferences, which are supervised by social service personnel and are attended by medical students, house officers, fellows, nurses, and laboratory technologists. Environmental factors, family relationships, and economic problems of the families of selected infants are discussed at each meeting. The goal of these conferences is to assess the infant's home environment before he is discharged and to apply community resources to the alleviation of existing problems. It is not unusual to defer discharge of an infant until our social workers have attempted to minimize the problems that may jeopardize his health at home. Medical aspects of the hospital course are related to the home environment that awaits the baby in question. All available personnel are encouraged to attend. The importance of total infant care plus social concern is effectively projected by the nature of the discussions during these sessions.

Laboratory technologists should attend all training sessions along with nurses. They thus acquire perspective regarding the importance of their role in the successful operation of the unit and an understanding of the clinical significance of the data they produce every day.

Training programs for medical students, house officers, and fellows are a part of the curriculum of the school of medicine. The fully staffed unit should also sponsor refresher courses for practicing physicians.

Although these training programs must necessarily be diverse if they are to serve the needs of all types of personnel, they are unified by their emphasis on each staff member's importance to the intact survival of sick infants.

REFERENCES

Committee on Perinatal Health: Toward improving the outcome of pregnancy, White Plains, N.Y., 1976, The National Foundation–March of Dimes.

Davies, P. A., and Stewart, A. L.: Low-birth-weight infants: neurological sequelae and later intelligence, Br. Med. Bull. **31**:85, 1975

Desmond, M. M., Rudolph, A. J., and Phitaksphraiwan, P.: The transitional care nursery: a mechanism for preventive medicine in the newborn, Pediatr. Clin. North Am. **13**:651, 1966.

Desmond, M. M., Rudolph, A. J., and Pineda, R. G.: Neonatal morbidity and nursery function, J.A.M.A. **212**:281, 1970.

Gluck, L.: The newborn special care unit: its role in the large medical center, Hosp. Pract. **3**:33, 1968.

Gluck, L.: Design of a perinatal center, Pediatr. Clin. North Am. **17**:777, 1970.

Lucey, J. F., editor: Problems of neonatal intensive care units, Report of the Fifty-ninth Ross Conference on Pediatric Research, Columbus, Ohio, March, 1968, Ross Laboratories.

Lucey, J. F.: Why we should regionalize perinatal care, Pediatrics **52**:488, 1972.

Organization for perinatal care. In Gluck, L., editor: Clin. Perinatol. vol. 3, Philadelphia, 1976, W. B. Saunders Co.

Schlesinger, E. R.: Neonatal intensive care: planning for services and outcomes following care, J. Pediatr. **82**:916, 1973.

Segal, S.: Neonatal intensive care: a prediction of continuing development, Pediatr. Clin. North Am. **13**:1149, 1966.

Segal, S., and Pirie, G. E.: Equipment and personnel for neonatal special care, Pediatr. Clin. North Am. **17**:793, 1970.

Silverman, W. A.: Intensive care of the low birth weight and other at-risk infants, Clin. Obstet. Gynecol. **13**:87, 1970.

Stewart, A. L., and Reynolds, E. O. R.: Improved prognosis for infants of very low birth weight, Pediatrics **54**:724, 1974.

Swyer, P. R.: The regional organization of special care for the neonate, Pediatr. Clin. North Am. **17**:761, 1970.

Tennessee Perinatal Care System, Guidelines for regionalization, hospital care levels, staffing and facilities, Nashville, 1978, Tennessee Department of Public Health, Division of Maternal and Child Health.

Index

B

Bacitracin, ointment containing, for treatment of conjunctivitis, 329

Bacteria as cause of perinatal infection, 317-318, 319-320

Bag resuscitator in resuscitation of infant, 74

Ballard score for estimation of gestational age, 113-114

Bands
  amniotic, 162
  annular, 162

Barbiturates
  as cause of respiratory distress, 263
  fetal and neonatal disorders and, 40

Base excess or deficit in acid-base balance, 174-175

Bases, and acid-base balance, 169

BB lights in phototherapy for hyperbilirubinemia, 296

Beds, radiant-heated, in nursery, 99-100
  heat shields, 99, 100
  insensible water loss from, 100

Benzalkonium chloride as source of postnatal infection, 321, 339

Betamethasone in prevention of hyaline membrane disease, 233

Betamimetic tocolytics, fetal and neonatal diseases, 41

Biliary obstruction (biliary atresia), 293
  neonatal jaundice and, 289, 293

Bilirubin
  in assessment of fetal status, 11-12
  encephalopathy; *see* Kernicterus
  in normal neonate, 284-287
    formation of, 285
    in liver, conjugation and excretion of, 286
    physiologic jaundice, 286-287
    in plasma (albumin binding), 285-286
    types of, 284-285
      conjugated, 284, 285
      unconjugated, 284, 285, 291

Birth weight
  distribution according to gestational age, 105
  maintenance volumes of fluid and, 190
  relationship to gestational age, 103-137
    classification of infants, 104-107
    intrauterine growth acceleration, 135-136
    intrauterine growth retardation, 116-128
      physical findings of, 125-128
    outcomes of small-for-dates infants, 130-133
    postmaturity, 134-135
    postnatal estimation of gestational age, 109-116
    predisposition to neonatal illness, 126-130
    prematurity, 133-134

Birth weight—cont'd
  relationship to gestational age—cont'd
    prenatal estimation of gestational age, 107-108
  relationship to neonatal mortality, 130

Bladder of newborn, 159

Blood flow, increased pulmonary, and redistribution of cardiac output, 202-205
  pulmonary-systemic pressure relationships, 202-203
    fetal aortic blood pressure lower than pulmonary artery pressure, 202
    pulmonary artery pressure higher than aortic pressure, 202-203
  venous admixture, fetal sites of (right-to-left shunt), 203-205
    closure of ductus arteriosus, 203-204
    closure of ductus venosus, 204-205
    closure of foramen ovale, 203

Blood group antigens, 269-270

Blood group factors, 269-270

Blood loss as cause of anemia, 275-278
  postnatal, 277-278
  prenatal, 275-277

Blood pressure of newborn, 157-158
  maintenance of, in hyaline membrane disease, 230-231

Blood sampling
  fetal, in assessment of fetus, 23-24
  sites of, in hyaline membrane disease, 215-216

Body composition, 177-181
  solids, 177
  solutes, 177-180
  water
    distribution among compartments, 177-178
    exchange between compartments and osmolality, 180-181
    extracellular, and solutes, 177, 178-179
    intracellular, and solutes (ICF), 178, 179-180
    solids and, 177
    solutes and, 177-178

Body heat, maintenance of immediately after birth, 78

Body temperature, decreases in, and hyaline membrane disease, 209

BPD; *see* Bronchopulmonary dysplasia

Brachial plexus palsy, 62

Brain
  congenital malformations of, as cause of neonatal seizures, 349
  flow of cerebral spinal fluid through, 351, 352

Brain-sparing pattern in intrauterine growth retardation, 119

Branchial cleft cysts, 153

Tolazoline
  in treatment of meconium aspiration, 241
  in treatment of persistent pulmonary hypertension, 238
Tolbutamide
  as cause of neonatal hypoglycemia, 305
  fetal and neonatal disorders and, 42
Total body water (TBW), 177
Touch, in establishment of parent-infant attachment, 355
Toxemia and intrauterine growth retardation, 121
Toxoplasma gondii as cause of perinatal infection, 36, 319, 335
Toxoplasmosis, 335
Tracheal intubation, procedure for, in resuscitation of infant immediately after birth, 75-76
Tracheoesophageal fistula, 258-260
Transcutaneous oxygen tension measurement (tcP$_{O_2}$) in oxygen administration, 216-217
Transfusion
  exchange; *see* Exchange transfusion
  fetofetal, and prenatal blood loss, 275-276
  fetomaternal, and prenatal blood loss, 275
Transient tachypnea of newborn, 240
Trauma of labor and delivery, 56-66
  physical signs of, 56-66
    central nervous system, 60-61
    fractures, long bone, 59-60
    hemorrhage into abdominal organs, 65-66
    nerves, peripheral, 62-65
    ocular, 61
    skin and subcutaneous tissue, 56-58
    skull, 58-59
Treatment
  antimicrobial, for perinatal infection; *see* Antimicrobial treatment for perinatal infection
  of hyaline membrane disease, 211-232
    acid-base, 229
    blood pressure and hematocrit, maintenance of, 230-231
    fluid therapy, 229
    oxygen administration, 224-229; *see also* Oxygen administration in hyaline membrane disease
    oxygen therapy, 211-224; *see also* Oxygen therapy in hyaline membrane disease
    thermal environment, proper, provision of, 229-230
    umbilical vessel catheterization, 231-232; *see also* Umbilical artery; Umbilical vein
Tuberculosis, fetal, 320
Turner's syndrome, 153
Twin transfusion, 124-125
Twins, 66

U

Ultrasound in fetal assessment, 25-31
  gray-scale images, 28-29
  real-time imaging, 29
Umbilical artery, 159
  catheterization in hyaline membrane disease, 231-232
Umbilical cord, 4, 159
  blood loss and, 275
  clamping of, and blood loss, 276
  impaired blood flow through, 53-54
Umbilical vein catheterization in hyaline membrane disease, 232
Umbilical perforation as hazard of exchange transfusion, 272
Uridine diphosphate glucuronic acid (UDPGA) and hyperbilirubinemia, 286
Urinary tract, infection of, 328-329
Urine, in assessment of fluid and electrolyte status, 188, 189-190
Uteroplacental insufficiency (UPI), 18, 19

V

Vaccinia virus as cause of perinatal infection, 318
Valium; *see* Diazepam
Varicella-zoster as cause of perinatal infection, 318
Variola poxvirus as cause of perinatal infection, 318
Vascular disease, maternal, and fetal asphyxia, 55
Vascular spasm and hyaline membrane disease, 206, 207
Ventral suspension in estimation of gestational age, 110
Vernix caseosa in postmature infant, 134
Viral infections, specific, 331-335
  consequences of, to fetus and neonate, 331
  cytomegalovirus (CMV), 331, 332-333; *see also* Cytomegalovirus
  herpesvirus, 331, 333-335; *see also* Herpesvirus
  rubella, 331-332; *see also* Rubella
Viruses as cause of perinatal infection, 318, 321
  vertically transmitted, 318
Vitalite in phototherapy for hyperbilirubinemia, 296
Vitamin D, excessive, fetal and neonatal disorders and, 42
Vitamin E, deficiency of, and hemolytic anemia, 274
Vitamin K
  deficiency, 278-279
    and diffuse scalp hemorrhage in newborn, 56-57
  excessive, fetal and neonatal disorders and, 42
  and hyperbilirubinemia, 291
  treatment of hemolytic anemia, 274